Innovative Staff Development in Healthcare

Renate Tewes
Editor

Innovative Staff Development in Healthcare

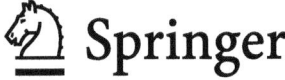
Springer

Editor
Renate Tewes
Crown Coaching International
Dresden
Saxonia
Germany

This book is an adaption of the original German edition „Innovative Personalentwicklung im In- und Ausland" by Renate Tewes and U. Christiane Matzke, published by Springer-Verlag Germany in 2021.

The translation of some chapters was done with the help of artificial intelligence (machine translation by the service DeepL.com). A subsequent human revision was done.

ISBN 978-3-030-81985-9   ISBN 978-3-030-81986-6   (eBook)
https://doi.org/10.1007/978-3-030-81986-6

© The Editor(s) (if applicable) and The Author(s), under exclusive license to Springer Nature Switzerland AG 2022
This work is subject to copyright. All rights are solely and exclusively licensed by the Publisher, whether the whole or part of the material is concerned, specifically the rights of reprinting, reuse of illustrations, recitation, broadcasting, reproduction on microfilms or in any other physical way, and transmission or information storage and retrieval, electronic adaptation, computer software, or by similar or dissimilar methodology now known or hereafter developed.
The use of general descriptive names, registered names, trademarks, service marks, etc. in this publication does not imply, even in the absence of a specific statement, that such names are exempt from the relevant protective laws and regulations and therefore free for general use.
The publisher, the authors, and the editors are safe to assume that the advice and information in this book are believed to be true and accurate at the date of publication. Neither the publisher nor the authors or the editors give a warranty, expressed or implied, with respect to the material contained herein or for any errors or omissions that may have been made. The publisher remains neutral with regard to jurisdictional claims in published maps and institutional affiliations.

This Springer imprint is published by the registered company Springer Nature Switzerland AG
The registered company address is: Gewerbestrasse 11, 6330 Cham, Switzerland

Contents

1 Introduction: Innovative and Courageous Human Resources Development in the Healthcare Sector 1
U. Christiane Matzke

Part I We Love the Challenge: Culture Change

2 Engaging Hearts and Minds to Advance Relationship-Based Cultures 23
Mary Koloroutis, Susan Wessel, and Jayne Felgen

3 Establishing Innovation Culture in Nursing: Butterfly Effect 39
Yeliz Doğan Merih

4 Initiate Change Processes via the Development and Introduction of Leadership Guidelines: A Systemic Approach 57
Ute Grießhaber-Paule and Bernhard Heuvelmann

5 Pearls of Wisdom: The Evolution of a Healing Healthcare Model 85
Emily Nowak and Valerie Lincoln

6 A Strategically Engaged Programme of Person-Centred Culture Development in Health Services: The Courage of the Irish! 101
Brendan McCormack, Lorna Peelo-Kilroe, Margaret Codd, and Debbie Baldie

7 Developing Practice Together with the University: Changing Health Care to Be Evidence-Based and Person-Centred 115
Renate Tewes, Irén Horváth, and Lydia Ulrich

Part II We Are Bold: Emotional Intelligence Pays Off

8 empCARE: An Empathy-Based Relief of Strain Training for Carers 129
Ludwig Thiry and Vera Lux

9 WellBeing at the Workplace: The Urgency and Opportunity........ 143
   Mary Jo Kreitzer

10 Stress Was Yesterday! Revitalising Care Is Today,
    by the Adoption of HeartMath® Interventions
    in Nursing within the National Health Service
    (NHS) UK: Facing the challenges 157
    Sue Ann Smith and Gavin John Andrews

Part III We Are a Dream Team: Interprofessional Collaboration

11 Agile Working and Leading: New Approaches
    for Cross-functional Expert Teams in the Context
    of Precision Oncology 169
    Sylvia Bochum, Christian Fegeler, and Uwe M. Martens

12 TeamProcessPerformance (TPP) in the OR with Gung Ho 181
    Thomas Roehrssen and Klaus Wohlmeiner

13 Interprofessional Training Wards: Transcending
    Boundaries—Learning and Working Together 199
    Christine Straub, Sebastian Bode, Lukas Nock, and Irina Cichon

14 Interprofessional Teaching and Learning in Germany:
    The "Operation Team" Support Program 213
    Lukas Nock and Irina Cichon

Part IV We Are Future: Innovative Staff Development

15 Bold Future of Human Resources Development in Healthcare 223
    Renate Tewes

Introduction: Innovative and Courageous Human Resources Development in the Healthcare Sector

U. Christiane Matzke

1.1 Healthcare in the Twenty-First Century

In this century, globalization presents the health care system with unprecedented challenges but also offers new opportunities and a variety of solutions.

The corona pandemic hit the world globally and in real terms like no other crisis in recent decades. The political handling of the crisis was very diverse. That is to say, the health systems in the world are very differently positioned, especially as the globalized economic markets and supply chains came to their limits. Not only vulnerable health systems were severely affected but the pandemic also subdued rich industrialized countries, resulting in numerous deaths.

The pandemic indicates that global health crises can only be solved by transcending sectoral and national boundaries. The same is to say for the preservation of our planet or economic growth that incorporates social justice and ecological limits. In the last 10 years, Germany has made an unmistakable contribution to the discourse by clearly positioning itself in the field of global health policy and strengthening the WHO. Since 2016, for example, the Federal Government of the Federal Republic of Germany has been funding the Global Health Protection Programme (GHPP) in cooperation with 39 partner countries and the WHO with a focus on supporting epidemic prevention measures [1].

In 2015, the global community adopted the UN 2030 Agenda with a total of 17 Sustainable Development Goals (SDGs). Through the 2030 Agenda for Sustainable Development the global community has set itself the task of shaping global economic progress by 2030 in accordance with social justice and within the Earth's ecological limits (United Nations https://sdgs.un.org/goals).

U. C. Matzke (✉)
Organizational Development and Nursing Management, SLK-Kliniken Heilbronn GmbH, Heilbronn, Germany
e-mail: christiane.matzke@slk-kliniken.de

© The Author(s), under exclusive license to Springer Nature Switzerland AG 2022
R. Tewes (ed.), *Innovative Staff Development in Healthcare*,
https://doi.org/10.1007/978-3-030-81986-6_1

Health is one of the 17 global Sustainable Development Goals (SDGs), "Ensure healthy lives and promote well-being for all at all ages." Among this, sub-goals are formulated that cover health care for all, reduction of communicable and non-communicable diseases, mental health and sexual and reproductive health and rights services, prevention and treatment of substance abuse and excessive alcohol consumption to management of global health risks as well as reducing the number of diseases caused by environmental strains. Other SDGs are closely related to the goal of healthy lives for all because they have a significant impact on health outcomes. For example, education (SDG4), food security (SDG2), water and sanitation (SDG6), gender equality (SDG5), and related improvements in sexual and reproductive health and climate change mitigation (SDG13) all contribute to improving health and can be understood as health-related Sustainable Development Goals.

Ultimately, the success of the 2030 Agenda in achieving sustainability will depend on how we succeed in thinking, acting, and in particular, cooperating across sectoral and national boundaries. As can currently be seen in the vaccination strategies and debates to combat the COVID-19 pandemic among countries, all countries are equally called upon to act beyond their own interests and to cooperate with each other. While the industrialized countries claim the available vaccines for themselves or within the European Union, fragile health systems in Africa, Asia, or Southeast Europe are left behind. People are largely at the mercy of the virus, and there is usually a lack of very basic equipment in the health care of the population.

In addition to the challenges of globalization, there are also promising approaches to solutions where everyone that is part of the world community could participate in for improved health. Greater international networking has succeeded in anchoring health issues internationally, while increased mobility, new communication options and technologies, and the rapid development of digitalization have simplified access to information, medicines, and diagnostic and therapeutic options.

However, in order to cope with current and future global health crises, everyone needs to be aware that these challenges can only be met collectively, in the sense of "the commons," i.e. sharing and democratically managing as a (world) community. Elinor Ostrom, who was the first woman to receive the Nobel Prize for Economics in 2009, proved that this is not an idealistic fantasy. She was able to prove, based on a worldwide collection of data, that everywhere in the world, from communal pastures in Switzerland to shared fields in Japan or irrigation farms in the Philippines to communally used water supplies in Nepal, the idea of commons, in the sense of communal management, works. This does not lead to a tragedy in which individuals gain an advantage and thus all perish as Garrett Hardin postulated in his article "The Tragedy of the Commons," which received much attention in the twentieth century [2], but rather success which is based on the fact that people communicate within a community [3:342].

The authors of this book "Innovative Human Resource Development in Health Care" are convinced that communication, overcoming external and mental boundaries, cooperation on all levels and between all areas as well as networking provide the real ground for sustainable innovations.

Innovation in Healthcare

▶ Some of the most important innovations do not come from new technologies, but through other ways of working together and reorganizing work.
Tom Malone, MIT

Every reader will be able to envision what it means to be courageous. Especially in the very hierarchically organized world of health care, everyone will have thought about whether more courage would not have been necessary in one situation or another instead of ducking away or running with the mainstream.

At this point, we will take a closer look at the concept of innovation, first in general and then with a focus on innovations in the health care sector.

Innovation is one of the buzzwords of our time, sometimes we ask ourselves: What is actually still innovative? There are very similar products or developments in the sense of *"copy and paste,"* which are rather imitations and are advertised in marketing with "Best Innovation 2020" and other slogans. Real discoveries or inventions of our ancestors probably went differently. Nevertheless, innovations have never been in such demand to solve the ever faster and more complex problems in this world.

Innovation (*Innovatio* late Lat.) means renewal or change. In economics, innovation refers to a (complex) innovation associated with technical, social, and economic change. So far, there is no universally valid approach to innovation or accepted definition of the term innovation. Nevertheless, all attempts at definition are concerned with the characteristics of first of all, novelty or (initial) innovation of a thing or a social mode of action and secondly, a change, a transformation, i.e. the idea alone is not enough. Innovation must be discovered or invented, introduced, used, applied, and finally institutionalized (cf. wirtschaftslexikon.gabler.de).

- "We will not be able to maintain our efficient healthcare system with less, but only with more innovations." This was said by the then Federal Minister of Health Hermann Gröhe in 2016 at the "Health Policy Dialogue" in Bochum [22]. In fact, we in Germany ask ourselves far too often and debate for an enormously long time whether we should dare to take a leap forward in innovation or rather put the brakes on. Hermann Gröhe puts it in a nutshell: "We will need innovations for the big challenges. We have to become more courageous." The major drivers of innovation in the healthcare system continue to be demographic change, the increase in chronic and, in some cases, rare diseases, and mechanization and digitalization (www.aerzteblatt.de 14.10.2016).

This is also confirmed by Roland Berger's annual German hospital study. In 2018, more than 70% of managers said they cooperate with medical technology companies from which they expect ideas and innovations for the further development of hospitals. This is not surprising, considering that medical innovations in the German healthcare system were already strongly driven by rapidly developing high-tech medicine in the twentieth century. The possibilities of digitalization will change healthcare in all sectors enormously and carry a high innovation potential both in terms of the development of examination and treatment options, as well as hospital managers expect this to lead to an even more significant internal increase in efficiency, increase in liquidity, and improvement in economic results (rolandberger.com).

The success stories of innovations in the healthcare sector essentially relate to achievements in technology, the rapid development of new technologies such as biotechnology, genetic diagnostics, robotics, sensor technology, electronic patient files, the use of drones or assisted living systems. On the one hand, progress is rapid, while the openness of the players towards technological innovations is still very restrained. What is little known is that nursing professionals also play a decisive role in the development of technological innovations. For example, a clinic in Istanbul has been training its nursing staff to produce innovations since 2012 and has since been able to register over 50 patents (see chapter by Yeliz Dogan Merih in this book).

Innovations can be expected to benefit the user, i.e. first and foremost the patient, and also to increase the productivity of staff. With the advancement of digital possibilities such as telemedicine, artificial intelligence, apps, and remote treatment, efficiency can be further increased even over long distances, e.g. in rural care areas. While, for example, a community health nurse visits the patient on site, carries out an initial assessment of the state of health and assessments, a doctor is later connected via video conference and contact is established with the patient in order to create a joint therapy plan in interprofessional discourse, which can then be implemented on-site.

Medical technology companies have also recognized the need for process optimization in the hospital landscape over the past 20 years and have entered into cooperative ventures with healthcare facilities with numerous optimization projects that are based purely on industry and technology logic. Nevertheless, it has become increasingly apparent in recent years that the healthcare system, which has been trimmed for efficiency, is reaching its limits. For the first time, patient growth rates in German hospitals are stagnating [19].

The shortage of skilled workers is intensifying all over the world due to the foreseeable demographic development.

- New technologies, in particular digitalization and robotics, may be able to cushion the increasing shortage of skilled workers to some extent. Nevertheless, direct physical examination, treatment, care, and, above all, attention will only be able to promote healing in the future if people act and assist.

For about 15 years, most health care systems in industrialized countries have followed the logic of economically driven and technically privileged efficiency thinking. Initially, there is nothing to be said against making procedures and processes more efficient in the interests of the patient, solving interface problems, and thus shortening waiting times. However, a discrediting of all solution strategies has crept in with it, which sensibly sometimes detours and goes along with continuous effort and is reasonable in the sense of a lasting healing process. Through this logic, emotional, social, and relationship-oriented solution strategies are also devalued. In her great statement "Courage in Nursing," Marie Manthey [4] brings the dangers of such a disbalance in the actions of the patient-oriented health care professions to the point (here related to the nursing professions, but equally valid for the medical profession):

▶ If we lose the balance of the technical and relational aspects of our work, putting the technical way out front, we necessarily put the relational aspects far behind. That means putting people-the very reason for the work of nurses-second (or third or fourth) to tasks [4:2].

We can say that this is not a dream of the future, but rather has already become a real conflict in the everyday actions of the health professions. In this context, Giovanni Maio argues that the health professions must defend their identity and that this requires a return to values such as patience, caution, reflexivity, and humility, without which care for people is not possible. It is the real challenge to a humane health care system, because for most health professionals this was and is the real driving force for choosing a health care profession (cf. [5]).

It is the so-called soft solution strategies and, in the case of staff, the "soft skills" used that have been shown to mobilize self-healing forces and contribute to a more sustainable recovery process (see [5] and Tewes in Chap. 4). New technologies are innovations in health care that have enormously advanced medical options for action, from significantly greater accuracy in diagnostics to minimally invasive surgery procedures that are gentler on patients or personalized medicine (see Bochum et al. in this book), which enables, for example, pharmacogenetics or tumor therapy tailored to the genome. Thus, it is not technological progress per se that should be viewed critically, but rather the changing attitude to the world and thus to the understanding of healing. Maio [5] notes that the "entry into the technical age is an expression of a society that values calculability and gives preference to strategic-controlling action over the inner attitude of letting things happen..." or letting things develop, letting things heal, which is not the case in every case, but every now and then, especially when conservative therapies are preferred over surgical procedures that are initiated too quickly, e.g. endoprosthetics or tumor therapy. This would be more beneficial in the long term, both medically and economically.

In the end, as is usually the case, it is a matter of being aware that we may be subject to an euphoria about technology, which obscures our view of alternative solutions, and that a blanket criticism of technology does not do justice to the challenges and possibilities of technology for medicine. Ultimately, it will be important to take a critically reflective approach to ensure that technology is not rashly used as a solution to problems that cannot be solved technically, but rather socially, physiologically, and psychotherapeutically or through care (cf. [5]).

The demographically induced changes confront the actors in the health care sector with unprecedented challenges in their daily work and require new approaches to design and management. Innovative competence is thus becoming an increasingly important requirement in the healthcare professions. For those involved, it is not so much a question of developing new technologies, but of approaching innovative technologies with courage and an open mind and applying them for the benefit of patients and the community. Further potential for innovation in the health care professions can be leveraged in the way prevention, treatment, and or palliative processes are designed, as well as in communication and cooperation with the respective users of health care services such as patients, clients, residents, or schools. Emotional competence has long since ceased to be a "nice to have" for the health care professions, but is indispensable for working with (vulnerable) people. Last but not least, the strongest potential for innovation in healthcare, which is still largely untapped, is quality-oriented interprofessional cooperation (cf. [6]).

The understanding of innovation, which has so far focused on new technologies and digitalization, must be expanded to include a social and organizational perspective for the health care sector in particular and equally for the working world of the future.

The Health Care System from an Innovation System Perspective

Until now, innovation research has hardly played a role in the discourse on the need for reform and the sustainability of health care systems.

Up to now, innovation in the health care system has been directed primarily towards the development of high-tech medicine and thus towards the achievements of medical technology and pharmaceutical technologies. In recent years, this industry-based thinking has been linked to the idea of efficiency-enhancing process optimization, which permeates all health care structures and is ultimately guided by the primacy of the economization of the health care system. For the most part, these projects lack a systemic approach; rather, they are thought of and acted upon in the classic cause-and-effect pattern in a linear fashion. However, it is nowadays known that innovation processes do not simply proceed in a linear fashion; rather, they are characterized by a multitude of feedbacks between the individual activities and actors involved, who in turn do not act in a vacuum but under certain framework conditions, interact with each other and, if necessary, form networks. This results in the necessity to conceptualize innovation as a system process. According to Chaminade and Edquist [7], an innovation system includes: "all important economic, social, political, organizational, institutional, and other factors that influence the development, diffusion, and use innovation."

In 2013, the Hans Böckler Foundation in Germany funded a study to analyze the healthcare sector from an innovation system perspective. The study was carried out by the Fraunhofer Institute for Systems and Innovation Research and for the first time, in Germany, systematically investigated the question of which characteristics

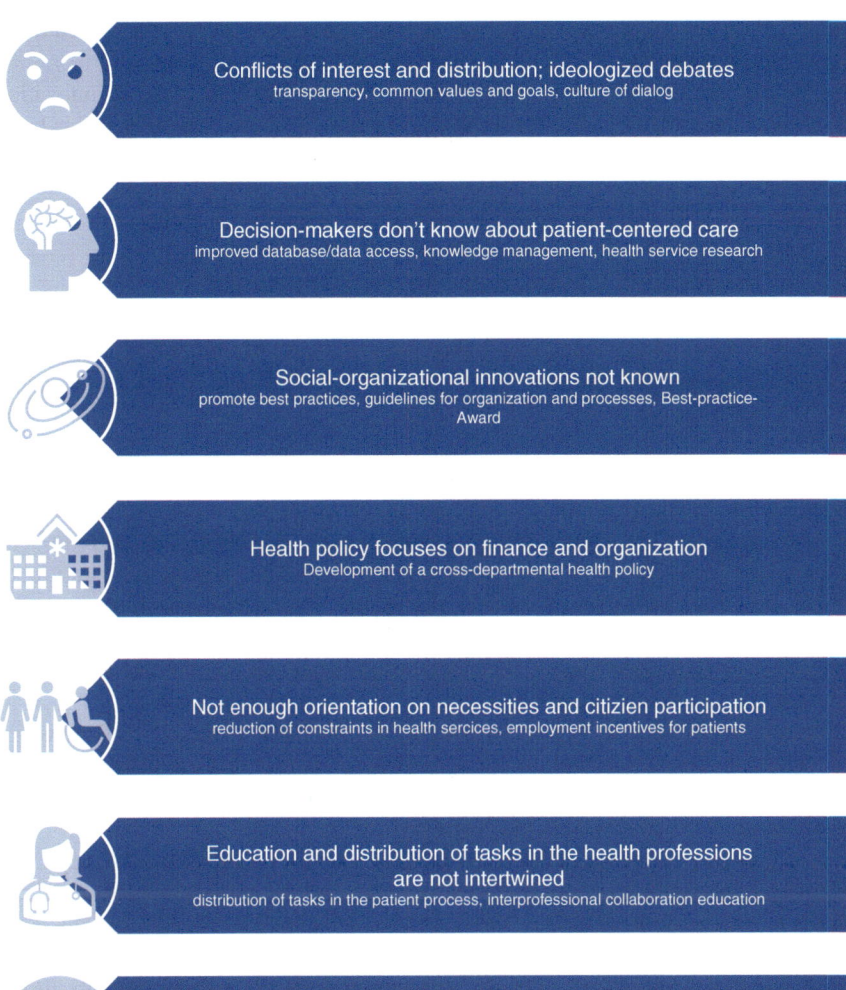

Fig. 1.1 Innovation potentials and opportunities for action in the healthcare sector. (Based on [8:272], own illustration)

and structures can be identified that limit innovative capacity in the health care system or in which there is still untapped innovation potential (cf. [8]). As a result, the researchers were able to elaborate eight theses on improvement and innovation potentials in the German healthcare system and present a variety of possible courses of action for discussion. What is significant about this study is that the previously rather neglected view of social-organizational innovation potentials could be elaborated.

It is precisely this perspective that we need to adopt if we want to approach human resources development in the healthcare sector in an innovative and courageous manner. Figure 1.1 provides an overview of the eight innovation potentials identified (based on [8]) and describes various options for action with which these potentials could be raised.

The possibilities for action elaborated by Heyen and Reiß from an innovation system perspective are explained in practical terms in various chapters in this book with regard to their significance for modern personnel development in the health care sector.

1.2 Personnel Development Yesterday and Today

▶ We can't solve problems by using the same kind of thinking we used when we created them.
Albert Einstein

Personnel development is now increasingly recognized by those responsible in healthcare facilities as a strategic success factor, because it supports the ability to develop and adapt in a rapidly changing working world. Although it has long been known that good personnel development promotes the long-term retention of employees, increases motivation and performance potential, and thus increases work productivity, the budgets for personnel development in health care facilities are known to be many times smaller than in industrial and commercial enterprises, without giving concrete figures here.

According to Becker [9], human resource development includes "... all measures of education, promotion and organisational development that are planned, implemented and evaluated in a targeted, systematic and methodical manner by a person or organisation to achieve specific purposes" [9:3].

For Becker, personnel development refers to an educational concept that relates to the entirety of a person who is in a permanent development process. In this understanding, it is not only a matter of pure knowledge transfer as it is still found in some health care institutions today in the sense of in-house further and continuing education. Analogous to the changing concepts in the vocational training courses of the health care professions, personnel development today is directed towards the development of holistic professional action competence.

Vocational action competence has been further developed by Rosenstiel and Erpenbeck since 2007 as a fixed concept and as a goal of modern vocational training (cf. [10]). In the meantime, not only have vocational training curricula been developed in a competence-oriented manner, but professional action competence has also arrived in the world of work. This is not surprising, because while classical qualifications are understood as certified, formal knowledge and are usually proven by examinations, competence development aims at the fundamental disposition of actions. Figure 1.2 shows the four levels of competence according to Arnold and Erpenbeck.

Fig. 1.2 Levels of the concept of competence according to Arnold and Erpenbeck [11]

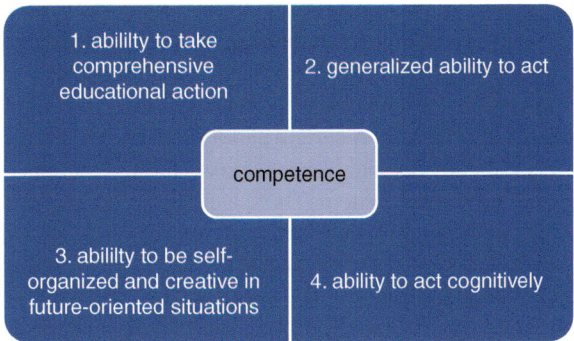

Competence as part of the **ability to act comprehensively in education is** often related to Humboldt's ideal of education. Humboldt ascribes education to the autonomous individual who produces himself by acting. Today we would speak of self-organization and self-efficacy.

Competence, understood as **generalized ability to act, is** described in the European and the German Qualification Framework, as well as in the new Nursing Professions Act (PflBG of 17.7.2017), which has been implemented in Germany since 1.1.2020. Generalized or comprehensive ability to act means here that from individual, specific observations (including linguistic data), thought and action processes are initiated, from which generally valid principles of a situation can be worked out, which can then be used again concretely for future situations and vice versa.

Competence as the **ability to act in a self-organized, creative manner in (future) open situations** is now widely accepted by vocational education and training, as well as by companies and organizations.

Understanding competence as the sole **ability to act primarily cognitively** is the basis of various comparative studies, such as the Programme for International Student Assessment (PISA). However, this understanding of competence excludes important motivational or affective aspects for successful action and is thus viewed critically. This is because there can be no competence without a motivational or emotional penetration of knowledge (cf. [11]).

- In health care, where it is also immanently about relationship work with the patient, the resident or the colleague, often with ethical references, an understanding of competence is to be preferred as Stangl formulates it in 2019 in the Online Lexicon for Psychology: "The concept of competence integrates not only knowledge and action, but also includes interests, motivations, value attitudes and social readiness" (https://lexikon.stangl.eu/).

Interest in interprofessional collaboration has increased enormously in the last 10 years, both in practice and research in the healthcare sector. Since around 2010, the topics of "interprofessional collaboration (IPC)" and "interprofessional education (IPE)" have increasingly been encountered at specialist congresses or in the specialist literature. A certain enthusiasm seems to have broken out that both quality and efficiency potentials can be raised through better cooperation between all actors in the health care system. There is no universally accepted definition yet, the WHO defines IPC as follows: "Interprofessional Collaboration occurs when two or more individuals from different backgrounds with complementary skills interact to create a shared understanding that none had previously possessed or could have come to on their own." "In addition, the WHO designates two further characteristics in its definition: Interaction and shared understanding of roles [23]. IPC, understood systemically, is more than the sum of the individual competencies of the professionals involved, it is about more than coordination, cooperation, and communication. At its best, it is about creating something new, which is beneficial for the client or patient and, where appropriate, even for the staff member. Effective interprofessional collaborative practice (ICP) goes beyond merely working together in a friendly manner and, if possible, "always at eye level," as is called for in many cases. Of course, good teamwork creates a better working atmosphere and thus greater staff and patient satisfaction. But we now know how important IPC is for the outcome of patient care. Numerous treatment errors occur due to poor communication and collaboration (see [12], among others). Increasing specialization and multimorbidity also require IPC more than ever, as does cross-sectoral care in different settings.

Health care systems that are subject to short-term economization through constant efficiency increases and process optimization are under increasing pressure to accelerate and are losing sight of the issues that give health care professions their identity, such as "helping others in need in a person-centered and professionally competent manner" and the related relationship work.

Communication venues and times such as joint rounds, case discussions, or further development as an interprofessional team on a ward or in a functional area fall by the wayside. Similarly, continuous communication and an exchange of information about the patient's progress between the different care settings take on a subordinate importance. New digital platforms, which have largely yet to be implemented, promise at least a better, and above all faster, case-related exchange of information.

All these are indications of necessary structures. These alone do not ensure a high quality of communication and a culture of cooperation. Communication thrives on the resonance of the communicators. In an accelerated world, as it is especially evident for patients and residents in the health care system, an expanded, even a specially trained communication competence is needed in order to generate resonance at all. Hartmut Rosa [13] points out that acceleration as a countermovement does not require deceleration, as is so often called for among health care professionals. Resonance requires mindfulness, attention, and concentration in the here and now. The civilized, mature human being, as a (self-)conscious being, is a shaper of his environment, no matter how challenging its framework conditions and developments may be.

The spotlight of an innovative and courageous personnel development in the health care sector must therefore be directed more than ever on the (value) attitudes of both managers and individual employees, their experience of self-efficacy, their sense of meaning, and their responsibility for a common cause.

New Requirements for the Personnel Development of the Future

▶ Thus our times present us with challenges that are as new as the changes in reality that they produce. Our response can only be: We must open our thinking to the new realities and their future development. We have to think in completely new dimensions. It is a matter of a New View and thus of an innovative achievement which must not only have the things of our living environment as its object, but our own thinking.
Kurt Biedenkopf [20]

The major drivers of an already emerging change in society and healthcare are clear: the effects of demographics, globalization, the knowledge society, climate change, digitalization, and new technologies affect the working world in all sectors equally. More than ever, organizations are challenged to quickly and thoroughly grasp the demands placed on them today and in the future, and to develop responses that do not merely combat symptoms in the short term, but rather take into account the essential factors for sustainable change. A mechanistic understanding of organization, in which the organization is seen as a machine that can be built up, converted and dismantled, leads to a dead end today. A purely people-oriented approach, which sees the organization as a group of people whose mindset and behavior must be changed according to requirements, is also obsolete. The closest approach would be the basic assumption that organizations are to be understood as social systems that are to be stimulated by interventions to change patterns, structures, and attitudes (cf. [14]).

In this context, corporate learning as well as self-directed learning in a learning organization is gaining new importance. In many places, today's personnel development cannot keep pace with the rapid and fundamental changes in the so-called VUCA world. While sustainable forms and processes of work, characterized by agility, self-organization, flexibility, and a focus on meaning, have long been established, especially in industrial and commercial enterprises, most health care institutions, and thus also their personnel development, are still stuck in the twentieth century with their structures, hierarchies, standardized structure and process specifications, one-dimensional performance measurement systems, standard seminars, annual training, and continuing education catalogs detached from the work process.

> - VUCA is an acronym that refers to "volatility," "uncertainty," "complexity," and "ambiguity." This is used to describe supposedly challenging characteristics and conditions of business management in the modern world. The term was introduced at the United States Army War College in the early 1990s. It was initially used to describe the multilateral world after the end of the Cold War. Later, the term spread to other areas of strategic leadership.
> - While VUCA describes the issues, the terms "vision" (vision), "understanding" (understanding), "clarity" (clarity), and "agility" (agility) also stand as an acronym for dealing with and surviving in the VUCA world (see Oliver [15]).

In order to meet the requirements of a flexible expansion of competencies in an agile and complex world of work, it is necessary to establish a new understanding of further education and training in which working, learning, and knowledge management are closely linked. The workplace-based learning that was already propagated in the 1990s, for example, in skills labs or learning workshops, as well as workplace-based learning in quality circles, learning islands, or school stations, is experiencing a renaissance here.

In the future, lifelong learning will have to consist of a meaningful combination of company learning and work processes. Learning belongs to the responsibility of the employees and the offers are also to be aligned with the needs of the employees in addition to the needs of the company. This is accompanied by a change from a supply-oriented to a demand-oriented personnel development. Among other things, employees are called upon to self-direct their learning processes ("employee-lead-learning"). In addition, an adapted learning and corporate culture ("learning organization") as well as the reorganization of the roles of all participants are required. Modern personnel development is required to translate strategic corporate decisions into competence requirements at an early stage and to transfer them into qualification concepts. Here, personnel development has a decisive value-creating function. Whether implementation processes in companies can be advanced quickly and successfully is directly related to the rapid implementation of adapted (self-)learning offers. Here, however, healthcare companies are also required to provide the necessary infrastructure, such as mobile learning, Internet access for employees, webinars, databases, videos.

The growing importance of self-responsible and self-directed learning must first be learned by employees. For this reason, personnel developers and managers should always also see themselves as learning coaches, establish mentoring concepts, and establish necessary offers that enable this form of learning.

Last but not least, the establishment of modern personnel development can only succeed if the company management defines a new demand-oriented learning architecture and learning culture in the company as a strategic goal and sustainably demands and promotes it across all levels. This also means that company management and personnel development must first overcome the traditional separation of the worlds of work and learning in their thinking and actions.

1.3 Practical Projects of Innovative Personnel Development

After the theory-based introduction, the next section introduces the practical projects of innovative personnel development.

We Love the Challenge: Culture Change

In the modern working world, a culture of working together is becoming increasingly important. The complex challenges can no longer be mastered with lone warriors. Nevertheless, the healthcare sector still often has a traditional hierarchical understanding of business and management. For example, the separation of the three pillars of doctors, nursing, and administration can still be found in most institutions. Many roles have not changed for decades; today, for example, we still find the type of chief physician who rules his "principality" as an "autocrat" and defends it with all his might. In nursing, on the other hand, the altruistic motif of the self-sacrificing helper is still deeply rooted and often comes into conflict in everyday life with challenges that, as a professional nurse, require enhanced competencies such as process control, communication and relationship building, prioritization, and self-organization. This is what nurses have been working on for decades and tends to present their profession to the next generations from an attitude of frustration. Measured against the real shortage of skilled workers, which represents a risk that can hardly be controlled in both occupational groups, it is urgently necessary for both occupational groups to reflect on their identity again and to actively participate in the design of sustainable working conditions from a positive attitude of values. The book describes two different approaches to successfully implement the focus on relationship-building in health care: the European Person-centred Care Programme, which was developed in Ireland, and the Relationship-Based Care Programme from the USA. Brendan McCormack and his team have succeeded in bringing about change processes in health care through a close integration of theories and practice. The focus of change (practice development) is on person-centered care. The change processes of the teams are accompanied by a coach, who on the one hand provides professional evidence-based knowledge and, on the other hand, motivates the team to engage in the process of cultural change. The focus is on the self-determination of the team. The coach introduces the suggestions and the team decides how they want to proceed. Self-reflection on one's own activities is an absolute must in order to adopt new behaviors and integrate new procedures. The coach therefore needs nursing research knowledge and a high level of social competence in accompanying these teams. The Protestant University of Applied Sciences in Dresden (ehs) offers a course of study in practice development to accompany this activity, in which precisely these competencies are learned. In this book, Tewes et al. describe how, on the one hand, the evidence base is promoted through own smaller research projects and, on the other hand, social skills are trained in the simulation laboratory with the help of actors.

From the USA, the Relationship-Based Care (RBC) program is well known, which aligns the entire culture of an organization to real encounters with a variety of trainings. First the encounter with oneself, then the encounter with colleagues, and finally the encounter with patients. With RBC, clinics are guided on the path to becoming a Magnet organization. The successes of this program are presented every 4 years at a symposium where clinics describe their culture change processes. This will involve all hospital staff in interprofessional groups, as Sue Wessel and her colleagues describe powerfully in this book. For example, the authors report on their successful training programs "See me as a person" and "Re-Igniting the spirit of caring" in this book. This is roughly how ward teams can be introduced to attitude work, by working with the question of "why." Why do I work in this clinic? Why do I work in this team? Why do I work in this profession? All questions that ask about meaning. According to Fink and Möller [14], meaning has two equally significant aspects in relation to companies. The emotional-individual aspect aims at "my work motivates me and gives me energy. I look forward to going to work every day, feel appreciated there." The factual-content aspect asks about the "what for" of the company, its ultimate goal. It provides orientation and guides fundamental decisions. Especially in the increasingly complex and turbulent world of health care, it is necessary to reflect again and again on the meaning and purpose of one's own actions and to use meaning as a navigational aid. However, the coherence of the experience in everyday life is decisive. If, for example, the mission statement says "The patient is the focus" and at the same time the length of stay is reduced with all possible force because there are bed shortages, then there will be conflicts of objectives for the employees and ultimately every mission statement will have missed its mark. The Purpose Drive Organization puts "purpose" at the core of an organization. Fink and Möller explain in detail and on the basis of organizational research and systems theory the importance of purpose for sustainable companies. They justify this with the elementary importance of meaning for the functioning of all kinds of social systems and thus also of organizations. Especially those who reckon with more complexity should focus on meaning and ask "why." Sense is necessary for a system to communicate and decide, to show direction. Sense connects people and organizations; it couples mental and social systems. Sense evolves evolutionarily as events unfold. And depending on what proves itself will continue to exist or not (cf. [14]). Cultural change cannot be ordered, cannot be decided, because cultures are unique because there is always an explicit or implicit reference to their own history in and with the organization. Luhmann writes on this "The dependence on one's own history individualizes the system. Even within an organization there can be different organizational cultures that react differently to the same measures" [16:80ff]. In this book, Grießehaber and colleagues describe how such a cultural change can succeed with their systemic approach of raising awareness and implementing leadership values.

When it comes to culture change in healthcare organizations, as in the first block "We love the challenge," the authors have used exactly this insight for their projects. Every change needs a close look at the respective cultures. By asking the question of the meaning of the project, they generate orientation and navigation assistance for all project participants, and in this way they promote the intrinsic motivation and cooperation to courageously shape innovation, which should not be underestimated. In Turkey, nursing professionals were trained to systematically "produce" innovations, which has now resulted in more than 100 patents. With this success, Yeliz Dogan Merih shows in this book how human resource development and employee motivation can succeed. Nowak and Lincoln qualify nursing professionals in the USA in a variety of integrative methods, such as acupressure, therapeutic touch, music therapy, aromatherapy, etc., and promote motivation through an increase in autonomy. Nurses are able to self-diagnose and order and implement appropriate integrative therapies.

Whether it is about relationship building, leadership, strategy processes. Through introducing a person-centered culture in healthcare or the development of a Healing Healthcare Model, the whole interacting system is always in view and the authors show their own systemic-autonomous matured attitude with which they face change (cf. [17]).

We Are Bold: Emotional Intelligence Pays

The institutions of the health care system are extremely rational and cognitively oriented due to the dominance of a science-based medicine and economization in the past decades. At the same time, the system of a hospital, for example, in which people are born, healed, suffer, cared for, or die every day, to take only the stories of patients and the professional groups close to the patients into consideration, are emotionally heated systems. Renate Tewes points out in detail in the chapter what effects this has on the people working in them. Numerous studies, e.g. Karin Kersting [18] "Coolout in care," prove that the lack of emotional work of relatives in health care professions can lead to a loss of empathy, bitterness, and even aggressive behavior and acts of violence towards those in need of protection.

> - If we consider that health institutions should generally be places of healing, health-promoting quality of life, and an environment for people who are ill and/or in need of care, then this cannot succeed if feelings are already suppressed, rejected, ridiculed, or devalued by managers.

Here, too, the reality for the employees shows a clear conflict of objectives between guiding principles that focus on the well-being of the patient and the managers or personnel developers who do not enable their employees to deal with their own and their patients' feelings in a (self-)reflective and professional manner. A still frequently encountered behavior among managers in the health care sector is that unpleasant topics are gladly tabooed or simply smiled at and devalued. This is downright dangerous in view of our current findings in neurobiology and neurophysiology, which have meanwhile proven the direct interaction and interplay between mind, feelings, and body and their effect on a person's well-being and health. All the more gratifying are various approaches that the authors have really courageously brought to the reality of health care.

It is high time that all these issues are taken seriously and addressed in healthcare facilities. Because it is worrying when, for example, the health report of the Technicians' Health Insurance Fund in Germany 2019 reports that geriatric and nursing staff are burdened with 8 days per year higher incapacity to work than in other sectors, higher demand for medicines, and a higher rate of mental illness Technicians [21]. All this causes high economically relevant costs in addition to the suffering for those affected. Therefore, yes: Emotional intelligence also pays off in the truest sense of the word.

Concepts such as those presented in this book, by Sue Smith and Gawin Andrews: "Stress was yesterday! Revitalizing care through Heart Math interventions," "EmpCare—an empathy-based relief training for caregivers" by Ludwig Thiry and Vera Lux as well as "Wellbeing in the workplace pays of" by Mary Jo Kreitzer show in a remarkable way, which (self-) effectiveness for patients, care recipients, and employees of the health care professions, a modern personnel development and leadership can achieve workplace-related and workplace-bound.

We Are a Dream Team: Interprofessional Collaboration

▶ The more dynamic and complex the business is, the less individual actors are able to make meaningful decisions on their own and the more important cross-hierarchical cooperation becomes [19:7].

And yet the players in clinics, practices and care facilities still work largely side by side with their own professional logics, which are mostly at cross purposes to the actual patient process. In addition, interface problems, for example, between functional departments and wards or logistical departments, are part of the everyday organizational challenges. And the principle in the hospital is then often: It's always the others who are to blame. Last but not least, the breaks in care for patients between the various sector boundaries of the health care system are also characterized by a coexistence rather than a cooperation for the benefit of the patient. The treatment and care of patients in health care institutions and cooperation in the interprofessional team is still hampered by the pursuit of self-interest or group interests.

- The vision would be that all employees of a health care facility, from the managing director to the cleaning staff, would be inspired to do everything possible so that patients can recover or their suffering can be alleviated in a health-promoting environment. This could develop into the spirit of a facility that radiates both internally and externally.

Well-intentioned management slogans such as "We're all in the same boat" or glossy brochures no longer win over employees. Cultural change must be more profound, authentic, transparent, and honest, and it starts with the managers.

Numerous health congresses and publications focus on the topic of interdisciplinary and interprofessional cooperation (IPC) and the interaction of different health care institutions. Although all players in the health care system are aware of it, the reality is completely different. This is becoming an increasingly pressing problem, not last because it is bound to deter any new blood for both doctors and nurses. As described above, cultural change cannot be ordered, it has to be worked out in the long term and evolutionarily in a participatory manner, then repeatedly re-examined and corrected. Udo Schuss and Reiner Blank [6] emphasize in their book "Qualitätsorientierte interprofessionelle Kooperation (QuiK)" that first order changes have already prevailed in health care institutions for many years, not least through numerous certifications in the sense of a continuous improvement process (KVP). In this sense, strategies and processes follow logically linear thought patterns and process chains. What must now take place is a transformation that shakes the foundations, the core of a system or an organization, as a second-order change. A radical transformation shakes the identity of the organization and requires appropriate preparation, good crisis management, and follow-up work (cf. [6]).

It stands to reason that interprofessional cooperation should be experienced and positively experienced by future professionals at an early stage during the socialization of trainees and students. In the practical fields of training, interprofessionality as an attitude and competence has so far been neglected. Here, too, the next generation is tied to its own professional group and learns how not to do it. With its "Operation Team" funding program, the Robert Bosch Stiftung has supported best-practice projects for several years that develop and test cooperative models in the training of physicians, nurses, and therapy professions. In their article "Interprofessionelle Ausbildungsstation: Grenzen überwinden-Zusammen lernen und arbeiten" (Interprofessional Training Station: Overcoming Boundaries: Learning and Working Together), Christine Straub, Sebastian Bode, Lukas Nock from Freiburg University Hospital, and Irina Cichon from the Robert Bosch Stiftung describe how learning can be integrated into the working world and how the protagonists can work together as a team to find the best possible solutions for patients.

Thomas Röhrßen and Klaus Wohlmeiner have gone beyond the process optimizations in the expensive operating rooms that have been common in German clinics to date and have focused on communication and cooperation in the team, from which a different performance emerges than in lone warriors. The project thus goes into much more depth and is an exemplary process of the courage it takes to tackle transformation in an organizational unit and yet it is worth taking on the effort.

In this book, Bochum et al. describe how interprofessional collaboration is the crucial basis for successful activity at the Institute for Personalized Medicine (MOLIT). The more individualized the healthcare system responds to the needs of the patient, the closer all the professional groups involved must work together.

1.4 Conclusion

Renate Tewes will conclude the book with her chapter "future perfect-innovative staff development" and will thus open the door to a possible future of staff development that we may not yet be able to imagine in all scenarios. In doing so, she does not take off into dreamy fantasy worlds, but rather describes in a basic and systematic way the central challenges that staff development in the healthcare sector will have to overcome in the future, develops approaches to solutions for this, and presents the necessary core competencies for staff working in the healthcare sector.

The combination of all the contributions presented here shows that the topics of innovative personnel development are on the agenda of health care institutions in a similar way internationally. As diverse as the approach and implementation of the individual projects may be, they are all characterized by a high degree of creativity, initiative, social-organizationally understood innovation, and courage. We would like to take this opportunity to thank all the contributors to our book for their exciting contributions, their perseverance with us. We wish them continued courage, always good small and big ideas for the health of all.

It's good to have courage.

References

1. Federal Ministry of Health (BMG). Global health policy challenges. 26 March 2021. https://www.bundesgesundheitsministerium.de/themen/internationale-gesundheitspolitik/global/globale-herausforderungen-der-gesundheitspolitik.html. Accessed 25 April 2021.
2. Hardin G. The tragedy of the commons. Science. 1968;162(3859):1243.
3. Bregmann R. Basically good. A new history of humanity. Hamburg: Rowohlt; 2020.
4. Manthey M. Courage in nursing. 2020. https://chcm.com/thought-leadership/courage-in-nursing-using-core-truths-to-create-a-better-world/. Accessed 30 Aug 2020.
5. Maio G. Values for medicine. Why the healing professions must defend their identity. Munich: Kösel; 2018.
6. Schuss U, Blank R. Quality-oriented interprofessional cooperation (QuiK). Nurses and physicians in focus. Bern: Hogrefe; 2018.
7. Chaminade C, Edquist C. From theory to practice: the use of systems of innovation approach in innovation policy. 2006. https://www.researchgate.net/publication/254420173_From_theory_to_practice_the_use_of_systems_of_innovation_approach_in_innovation_policy. Accessed 12 May 2020.
8. Heyen NB, Reiß T, et al. Das Gesundheitswesen aus Innovationssystemperspektive: Acht Thesen und Handlungsmöglichkeiten. Social Prog Independent J Soc Policy. 2014;Part 1:10/2014: 246–52. Part 2: 11/2014: 267–76.
9. Becker M. Personalentwicklung. Education, promotion and organizational development. sixth revised and expanded ed. Stuttgart: Schäffer-Poeschel; 2013.
10. Erpenbeck J, Rosenstiel L, Grote S, Sauter W (eds). Handbuch der Kompetenzmessung. Recognizing, understanding and assessing competencies in operational, educational and psychological practice. 3. rev. and extens. Auflage. Stuttgart: Schaeffer-Pöschel; 2017.
11. Arnold R, Erpenbeck J. Knowledge is not competence. Dialogues on competence maturation. Baltmannsweiler: Schneider Verlag Hohengehren; 2014.
12. Gerbera M, Kraft E, Bosshard C. Interprofessional collaboration from a quality perspective. Swiss Med J. 2018;44. https://saez.ch/article/doi/saez.2018.17276. Download pdf file on 30 Aug 2020.

13. Rosa H. Resonance. A sociology of the world relation. 3rd ed. Berlin: Suhrkamp; 2020.
14. Fink F, Moeller M. Purpose driven organizations. Meaning-self-organization-agility. Stuttgart: Schäffer-Poeschel; 2018.
15. Bendel O. Defining VUCA. 2019. https://wirtschaftslexikon.gabler.de/definition/vuca-119684. Accessed 20 Aug 2020.
16. Luhmann N. Organisation and decision. 3rd ed. Wiesbaden: Springer; 2011. p. 80ff.
17. Permantier M. Attitude decides. Shaping leadership and corporate culture for the future. Munich: Franz Vahlen; 2019.
18. Kersting K. Coolout in the nursing professions. A study on moral desensitization. Frankfurt/Main: Mabuse; 2011.
19. Berger R. 2018. www.rolandberger.com/publicationen/Krankenhausstudien 2018; 2019 and 2020. Accessed 20 July 2020.
20. Biedenkopf K. Dimensionen von Innovationen. In: Bührlen B, Kickbusch I (eds) Innovationssystem Gesundheit: Ziele und Nutzen von Gesundheitsinnovationen. Results of the first MetaForum on Innovations in the Health System. ISI-Schriftenreihe Innovationspotentiale. Stuttgart Fraunhofer IRB; 2008.
21. Die Techniker. Health report 2019. Care case care industry? This is how Germany's caregivers are doing. 2019. https://www.tk.de/resource/blob/2066542/2690efe8e801ae831e65fd251cc77223/gesundheitsreport-2019-data.pdf. Download pdf-Datei 27 Aug 2020.
22. Gröhe H. Innovationen im Gesundheitswesen -Wir müssen mutiger werden. 2016. www.aerzteblatt.de from 14 Oct 2016, https://www.aerzteblatt.de/nachrichten/70910/Innovationen-im-Gesundheitswesen-Wir-muessen-mutiger-werden. Accessed 8 June 2020.
23. World Health Organization. Framework for action on interprofessional education and collaborative practice. Geneva: WHO; 2010. p. 6. https://apps.who.int/iris/bitstream/handle/10665/70185/WHO_HRH_HPN_10.3_eng.pdf;jsessionid=45BB7F23409F0A10FA2B8B9447458D03?sequence=1. Download 30 Aug 2020.

Part I

We Love the Challenge: Culture Change

Engaging Hearts and Minds to Advance Relationship-Based Cultures

Mary Koloroutis, Susan Wessel, and Jayne Felgen

2.1 Creating a Culture of Caring

New strategies were needed to help healthcare organizations achieve excellence in quality, safety, patient and caregiver experience, and financial health. These outcomes have been cited as essential elements for health care quality by the Institute of Healthcare Improvement in their quadruple aim [1, 2]. We have supported these goals by translating relational competence and caring into practical, repeatable behaviors. Clinical and technical competence without relational competence is not professional practice. This belief underpins the philosophy of Relationship-Based Care™[1] [3–7]. Relationship-Based Care (RBC) focuses on the improvement of three caring relationships: relationship with self, relationship with colleagues, and relationship with patients and their families. RBC has been implemented in all types of health care settings and for all disciplines and services. The innovative project we share describes the impact of two workshops that are instrumental in the formation of RBC cultures.

---

[1] Relationship-Based Care™ is a registered trademark of Creative Health Care Management. All Rights Reserved.

M. Koloroutis · S. Wessel (✉) · J. Felgen
Creative Health Care Management, Eden Prairie, MN, USA
e-mail: mkoloroutis@chcm.com; swesselrn@comcast.net; jfelgen@chcm.com

2.2 Beliefs About Innovative Learning

Health care staff members often report feeling depleted and overwhelmed by rapid change and a heavy focus on efficient task completion. Two innovative educational workshops focus on revitalizing staff members and bring back the joy and meaning of their work. Our experience has taught us that education must engage the heart and mind and convey an authentic respect for the work of human caring and for the staff members who fulfill this work. The workshops are an invitation to reflect on one's practice and are conducted through experiential learning methods. The learning methods open participants' minds to new ways of thinking and being. Therefore, these workshops stand in sharp contrast to mandatory education, which often emphasizes didactic presentations and compliance. These workshops are designed with the adult learning principle that learning should be grounded in respect for the wisdom of the learner [8].

Our approach is to create space for reflection and a sense of psychological safety so that participants can share openly. Exercises are designed to access the right brain (the creative side) as well as the left brain (the analytical side). Learning is promoted through humor and creativity. In addition, structured reflection and journaling allow participants time with their own thoughts and time to wonder about and access their emotions through written work and/or artistic expression. Storytelling is employed to engage participants' hearts and to build a sense of common connection and community.

A feature of the workshops that has been instrumental in achieving mindful speaking and deep listening is circle practice, as described by Christina Baldwin and Ann Linnea [9]. The two innovative workshops described in this chapter use the practice of meeting in a circle at the beginning and end of each day. Circle practice provides a way for each person to share what is on their mind and heart in response to the facilitator's reflective questions. Learning becomes shared and amplified within the circle through the deep listening of everyone in the group. Participants begin to know each other simply as people, without the influence of titles, roles, and rank that often characterize our work settings.

The teaching methods that underpin the curricula are designed so that each idea is first described conceptually (and briefly), then brought to life with a story or anecdote, and finally, applied by participants in an exercise. Exercises may include journaling, self-assessments, storytelling, or creative artwork, to name only a few. This cycle of learning enables participants to internalize the concepts in a way that is meaningful to them.

2.3 How to Achieve Relationship-Based Care

The two innovative workshops highlighted here have proven instrumental in forming RBC cultures. The current national emphasis on patient-centered care, employee engagement, and professional practice has led many US health care organizations to choose RBC, particularly those seeking Magnet™[2] designation.

---

[2] MAGNET®, Magnet Recognition Program®, ANCC Magnet Recognition®, Journey to Magnet Excellence®, Pathway to Excellence® Program, Pathway to Excellence in Long Term Care®, Demographic Data Collection Tool®, and DDCT® are registered trademarks of the American Nurses Credentialing Center (ANCC). Practice Transition Accreditation Program™ and PTAP™

Relationship-Based Care is a philosophy, an operational blueprint, a model that supports professional practice, and a way of being. It promotes a healing culture in health care organizations by focusing on three key relationships: the relationship with self, with colleagues, and with patients and their families [5, 6, 10]. It has been implemented by organizations in all types of clinical and nonclinical departments and settings. The RBC model includes eight dimensions that create a culture of excellence and that correlate with positive outcomes in quality, safety, patient and staff satisfaction, and financial health [2].

2.4 Dimensions of Relationship-Based Care [10]

- **Patient and Family at the Center**
- Structures, processes, and relationships are developed to support each caregiver's ability to provide attuned, compassionate, high-quality care. All systems and services align with the patient's and their family's needs and priorities.
- **Healing Culture**
- A healing culture holds patients, families, and all who work in health care with respect and dignity. All staff members are supported in learning and reaching their full potential and are valued for their contribution to the health and healing of patients. Therapeutic relationships and a calming physical environment are core components of healing cultures.
- **Leadership**
- Leaders cultivate a shared vision, inspire and model healthy relationships, and empower the people closest to the work to continuously improve their own structures, processes, and relationships. Leaders enhance staff capacity by nurturing growth and learning. They hold the well-being of patients, families, and staff members as their highest priority.
- **Teamwork**
- Teamwork requires people from all disciplines and departments to define and embrace a shared purpose, proactively communicate, and work together with trust and mutual respect. Consistent and visible teamwork is essential to the provision of high-quality, safe care, and psychological safety which is essential to good teamwork.
- **Interprofessional Practice**
- All clinical professionals are respected and valued for their unique expertise and full scope of practice. Clinical practice is grounded in research, professional standards, and ethics. Diverse perspectives are essential for effective collaboration and optimal patient care and outcomes.
- **Care Delivery**
- The patient care delivery system is the infrastructure for organizing care. Care processes are designed to support a named primary caregiver for each discipline

---

are trademarks of the ANCC. The products and services of Creative Health Care Management are neither sponsored nor endorsed by ANCC. All Rights Reserved.

in accepting individual ownership for forming a therapeutic relationship with the patient and family and leading care for their discipline. Fragmented processes are replaced with systems that enable continuity of relationships and smooth transitions across the continuum of care.
- **System Design**
- Structures, processes, and relationships are continuously improved to bring quality, safety, effectiveness, and efficiency to patient care and the work environment. Incorporating the perspectives of patients and the community is essential for optimizing decisions.
- **Evidence**
- Evidence-based practice (integration of research, clinical expertise, and patient values) guides standards and provision of care throughout the organization. Measurable outcomes are identified and shared as evidence of achievement of the organization's mission and vision.

Health care leaders and caregivers are often asked to share what Relationship-Based Care means to them. A sampling of their words conveys the essence of this model and its ability to inspire organizations.

Relationship-Based Care is…

> ...a conscious action of intentional caring in all relationships within the organization that bring life to our mission and values every moment of every day.
> ~Director of Emergency Services

> ...an approach to care of self, colleagues, patients and families built on the uniqueness of that person. Relationships allow us to partner in a journey to trust, share and collaborate.
> ~Staff Nurse

> ...teamwork at its highest calling.
> ~Chief Operations Officer

> ...the foundation for every encounter in our organization. It helps us honor the privilege we have as healers during some of the most sacred moments in the lives of those we touch. First and foremost, people will remember how we made them feel. Simply stated, it's about relationships.
> ~Chief Nursing Officer

How Do We Find the Time?

In helping organizations implement RBC, we find that it is important to address a common misconception that causes staff members in all departments to be skeptical about embarking on this journey. This myth is that caring must involve spending more time with patients. Our study of best practices in compassionate and therapeutic relationships has shown that mindful and intentional caring does not take more time and can actually save time as patients' and families' fears are reduced and they feel heard by caregivers. Learning what is most important to patients can help clinical staff members prioritize what is most important and let go of things that are less important to patients and/or families. The two workshops highlighted in this chapter help staff members understand the essence of human connection, and that the most meaningful interactions can happen in the briefest moments.

2.5 Two Impactful Workshops

The two workshops, *Re-Igniting the Spirit of Caring* and *See Me as a Person,* create communities of learners who come together around their shared purpose of being part of something meaningful—something bigger than themselves. The curricula are built on the principle that human connection is healing, while isolation increases patient and staff-member suffering and leads to compassion fatigue and burnout in clinicians. Participants emerge from these programs with a deeper appreciation of each other's contributions to care and a greater understanding of themselves and their vital importance in the work of human caring [2, 11].

Workshop #1: *Re-Igniting the Spirit of Caring*

Early in the process of implementing Relationship-Based Care in an organization, groups of 30 staff members and their leaders attend a 3-day immersion experience built on the science of caring. This learning experience unfolds in four modules: (1) caring for self, (2) caring for colleagues, (3) caring for patients and families, and (4) transformational leadership. For each workshop, two facilitators use diverse learning methods that are highly interactive. They facilitate by modeling deep listening and inviting participant engagement rather than by a didactic teaching method.

The *Re-Igniting the Spirit of Caring* (RSC) workshop translates the three caring relationships—care of self, care of colleagues, and care of patients and families—into daily practice [10] (Image 2.1).

RSC grounds and renews members of the health care team in understanding the power and purpose of caring. Participants deepen their knowledge of and skills in caring for themselves, their colleagues, and patients and families.

The Caring for Self Module of *Re-igniting the Spirit of Caring*

The *RSC* curriculum starts with care of self as a precondition for establishing caring relationships with others, whether with colleagues or patients and their families. Concepts include:

- Who am I? (A self-awareness exercise).
- Vision for a fulfilling life.
- Balancing body, mind, and spirit.
- Managing energy and stress.

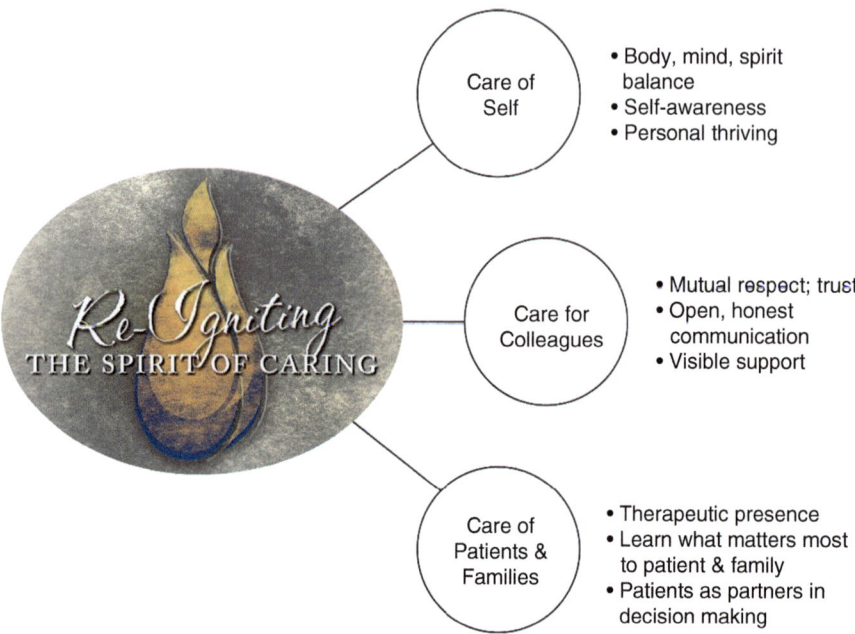

Image 2.1 Re-igniting the spirit of caring. (Source: Creative Healthcare Management)

One of the most impactful exercises in the self-care module is the exercise and reflection on well-being of body, mind, and spirit. After being introduced to the concepts, participants complete a self-assessment that includes evaluating their self-care practices in each realm (body, mind, and spirit). They notice in which area they have scored the highest, and which area is most in need of improvement. Then all participants are asked to stand in groups according to which area they scored the highest (body, mind, spirit, or balanced). The facilitator invites people in each group to share what they do that helps them be strong in the realm they scored the highest. This inevitably generates practical ideas that plant seeds for the final part of the exercise, which is quiet journaling. Following the standing discussion, participants journal about their commitments to themselves, including one idea they will implement to improve their self-care. This one idea is revisited later to reinforce the personal commitment to action.

The Caring for Colleagues Module of *RSC*

This second module encourages participants to reflect on what kind of co-worker they are and to understand the behaviors that foster healthy teamwork and colleagueship. The self-assessment and small group dialogue are framed around the ten *Commitment to My Co-Workers©* behaviors described by Marie Manthey, founder of Creative Health Care Management [10]. These behaviors resonate with staff members and the staff councils who have been charged with implementing RBC. The staff councils create action plans to implement the commitments in their units or departments. Three examples of these behaviors illustrate why they are so fundamental to healthy interpersonal relationships:

- I will talk to you promptly if I am having a problem with you. The only time I will discuss it with another person is when I need advice or help in deciding how to communicate with you appropriately.
- I will accept you as you are today, forgiving past problems, and ask you to do the same with me.
- I will remember that neither of us is perfect and that human errors are opportunities, not for shame or guilt, but for forgiveness and growth.

One of the most impactful exercises in the caring for colleagues module provides tools and an opportunity to practice healthy communication in which learners need to resolve an issue with a co-worker. Participants are provided with a respectful framework they can use to prepare for a difficult conversation. After they write how they plan to approach the conversation, they practice with one or two other partners, getting helpful feedback in this safe setting. Then, the group as a whole discusses what they learned as they practiced the challenging conversation.

The Caring for Patients and Families Module of RSC

The content regarding patients and families is designed to help participants get inside the varied emotions experienced by patients and their loved ones during a health care experience. In a small group exercise, participants are invited to share a personal story of caring. In groups of four, they share a time when they were a patient or the family member of a patient, and they recall the emotions they experienced during this time. This exercise is debriefed with the entire group as participants share the various emotions they noticed, both positive and negative. This exercise brings back to them what the experience of being a patient or family member felt like. In another exercise they reflect quietly on their own caring practices in a self-assessment and then are introduced to the practices that create therapeutic relationships. This content, which is from the book and workshop, *See Me as a Person,* [12] sets the stage for deeper work when they attend that workshop later as a way to sustain and deepen RBC.

The most impactful experience in the caring for patients and families module on the second workshop day involves small group experiences with former patients and family members who received care in that organization. Four to six former patients or family members are invited to share, in small groups, their experiences when receiving care. Listening deeply to these guests provides significant insights for the workshop participants. What they thought mattered most to patients or families is often not what they hear described. The insights from patients and family members provide ideas for giving care that participants can then incorporate into their personal practice and into action plans for implementing Relationship-Based Care.

The final workshop day sets the stage for taking caring practices back to the work setting. Small groups create a brief presentation that creatively demonstrates their vision for Relationship-Based Care in their own departments. These visions become part of their future work to apply best practices in caring relationships. All participants take their visions back to their work groups and create action plans for strengthening the three foundational relationships of RBC, relationship with self, with colleagues, and with patients and their families.

Designed for health care providers, ancillary staff members, and support team members, *RSC* inspires participants to reconnect with the meaning, purpose, and joy of their work and to be even more intentional in how they contribute to their organization in service to patients and families.

Workshop #2: *See Me as a Person*

See Me as a Person is an exploration of four practices that improve all relationships. The four therapeutic practices were introduced in the book, *See Me as a Person: Creating Therapeutic Relationships with Patients and Their Families*, by Mary Koloroutis, a nurse, and Michael Trout, a psychologist, in 2012. They developed these practices by discerning therapeutic principles, evidence, and best practices from an interdisciplinary lens. Nursing scholars in caring science such as Watson [13], Peplau [14], and Swanson [15] informed their work as did scholars in human connection, psychology, and infant-mental health [12, pp. 44–46]. Koloroutis and Trout deconstructed what happens when human connection and therapeutic care are at their best to develop the four therapeutic practices. Since then it has become clear that clinicians who also integrate the four practices into their lives outside of clinical settings experience improvements in all their relationships. The workshop is based on these practices so that staff members can more reliably apply them in their daily work.

The curriculum helps participants understand the human responses to illness, trauma, and crisis, which represent a non-ordinary state often accompanied by fear, pain, powerlessness, grief/loss, and difficulty coping.

The Four Therapeutic Practices: Attuning, Wondering, Following, and Holding

In studying the nature of therapeutic relationships and how they are developed, Koloroutis and Trout identified four essential practices that create just such a personal connection (2012). These practices form the basis of learning in *See Me as a Person* workshops [10] (Image 2.2).

Attuning. Attuning is often explained as "tuning in" to someone or "meeting people exactly where they are." When you tune in to someone, you will notice things about the person's way of being as well as any impact—positive or negative—that you may be having on the other person. You attune when you focus your attention on the well-being of the other person. Closely related concepts used in nursing are: *knowing and being with* [15], *transpersonal caring relationship* [13], and *therapeutic relationship and presence* [12, 14]. Attuning is grounded in empathy and compassion and puts the "how" to both.

Attuning is the foundational practice of therapeutic relationships. While attuning can happen in the absence of the other three practices, the other three practices

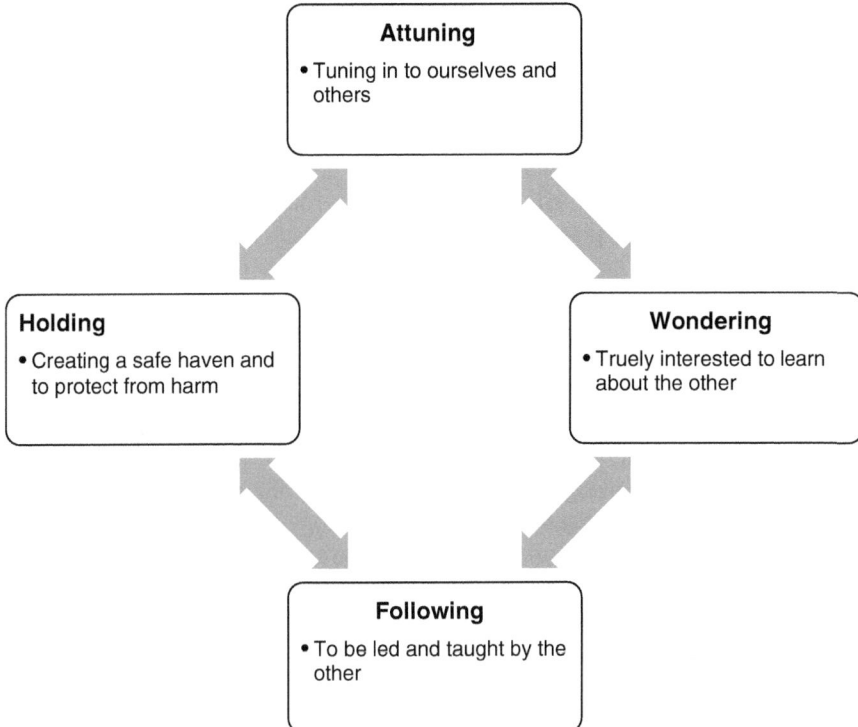

Image 2.2 See Me as a Person practices. (Source: Creative Healthcare Management)

cannot happen in the absence of attuning. Unless you are "tuned in" to someone, it is not possible to establish and nurture a healthy relationship.

Wondering. Wondering is a practice of discovery grounded in curiosity and genuine interest in the other. Actively wondering prevents you from making assumptions, rushing to judgment, or disconnecting from people prematurely. You become more scientific when you wonder. Wondering helps you resist hasty conclusions, welcome and seek new data, and imagine possible explanations beyond the apparent ones. When you wonder, you notice more and miss less.

Following. Following is the practice of allowing yourself to be informed and guided by the nuances of a person's words as much as by their content. When you follow, you allow your demeanor, words, and actions to be influenced by what you have observed about the other person. Following may mean sitting quietly for a moment with someone, offering a gentle touch, or providing that which you have learned is most needed at this moment.

Holding. Holding is a conscious decision to remember, affirm, and dignify what the patient or family member has taught you. You hold someone when you do what you said you would do. You hold when you remember the things people tell you and act on them. You hold when you listen without defensiveness. You hold when you provide knowledgeable and proficient technical care. Holding is also the natural result of attuning, wondering, and following. When you do all of these things, a reliable side effect is that you create a safe haven around the person.

Experiential Learning in Action

The diverse learning tools in *See Me as a Person* workshops are designed to help participants understand and internalize the four practices that create therapeutic relationships. A variety of methods such as videos, role play, application exercises with partners, and circle practice facilitate self-awareness and new skills that apply directly to any type of health care setting.

One of the most impactful exercises is based on research with infants that demonstrated the impact of attuned facial expressions by parents on the emotional development of infants. This research is relevant to the importance of attunement between caregivers and patients [12]. The experiences of being attuned and of being misattuned with another person are powerfully felt in an exercise that involves pairs of participants who engage with each other, first in strong attunement, and then being misattuned. Following this exercise, participants are asked to share situations in their day-to-day work that happen because someone was misattuned. This often leads people to share wonderful strategies they have used to overcome the barriers that impede our attuning to patients. Other exercises help participants practice ways of following the verbal and non-verbal cues of patients and families so that care is based on what matters most to them. Participants also learn therapeutic responses to anger, fear, grief, and pain.

The purpose of giving definition to the individual practices that comprise therapeutic care is to take the mystery out of what constitutes effective relationships. Through the study of the four therapeutic practices (attuning, wondering, following, and holding), authentic connection can be learned, reflected on, practiced, and mastered.

Sustaining and Deepening *See Me as a Person*

Organizational leaders are continually challenged with how to sustain and deepen caring relationships. To address these needs, Creative Health Care Management developed a digital platform, Creative Health Care Insight™, to support ongoing learning [16]. This platform contains assessment instruments based on relational competencies. Users gain valuable insights that enhance self-awareness about strengths and learning opportunities in relational behaviors. The assessments are accompanied by self-directed online learning modules to deepen understanding and application of therapeutic relationship behaviors that were included in the workshop.

Measuring the Impact of the Workshops

As we originally imagined how these two workshops would support Relationship-Based Care, we hoped participants would be inspired and re-energized about their personal impact on patients, families, and co-workers. We wanted participants to reconnect with the joy and meaning that originally brought them into the work of healing. In addition, we wanted those attending to be willing and able to translate the ideas they were learning into day-to-day action. This notion of translating caring into practical behaviors informed our choices of teaching and learning methods.

We captured the impact of the workshops through participant assessments immediately following each workshop, and we measured longer-term outcomes through departmental and organizational improvements in performance metrics [17–20]. As participants shared their very personal thoughts during circle, we could also immediately see whether we were touching the hearts of participants and whether they understood the concepts being taught. The evaluations at the end of each workshop asked how participants would change their practice as a result of what they learned (in addition to the more traditional evaluation questions).

Participants were charged with using the ideas from the workshops in their work implementing RBC. Many of those attending were members of department-based staff councils who were being educated and coached by our consultants as they developed comprehensive action plans for how they would bring RBC to life and measure the effectiveness of their plans. Each action plan was to include outcome measures that would show how effective their action plans were. Many times staff council members could find existing measures to use, such as an individual question on a patient survey or a staff survey.

We also watched closely the organization-wide metrics that the executive leaders followed. These measures generally reflected patient experience, quality, safety, employee satisfaction and retention, and ultimately the financial health of the organization. Every 4 years we held an international symposium to capture and show case the extraordinary results that our clients achieved. At these events, individual departments implementing RBC (generally including one or both of the workshops highlighted here) conducted poster presentations or live break-out sessions that demonstrated their innovations or explained their successes.

2.6 Quantitative Outcomes

Executive health care leaders identify key performance metrics as part of their strategic goals. Most often these metrics fall into four categories: (1) patient and family experience/satisfaction, (2) quality and safety, (3) employee and physician engagement/satisfaction, and (4) financial health. Relationship-Based Care is a blueprint for excellence that positively impacts all four of these categories [2]. Every organization that committed to implementing Relationship-Based Care has achieved positive results [5, 21]. As a part of RBC implementation, *Re-Igniting the Spirit of Caring* and *See Me as a Person* workshops are most directly linked with improved patient and family experience/satisfaction and employee engagement/satisfaction. We will share just a few of the most notable positive outcomes.

Patient and Family Experience/Satisfaction

Policies for health care reimbursement for a sizeable portion of the USA have begun to structure payments based in part on scores for patient experience. For this reason, stronger emphasis has been placed on how satisfied patients are with their health care experience. This has been a driving force for organizations to implement RBC.

- New York-Presbyterian/Columbia University Medical Center achieved the highest patient satisfaction score in their history (10 basis points above the national average) after implementing RBC with regular sessions of *Re-Igniting the Spirit of Caring*. Over 5 years, the mean scores improved in each of the 15 questions that evaluate patient satisfaction with nursing care in the Press Ganey Patient Experience Survey [18].
- Pennsylvania Hospital embraced *See Me as a Person* workshops as a part of implementing RBC to improve patient satisfaction, staff engagement, and professional practice. They reported significant improvement in their patient experience/satisfaction scores on Press Ganey surveys. Findings were: (1) Communication with nurses improved by 34%, (2) "Nurses treat with courtesy/respect" improved by 42%, (3) "Nurses listen carefully to you" improved by 50%, and (4) "Nurses explain in a way you understand" improved by 11% [20].
- The James Comprehensive Cancer Center of Ohio State University was awarded the prestigious Press Ganey Guardian of Excellence award for achieving an overall inpatient satisfaction score above the 95th percentile for four consecutive quarters. They credited Relationship-Based Care and their frequent sessions of *Re-Igniting the Spirit of Caring* for their success [19].

Employee Engagement/Satisfaction and Financial Health

Health care organizations have embraced recent evidence that there is a strong correlation between employee engagement and patient satisfaction and quality. They generally employ national survey companies to assess their employee engagement every year, and they closely monitor staff turnover by department.

- Faxton-St. Luke's Healthcare in New York improved their Press Ganey employee satisfaction scores from the 14th percentile to 60th percentile after system-wide implementation of Relationship-Based Care and extensive sessions of *Re-Igniting the Spirit of Caring* [22].
- Crittenton Hospital Medical Center, in Michigan, achieved a reduction in annual nurse turnover from 16 to 3% after implementation of Relationship-Based Care with *Re-Igniting the Spirit of Caring* workshops as a key part of their strategy [17].

2.7 Qualitative Outcomes

Initial evidence of the impact of the two workshops tends to be qualitative in nature. Immediate feedback is obtained from participants in their evaluations of the workshops. While over 98% of participants say they would recommend the workshops to others, their narrative responses reveal the most about how they experience the courses.

Verbatim Comments from *Re-Igniting the Spirit of Caring* Participants

Comments were collected as a part of the workshop evaluations following each session. These were collected anonymously to preserve participants' willingness to be honest.

- *This amazing and emotional experience has completely reaffirmed my commitment to my work and that nursing is truly a calling.*
- *I feel renewed and proud that I am part of an organization that invests in a program like this for me and my colleagues.*
- *I feel strong, and I am committed to continuing my positive outlook, even when others are being very negative.*
- *This has made me realize how important I am as a health care worker and how much positive influence I can have on people and my team.*
- *I realize how important it is to care for myself so I can be a compassionate caregiver for my patients.*
- *I was ready to hand in my resignation…I had written my letter…and now I don't want to leave. I'm renewed!*

Verbatim Comments from *See Me as a Person* Participants

- *See Me as a Person is the "how" to empathy. This is a breakthrough for me. I can now see how to teach it to my fellow physicians who struggle with empathetic connections.*
- *Thank you for focusing on human connection and not the scores and scripting.*
- *This was a wake-up call—and call to action to reignite the passion to create meaningful human connections that can assist the physical and emotional healing of our patients.*
- *Amazing reminder to stay present, as we always need to be.*
- *I can tell the differences in nurses who have taken the workshop and those who have not.*

- *I feel closer to everyone here. I learned from everyone, and I feel better prepared to communicate with my patients.*

It is not uncommon for participants to write notes to their executive leaders thanking them for bringing the workshops to their organization. We encourage one of the executive leaders to welcome participants on day 1, and they are also invited to the presentations on day 3 of *RSC*, in which small groups creatively act out their vision for taking the ideas back to their departments. This has proven to be an ideal way of helping leaders see firsthand the remarkable impact of their investment in the workshops and in RBC. Leaders consistently describe these programs as pivotal to opening hearts and minds and cultivating active engagement for true cultural transformation.

Implications and Lessons Learned

We gained important insights as we studied the outcomes of organizations and individual departments that applied the concepts and practices in *Re-igniting the Spirit of Caring* and *See Me as a Person*. These insights allow us to support and advise our clients on best practices to deepen and sustain their progress.

- Organizations must have an empowerment structure (such as staff councils) to design how the newly learned practices will be imbedded in day-to-day work systems. If there is no such structure, the initial inspiration and quantitative impact from caring practices are not likely to be sustained.
- Leaders should engage newly returning workshop participants in conversations about what they learned. Their ideas should be shared with colleagues and staff councils so they can become part of council action plans. In this way, leaders are actively nurturing the growth of participants who attended the workshops and supporting their staff councils.
- The Creative Health Care Insight™ online platform is useful for strengthening self-awareness and measuring perceptions of relational competence over time. This 360° assessment process includes a self-assessment as well as assessment feedback from peers, direct reports, and one's immediate supervisor. In addition, having e-learning modules available to reinforce the content is a helpful way to sustain and deepen caring behaviors through self-directed learning.
- Enculturating and embedding Relationship-Based Care takes intentional leadership and continuous reinforcement. Staff must be engaged in the process. If people are inspired and filled with hope from these workshops and yet nothing advances with the culture, it can create cognitive dissonance. The culture must continuously evolve to achieve the best quality, satisfaction, and staff engagement consistent with the principles in these workshops.

2.8 Closing Reflections

Re-Igniting the Spirit of Caring and *See Me as a Person* workshops create communities of learners who come together around their shared purpose of providing humane and compassionate health care. The experiential learning methods that participants experience have re-inspired and renewed their enthusiasm for the gifts of caring they bring to others. They feel seen and valued for their extraordinary work. This renewed passion motivates staff members and leaders to directly contribute their energy and wisdom in creating innovative changes and continuous improvement in their day-to-day work.

References

1. Institute for Healthcare Improvement (producer), Manchanda R (presenter). WIHI: moving upstream to address he quadruple aim [Audio podcast]. 15 Dec 2016. http://www.ihi.org/resources/Pages/AudioandVideo/WIHI-Moving-Upstream-to-Address-the-Quadruple-Aim.aspx.
2. Petry A, Wessel S, Perrizo C. Evidence that relationship-based cultures improve outcomes. In: Koloroutis M, Abelson D, editors. Advancing relationship-based cultures. Minneapolis: Creative Health Care Management; 2017. p. 225–44.
3. Felgen J. I_2E_2: leading lasting change. Minneapolis: Creative Health Care Management; 2007.
4. Koloroutis M, Felgen J, Person C, Wessel S, editors. Relationship-based care field guide: visions, strategies, tools and exemplars for transforming practice. Minneapolis: Creative Health Care Management; 2007.
5. Koloroutis M, Abelson D, editors. Advancing relationship-based cultures. Minneapolis: Creative Health Care Management; 2017.
6. Koloroutis M, editor. Relationship-Based Care™: a model for transforming practice. Minneapolis: Creative Health Care Management; 2004.
7. Manthey M. The practice of primary nursing. 2nd ed. Minneapolis: Creative Health Care Management; 2002.
8. Senge PM. The fifth discipline: the art and practice of the learning organization. New York: Currency and Doubleday; 1990.
9. Baldwin C, Linnea A. The circle way: a leader in every chair. San Francisco: Berrett-Koehler Publishing; 2010.
10. Creative Health Care Management. A quick guide to relationship-based care. Minneapolis: Author; 2017.
11. Koloroutis M. Reigniting the spirit of caring: inspiring through connection. In: Koloroutis M, Felgen J, Person C, Wessel S, editors. Relationship-based care field guide: visions strategies tools and exemplars for transforming practice. Minneapolis: Creative Health Care Management; 2007. p. 5240526.
12. Koloroutis M, Trout M. See me as a person: creating therapeutic relationships with patients and their families. Minneapolis: Creative Health Care Management; 2012.
13. Watson J. The human caring science. Sudbury: Jones & Bartlett; 2012.
14. Peplau H. Interpersonal relations in nursing: a conceptual frame of reference for psychodynamic nursing, Putnam; 1952.
15. Swanson S. Nursing as informed caring for the well-being of others. IMAGE J Nurs Scholarship. 1993;25/4:352–7.
16. Creative Health Care Management. (Producer). Creative Health Care Insight Platform Demonstration. [Webinar recording]. 2019. https://chcm.com/events/platformdemo/.
17. Creative Health Care Management. (2010). Transforming hospital culture with Relationship-Based Care™: Crittenton Hospital Medical Center brings intentional relationships to patient

care and ancillary and support services. https://chcm.com/wp-content/uploads/2013/04/Transforming-Hospital-Culture-with-RBC.pdf.
18. Persky G, Felgen J, Nelson J. Measuring caring in primary nursing. In: Nelson J, Watson J, editors. Measuring caring: international research on caritas as healing. New York: Springer; 2012. p. 65–86.
19. Tippett J. From striving to thriving: reflections of a mature relationship-based care culture. Keynote speech presented at the International Relationship-Based Care Symposium in Minneapolis, Minnesota; June 2017.
20. Wessel S. Impact of unit practice councils on culture and outcomes. Creat Nurs. 2012;18(4):187–92. https://doi.org/10.1891/1078-4535.18.4.187.
21. Nelson J, Watson J. Measuring caring: international research on caritas as healing. New York: Springer; 2012.
22. Dowling MA. Engaging the front line to improve patient care. Presentation at meeting of VHA, New York, Sept 2009.

Establishing Innovation Culture in Nursing: Butterfly Effect

3

Yeliz Doğan Merih

3.1 Introduction

In a world where technology is growing fast, investment of countries in innovation and research and development activities is the most important factor for them to increase their competitive power. Innovation is of great importance for countries to increase their basic development power. As a concept, innovation expresses both a process and a result. In the EU and the USA literature, innovation, as a process, is defined as "turning an idea into a marketable product, into a new or improved production or distribution method, or into a new social service method" [1–3].

In recent years, it has been noticed that there is a wide consensus, both among academicians and practitioners, about the necessity of being innovative in order to be effective and to survive. In this context, it is generally agreed that innovation is an important paradigm that can be used in the face of dynamic conditions. Conversely, hospitals, which are major institutions of the health sector, need to be innovative so as to provide sustainability and competitive power to better respond to the needs of health care workers and their partners. In view of this approach, during the last decade the importance of innovation with respect to the health sector has come to the fore, and academicians and practitioners have started to take more interest in this respect [3, 4].

In the light of the developments, nurses, who hold an important position among health care workers, have taken on an active role in the innovation process over time. This is because one of the most important building blocks of nursing education is to develop creativity in individuals. One of the first principles which is taught to nursing students at the first stage of their vocational education is "a nurse is

Y. Doğan Merih (✉)
Nursing Depertmant of Obstetrics Gynecology Nursing, Health Sciences University, Faculty of Hamidiye Nursing, SBÜ Zeynep Kamil Obstetricsand Children's Diseases Hospital, Innovative Nursing Association, Istanbul, Turkey

Turkey Institutes of Health Presidency, Istanbul, Turkey

© The Author(s), under exclusive license to Springer Nature Switzerland AG 2022
R. Tewes (ed.), *Innovative Staff Development in Healthcare*,
https://doi.org/10.1007/978-3-030-81986-6_3

creative" approach [5–7]. When changing health care different requirements are taken into consideration, the nursing profession needs members who are creative and investigative and who can produce and use knowledge. New inventions in many fields, such as health, will be possible by means of individuals using their creativity and starting the innovation process. In this process, bringing new approaches to innovation and care ranks among the requirements of the profession [7–9]. Innovation is of vital importance in improving and maintaining quality in nursing care. As stated in the ICN (2009) report, innovation in nursing practices plays an important part in coming up with information, methods, and services to promote health, preventing diseases, identifying and preventing risk factors, increasing health promoting behaviors, and providing better care and treatment [6, 10].

This part, which was planned considering the necessity of innovation in nursing, will include the place and importance of innovation in nursing, how innovation will be activated in the nursing profession, the stages of establishing innovation culture in nursing, and successful examples of innovative products.

3.2 The Place and Importance of Innovation in Nursing

In recent years, revolutionary developments in technology have resulted in important transformations in health sector by influencing the supply and quality of diagnosis and treatment services. Innovation, which has become the symbol of transition to creative economy in the information age, is the development process of new approaches, technology, and working styles. Innovation starts with a good idea; however, it goes on with more than a good idea. Innovation is the whole creative process which turns "the good" into something applicable. Everything that can be completed and achieved and that is promising can be a tool to improve health and prevent diseases and to improve health care management [3, 5, 10, 11].

Because of the changes and increase in disease types, the increase in social expectation and technological developments, new needs arise and these needs necessitate changes and novelties. The most influential health care workers that supply these changes to individuals, families, and the society and transfer these novelties to the society are nurses. Using innovative strategies in planning, presenting and evaluating nursing services is among the important factors that directly affect the quality of the service provided. Innovation in nursing practices plays an important part in maintaining and improving health, identifying risk factors, preventing diseases, and providing better nursing care [1, 12, 13].

Innovation process in nursing profession has kept its importance in the profession since the time when nursing came into existence. Florence Nightingale, who is regarded as the person who started modern nursing, pointed out to the necessity and inevitability change by saying "A better world worth living will not be offered to us, so we should work constantly to create such a world. Instead of complying with the world we should change it" [2, 5]. The concept of innovation entered nursing literature for the first time in the 1980s with the study titled "American Nurses Association: Reconstructing Nursing Curricula." In this study, it was stressed that nursing trainers should support innovative attempts, help students to develop critical thinking, problem solving, and research skills and that they should place more emphasis on contemporary teaching techniques by means of evidential education approach [2, 13, 14]. The International Council of Nurses (ICN) and the European Union (EU) declared 2009 as "the Year of Innovation" and set the goal of increasing the competitive power of countries and making scientific institutions open to all kinds of development. In recent years, there have been some developments in nursing education such as making practices be based on evidence, educating students by using simulation techniques in order to turn knowledge into practical skills, providing standardization in patient care, and increasing attempts to obtain accreditation. Each of these practices increases the critical thinking and decision making skills of nurses and enables innovation practices in nursing to be easier [5].

It is important that nurses should have an innovative mindset individually to display their "innovative" roles in their work environment. An individual having qualified education, being experienced in the field, having creative thinking skills, internalizing the problem, and being motivated to solve it are regarded as prerequisites for innovation to materialize. Another variable which is thought to be effective in successful innovation practices is an individual's internal motivation. Internal motivation is referred to as the experience of an individual to display his/her skills [6, 9, 15].

Nurses have to keep up with the constant change in order to achieve effective and desired results in providing service. At this stage, nurses are implementing new and creative activities to increase the quality in patient care. In the literature, it is mentioned that there is a positive correlation between innovation and healing. Nurses play a major role in transferring creative arts to patient care. Innovative thinking offer nurses new perspectives about how to care for patients. Creative nurses should come up with new and different ideas that will be beneficial for both organizations and practitioners. Innovation increases both problem solving skills of nurses and their entrepreneurship roles. Besides, creativity and innovation will lead nurses to be surprised by their potentials and to feel highly satisfied with themselves [14, 16].

3.3 Steps Toward Innovation in Nursing

Promoting innovation contributes both to improve the general health level of the society and to the economic situation of the health sector. However, innovation is not a process which develops spontaneously. One of the priorities of all governments is to mobilize the determinants of innovation in health sector and to increase the health level of the society [7, 9]. Because of complex functions that should be carried out together, governments support in innovation in health sector necessitates a comprehensive and integrated approach through strategic policy making and planning [17, 18]. In an institution the rate of innovative developments is directly related to the work environment that the management provides to the employees. In those institutions which are open to innovation and in which proper conditions are provided to employees to develop innovation, to think in an innovative mindset and to put these into practice, employees are more prone to innovation [1, 4, 19].

It is important that nurses should have an innovative mindset individually to display their "innovative" roles in their work environment. An individual's having qualified education, being experienced in the field, having creative thinking skills, internalizing the problem and being motivated to solve it are regarded as prerequisites for innovation to materialize [20, 21]. The basic steps of starting an innovation process in nursing consist of creating opportunities, generating motivation, supporting instructive processes, and designing models that will make the process designable. These steps will increase the participation of nurses in innovation process and enable nurses to be integrated into a cost-effective and high-grade health care system with clearly set goals [2, 5, 22, 23].

3.4 Activation Process of Innovation in Nursing: A State Hospital Example

The History and Service Process of University of Health Sciences (SBU) Zeynep Kamil Obstetrics and Children's Diseases Training and Research Hospital

Zeynep Kamil Hospital (ZKH), which is one of the long-established health institutions in Istanbul, was founded by Yusuf Kamil Paşa and his wife Zeynep Sultan in 1862 on their own landed property with the intention of providing health service to people free of charge. Zeynep Sultan was the daughter of Egypt Governor Kavalalı Mehmet Ali Paşa. The ZKH had 100 beds in the beginning and on top of the entrance door it was written "There is good health for people there." The hospital is the oldest one in the province of Üsküdar in İstanbul, and it has provided health service by now. Another feature is that it was the first private charitable institution. The ZKH, which has been providing health service for 150 years, has witnessed the birth of a full generation of İstanbul residents and many famous people. The tomb of Yusuf Kemal Paşa and Zeynep Sultan is in the yard of the hospital.

The ZKH has the characteristics of a brand and it is providing service in the fields of gynecology, obstetrics, and pediatrics. It is a hospital which has provided efficient service for many years, and it has broken grounds in its field. Zeynep Kamil Hospital was the first specialized hospital in our country. The first modern gynecologic surgery was performed in ZKH. The birth of the first quadruplet babies took place in ZKH. The doctor who managed this process was Halil Onultan and cesarean section was not used in the process. This event took part in world medical literature at the time. The first laparoscopic operations in gynecology were performed here. The first center in İstanbul for genetical diagnostics and in vitro fertilization was established here. The first Newborn Intensive Care Unit in Turkey was also established in Zeynep Kamil Hospital. Zeynep Kamil Medicine Bulletin has been published for 48 years, and the 37th Zeynep Kamil Gynecopathology Congress and International Innovative Nursing Congress are going on. Within the hospital, in addition to providing medical service, there is also career education for medical doctors in the fields of obstetrics, gynecology, pediatry, and pediatric surgery. Besides, many postvocational training practices with a certificate in the end are carried out successfully in ZKH.

One of the goals is to become a major national and international reference institution with the projects we have recently initiated. The ZKH has developed a pivotal identity in patient-centered and staff-centered services by providing the following services and projects for the first time in our country: The Oncofertility Project, Decreasing the Rate of Cesarean Sections, Vaginal Delivery After Cesarean Experiences, Üsküdar Model Project to Screen for and Prevent Cervical Cancers, Mother and Baby School, Baby-Friendly Newborn Intensive Care Unit, Fetal Echo Outpatient Clinic and Project, and Zeynep Kamil Practice and Innovation Center.

After the renovation period, the inpatient bed availability in ZKH has become 325, and it provides services in three building complexes in which there are clinics, emergency care service, intensive care service, and operating rooms-serving for 24 h and ambulatory care services are provided in five different departments. There are 234 nurses working. Seventy percent of the nurses in the hospital have bachelor's degree and 20% of them have a master's degree. Besides their successful practices in their profession, nurses also take an active part in quality processes. Patient and staff satisfaction levels, 92% and 81%, respectively, are quite high. Nurses in Zeynep Kamil Hospital are also trying to create an academic environment in the field. They established a scientific committee and recruited nurses who were willing to work in the committee. They encouraged these nurses to get a master's degree and invited experienced instructors to provide training to these nurses in the committee in order to enable them to be proficient in research processes. The leading nurses tried to increase their motivation by means of competitions which helped them to improve their scientific study skills and article writing skills. Also, they performed many scientific studies in order to have nurses bring novelties to patient care, to lower the cost of care, and to increase the quality of nursing service. The nurses attended scientific meetings and received awards. The Zeynep Kamil Hospital is among the pioneers of exemplary institutions in which nurses take an active part in scientific processes. The most important part in these processes is the innovation practices in nursing.

Innovation Practices in Nursing in Zeynep Kamil Hospital

The term innovation is described as developing and using new and different ideas. The importance of innovation in our lives is getting bigger. Especially, the innovations in the field of health make taking on more responsibilities and developing themselves obligatory for health care workers. In this process, bringing new approaches to innovation and health care is one of the vocational requirements. The nursing profession also gets its share from innovation and development processes.

Considering all these requirements, a project in SBU Zeynep Kamil Woman and Child Diseases Education and Research Hospital was started in 2012 to activate the innovation process in the nursing profession. An "Innovation Team" of 6 proficient people was established to take an active role in the process of innovation and of training and consultation of the nurses and to motivate them. The team consisted of innovative nurses who supported this process and aimed to provide the best service to our patients through their professional vocational approaches. The chair of the team was the director of the nursing services of the hospital. Thus, the support of the high executives was provided throughout the innovation practices and periods of change. The process started with the trainings. The trainings were prepared primarily for ZKH nurses. Trainings were integrated into in-service training programs. Web site announcements, training posters and guides, and trainings were made visible. All of the nurses were provided with efficient and applied trainings about the innovation process. In the workshops, innovative ideas were developed, prototyping the innovative idea, patent application process for the product, promotion, and advertisement of the certified product was applied. Nurses who have received first level training in this field participated in the application trainings. A total of 300 people participated in the trainings in groups of 10 people. Through applied workshops, the process was consolidated. At the second step, with the mentality of "The One Who Does Knows The Best," a project team was established, and it included nurses who provided service for 24/7 in this field. The project development team consisted of 7 people, the head of which was the director of nursing services, and the assistant was a research nurse and 5 other nurses competing in innovation training. Under the coordination of this team, clinical innovation mentor nurses were formed from 10 nurses who received formal and workshop trainings. These mentor nurses mentored their colleagues in their clinics in order to activate their innovation work individually and as a group in their innovation work. Thanks to these nurses, mentorship was provided not only in trainings but in all of the clinical processes as well. Integration of all innovation processes at work was achieved. Involvement of the nursing services director in coordination and in the innovative processes made the activation of the project in nursing services easier. Identifying the innovative medical products that our patients and we needed and developing them were the major steps in the project. Our main objective was to increase the quality of our services and to provide an accretion value for our country. This project, which was started in Zeynep Kamil Hospital, got the attention of many nurses in a short time and so many innovation trainings were conducted in different universities, schools, and hospitals with our project team. Many of our colleagues were made aware of the innovation process. This innovation light which started at Zeynep Kamil Hospital spread to many nurses throughout our country. After increasing the awareness about the topic, in order to make the process attractive competitions and symposiums were held under the coordination of Zeynep Kamil Hospital.

As part of the celebration events of the 150th year of ZKH, a prize competition, and a symposium called "Innovation in Nursing," which was the first in the field and which had the purpose of activating the process in the nursing profession were organized. The aims of the competition were introducing innovation to the nursing profession, decreasing the cost of care, and helping nurses exhibit new application examples which were practical, applicable, suitable for time-management techniques and which furthered improvement in clinical services. In the first year of the competition there were 29 applications from hospital in the fields covering all of the nursing practices, namely treatment services, care services, training and consultancy services, and nursing service records. Evaluations were carried out using scales based on scientific criteria. In 2013 the Innovation Team set out to make more colleagues be informed about our project. At this stage, our competition, under the leadership of the hospital, evolved to a scientific event that all of the nurses throughout Istanbul could take part in with their innovative application samples. In 2013, within the scope of celebration of the Nursing Week, the ZKH also organized "Innovation Symposium in Nursing" to activate the process and to increase the awareness of nurses about innovation. In this year, as a result of 50 applications throughout Istanbul, it was revealed that 16 applications had the characteristics of a discovery that could bring innovation to the field of nursing. In 2014, the innovation process was extended and became a scientific celebration that all of the nurses could attend during Nursing Week celebrations organized by Turkish Public Hospitals Institution. In the competition, 200 applications were made throughout Turkey, nurses from ZKH ranked the first with 33 innovative discoveries. In 2015, the symposium and the competition were organized in the hospital again, and there were 29 discoveries in the field of nursing in the competition. In 2016, in the symposium and the competition which were organized throughout Istanbul, 75 of innovative discoveries were presented, and 67 of those were from nurses working in Zeynep Kamil Hospital. In 2017, nurses from all over our country attended the symposium and the competition, which were organized under the leadership of the hospital. There were 130 innovative project applications for the competition, and 100 of them were from nurses in ZKH. Trainings, competitions, and symposiums were organized traditionally by this hospital for 7 years. "1st International Innovative and Nursing Congress," which had the characteristic of being a pioneer in our country, was organized in 2018. After the evaluations carried out during competitions and scientific meetings, some of the projects and papers were awarded, participating nurses were motivated, and awareness about the topic was ensured. It was elating that every year more and more nurses attended our competitions in which innovative application samples were new, applicable, and could increase the quality of nursing services, and that more and more nurses developed important innovations in our field.

During the innovation practices of the nurses in ZKH, 376 medical inventions which were beneficial for the health of mothers and babies were developed. We did not want these inventions to stay on paper. In order to put the projects into practice, we set out on a challenging journey, but the result was positive. In 7 years, there were applications for patents and useful models in order to protect the innovative inventions that were developed by nurses in the hospital. During this period, about 100 certificates for patents were acquired, certification process for some others is still going on. Some of these products are:

- Surgical instruments,
- Surgical needles with different protection mechanisms,
- Labor tracking devices,

- A post-natal anti-bleeding device,
- Newborn intensive care products—formula milk preparation device,
- A bed that teaches how to breathe,
- Crying sensor,
- Special blood collecting needles for the newborn,
- Blood transfusion devices, sliding beds to increase patient comfort,
- A bed that can change positions and give massages,
- A wearable iv holder and Foley-catheter holder that will support patient mobilization,
- Specific milking devices,
- Drug navigators, testing pens for drug safety,
- Multipurpose wheel chairs and controlled waste collecting devices. One of our biggest goals for the future is to be able to use the products that we have developed (Fig. 3.1).

The number of patents is an important criterion that shows the development level of countries. These innovations lead to an increase of value and have an important part in reaching the goals for evolution in Turkey. The nurses of this hospital see how they have been supporting this process well by obtaining patent specifications for inventions. Prototypes of some of the innovative products of our nurses were developed. After getting permission, trial processes were started for some of the

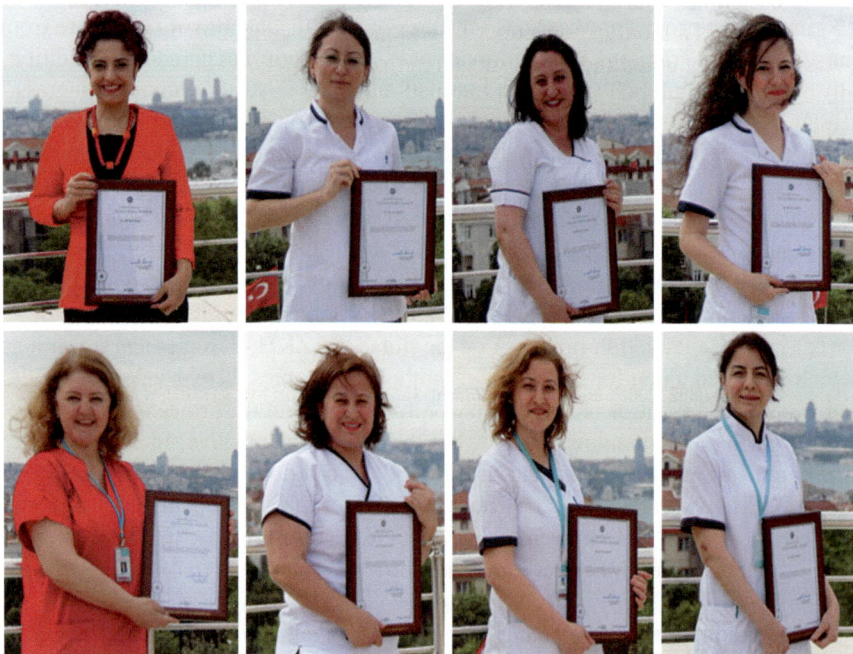

Fig. 3.1 Nurses with their patents

products. Then, we joined the team of Istanbul Aggregation of Health Industry (ISEK) for the products for which the process of certification was completed. Nurses from ZKH are the only ones who became members of this scientific team. Thanks to this participation, we got invitations from Istanbul Research and Development Fairs many times and we demonstrated the inventions so as to be able to put them into practice. In this way, nursing profession was made to be visible in the innovation process.

Our endeavors also caught the attention of media. After the news in media about the successful practices of nurses in the field of innovation, both motivation of our colleagues for the innovation processes was increased throughout the country and the inventions were publicized. At present, we are about to start to produce some of the inventions. We have received many awards for our achievements. We may start to use the inventions of our nurses in our service deliveries in a few years.

It was a tough but well-ending journey to activate the innovation process within nursing services. The nurses of Zeynep Kamil Hospital turned innovation into a culture into the hospital. However, not all hospitals are as lucky as ours. In fact, a lot of nurses in different institutions have innovative ideas but as they do not have guiding role models they cannot make their ideas come true and they limit themselves, therefore their inventions continue to stay as dreams. Our process started with continuous support. Innovative nurses of Zeynep Kamil Hospital became role models for our nurses and guided them. They were encouraged and motivated, trainings were provided, and a guide book called "Roadmap for Innovative Nurses" was written. The aim was to provide better service to our patients, support manufacturing process in our country and provide vocational development by spreading this innovation light to all our colleagues. In this process, professional trainings and implementation workshops are very important. We established the "Innovation Academy in Nursing," which is a pioneer in our country. Thanks to this academy, trainings in the innovation process became more professional, and prototype processes of innovative practices and inventions became more effective. Nurses from ZKH believe that the success in innovation will increasingly go on in this way (Figs. 3.2, 3.3, 3.4, and 3.5).

Fig. 3.2 Lockable stretcher for patient bed

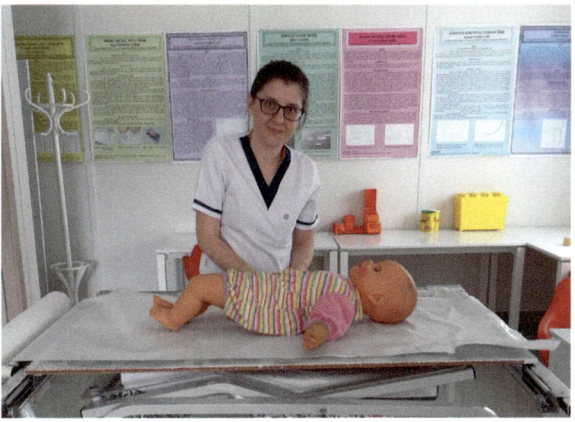

Photos of Nursing Innovations (Figs. 3.3, 3.4, and 3.5)

It is important to adopt an organizational culture in order for innovative practices in nursing to be widespread. Organizational culture is the combination of traditions and beliefs which differentiates an organization from another and which encompasses its life style. The more organizational values and beliefs are accepted and adopted by employees, the stronger the organizational culture may become. In this context, national societies and associations of nurses play an important role. This is because with their organizational culture national societies and associations of nurses are the key institutions that can best reflect organizational culture and support innovation. In order to make innovative practices in nursing more common, national societies and associations of nurses should structure their practices so that they can develop organizational innovation.

Fig. 3.3 Electropneumatic smart bed with micro cushions

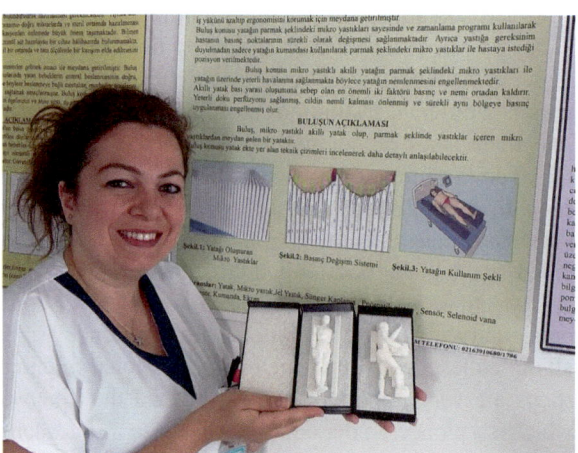

Fig. 3.4 Crying sensor

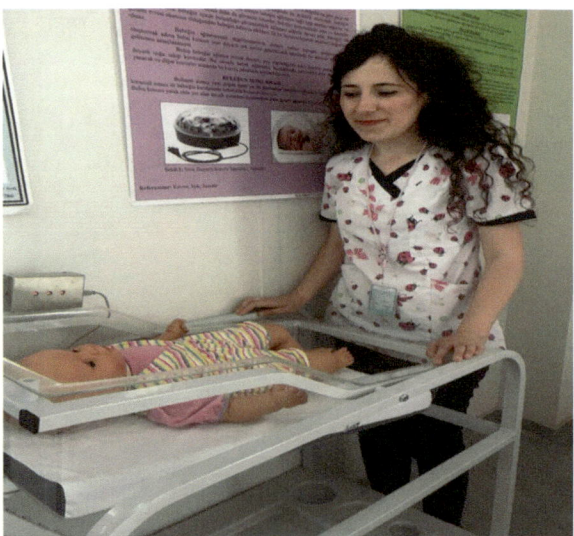

Fig. 3.5 Self-service table

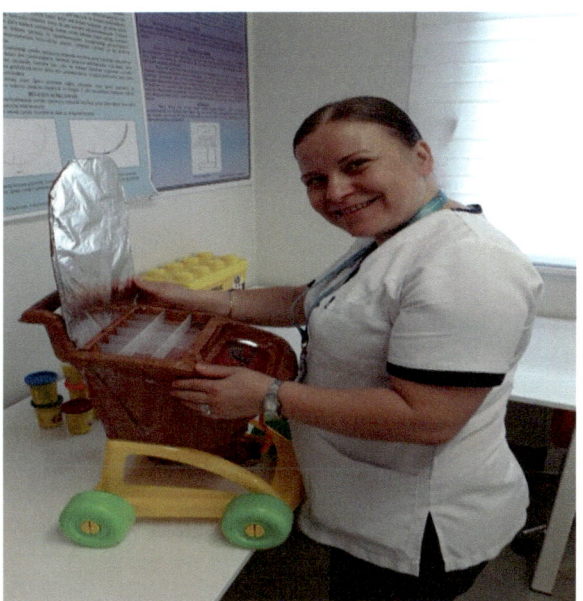

As the nursing innovation development team, we have expanded the innovation work further. After making innovation in nursing an institutional culture, in order to become role models for nurses, to encourage and motivate them, and to train them the "Innovative Nursing Association" was established on 18.05.2016. It was the first one in the sense of innovation in nursing and the headquarters was in Istanbul. The purpose of the association is to enable nurses to achieve effective and desired results, counseling them how to keep up with the changes and integrate innovation processes into their work, to promote health in nursing practices, to prevent diseases, to identify and prevent risk factors, to increase health-improving behaviors, and to support innovation in order to provide better care and treatment. Through this association, the work will be maintained and spread the success of ZKH to other nurses across the country (Fig. 3.6).

Innovative Product Examples Developed by the Nurses in Zeynep Kamil Hospital

As far as the concept of "Innovation in Nursing Care" is concerned, innovation plays an important part in nursing practices to promote health, to prevent diseases, to identify and prevent risk factors, to increase health promoting behaviors, and to develop new information, methods, and services so as to

provide better care. While nurses are providing an important and complicated service, which is health care, they also bear the responsibility of questioning the suitability and effectiveness of their services and of searching for the ways by which they can provide better and more cost-effective services. To take this responsibility nurses should be innovative, and they should initiate novelties and maintain them [4, 8, 24, 25].

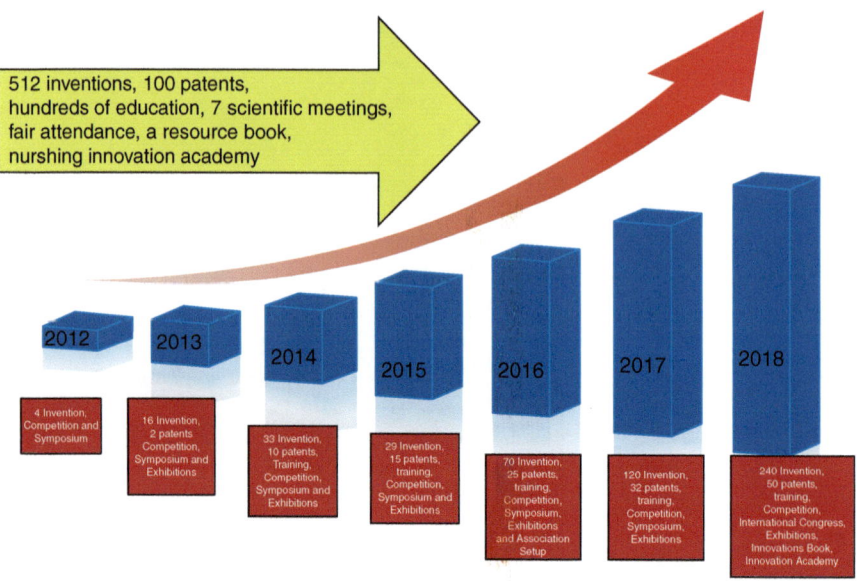

Fig. 3.6 Innovation journey of innovative nurses. (Source: Yeliz DOĞAN MERİH)

The following are new, different, and innovative product examples that the nurses in ZKH considered necessary in patient care and treatment so as to be able increase the quality in patient care, to bring new approaches to patient care, to lower the cost of care, and to increase the quality of nursing services.

Example 1: Developing a Wearable Holder Systems
Current Situation

Today, lots of holding apparatus such as movable iv holders and catheter holders that can be attached to bed are used in order to carry invasive treatment items and to provide comfort to patients. Because of their size and because they limit the patient and the staff during mobilization, they are not used willingly and this results in increasing the number of health care workers or patient accompanist to carry out this job. Because a patient already feels passive and dependent on others, mobilization with so many devices and health care workers increases the dissatisfaction of patients and decreases self-care power (Fig. 3.7).

The Purpose of the Invention

The purpose of the new holder is that by means of two different wearable holders that patients can put on by themselves, those patients who need someone only to carry invasive treatment apparatus will be provided with mobilization, and that self-care power of patients will be increased, thus both patient and staff satisfaction will increase.

Results (Fig. 3.8)

Evaluation

Fig. 3.7 Movable iv holder

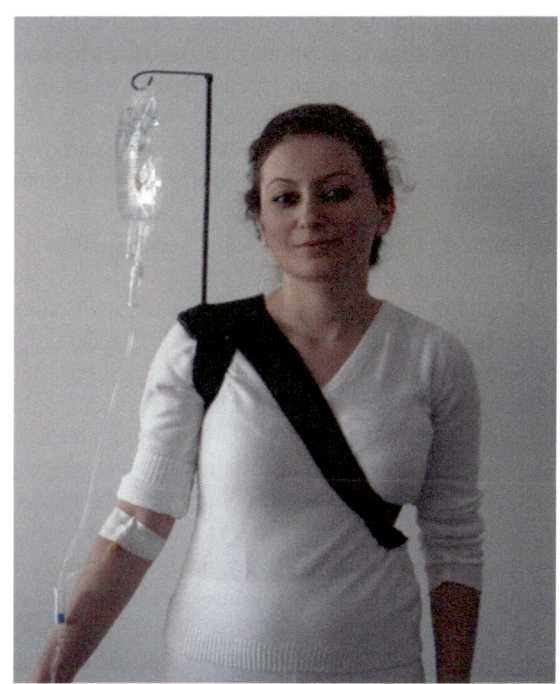

Fig. 3.8 Attached catheter holder

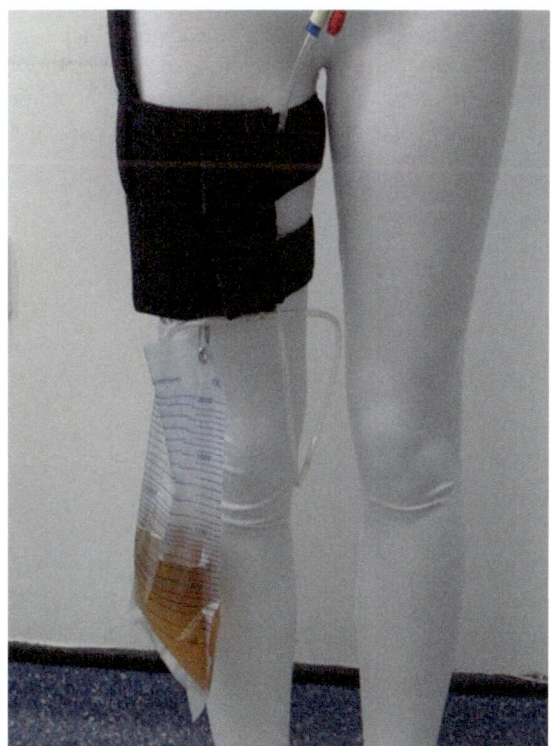

When the opinions about the new wearable holder systems were evaluated, it was seen that both patients and health care workers had positive opinions about them. Health care workers were especially happy because the new systems enabled them to save both workforce and time. Conversely, the patients were happy because their self-confidence increased and they were spared from cumbersome holders. The owner of the Invention is Asst. Professor Yeliz DOĞAN MERİH.

Example 2: Developing a Uterus Massage Belt
Current Situation

Obstetric hemorrhage is the most frequent and preventable cause for maternal death both in Turkey and in the world. In recovery units of delivery rooms in postoperative units after cesarean section operations, puerperants are trained about how to perform uterus massage in order to prevent atonic bleeding. Health care workers are also trained about this point. After giving birth, whether it is normal or cesarean section, mothers do not apply the uterus massage effectively because of residual effects of anesthesia and sometimes because of anxiety of pain. Also, because the number of health care workers is not enough, it is not possible to perform regular uterus massages by them. Today, in order to prevent atonic bleeding during the postpartum period, some kinds of massages are performed, but their frequency and their pressure cannot be measured precisely. There is not an existing device that can perform uterus massage in the known technique (Fig. 3.9).

Result

In order to ensure involution to prevent atonic bleeding, it is essential to give a controlled massage by means of a device which can be adjusted completely beforehand for the purpose of providing patient safety, comfort, and satisfaction. This invention, uterus belt, will be used to prevent atonic bleeding by giving a massage to the uterus of a puerperant through vibrations and to diagnose atonic bleeding at

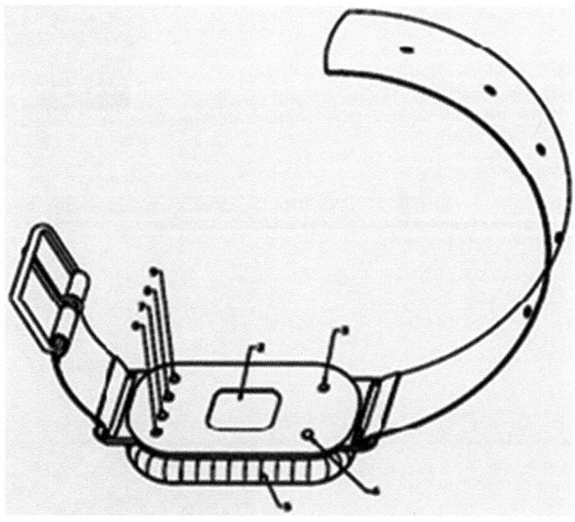

Fig. 3.9 Unterus massage belt

an early stage and to help treatment by controlling whether uterus contraction is enough. Also, if a physician orders it, this device will be used to prevent bleeding by means of its pressure adjusting air bag system that functions as a sandbag. The purpose is to detect insufficient contractions in the uterus and progression toward atony at the earliest stage by means of a lighted and audio alarm system and to take the necessary steps before the health of the patient is endangered.

The uterus massage belt was patented and registered in favor of İkbal ENGİN and Meltem SOYHAN.

Example 3: Developing a Surgical Needle with Controlled Safety
Current Situation

Three-fourths of injuries happening in hospital environments consist of wounds caused by sharp and penetrating instruments. One of the most important problems is blood-borne diseases such as AIDS hepatitis B, hepatitis C, which can be caused by sharp instruments. Although some precautions, such as using waste bins for sharp and penetrating instruments, using vacutainers with safety locks and using double layer gloves, full protection cannot be ensured. Research has shown that surgeons are mostly injured during suturation process and that this is due to the surgical technique because they support the tissue with their fingers while they are cutting or suturing. It has been revealed that surgical nurses and technicians are injured while they are giving sharp or penetrating instruments to surgeons or taking them back. In the existing method, there are no controllable systems to prevent injuries caused by surgical needles (Fig. 3.10).

Result

This invention was designed to prevent injuries caused by suture needles during the surgical operations of patients with communicable diseases. The main purpose is to protect health care workers from injuries caused by sharp or penetrating instruments during operations of patients with diseases that can be transmitted through blood. A needle with a blunt tip was designed for this purpose. This invention is a

Fig. 3.10 Surgical needle with controlled safety

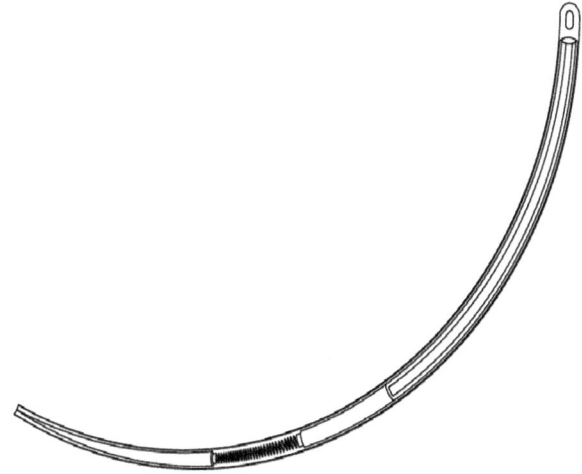

surgical suture needle that will be used during surgical operations, and it has three parts, namely front, middle, and back parts. The front part is placed in the middle part and it has a trigger mechanism which is activated by means of a safety lock. This invention protects health care workers from injuries caused by surgical suture needles and decreases the risk of catching blood-borne diseases such as AIDS, hepatitis B, and hepatitis C. This invention was patented and registered in favor of Msc. Ayşegül ALİOĞULLARI.

3.5 Conclusion

In order to be able to continue its existence in today's ever changing and developing world, the nursing profession should be open to change and development, form a firm unity, be stronger through continuous professional training, and increase the quality of service by making all existing information accessible to each member of the profession. At this stage, nurses should activate the innovation process, and they should shape the future of their profession by initiating professional change and development process.

Putting innovative nursing endeavors into practice through a national integrated strategy, determining which subsectors and value chain stages should be focused on in short, medium, and long term through analyses, creating global supportive domains in health sector, cooperating with international actors, and encouraging commercialization of research outputs will contribute to increase the competitive power of health sector and to establish the innovation culture in nursing.

3.6 What Others Can Learn from This Project

The basic steps of starting innovation process in nursing consist of creating opportunities, generating motivation, supporting instructive processes, and designing models that will make the process designable. These steps will increase the participation of nurses in innovation process and enable nurses to be integrated into a cost-effective and high-grade health care system with clearly set goals.

- It is necessary to increase innovation culture in work environments and develop "Positive Work Environments" in which innovative ideas can be discussed and the idea of being ready for change is supported,
- Enable nurses and other health care workers to have easy access to information, sources, and facilities in order to be able to develop innovation,
- Guide them to develop ideas,
- Organize competitions and activities to generate motivation with respect to innovation,
- Provide training about innovation, creative thinking, patent acquisition, prototype development and about the process of putting the idea into practice,
- Provide support in putting the ideas they have developed into practice,

- Present successful ideas to science world and by this way encourage other health care workers and strengthen professional scientific infrastructure,
- Organize national and international symposiums, conferences, and seminars about innovation and creativity,
- Establish professional associations and communities that support innovation process,
- Organize forums in which innovation is discussed and ideas are exchanged,
- Encourage organization of national and international certification programs,
- İntegrate innovative developments in science, technology, and industry into health sector and establish a national policy which has a systemic integration and continuity,
- İntroduce people who lead innovation in nursing and act as role models to nurses [2, 6, 20, 21].

The first step to establish and generalize an effective innovation culture in an institution is senior executives' adopting and encouraging it. Executive nurses have a special responsibility for creating an innovative perspective and practice environment for newly recruited nurses. Also, executive and leader nurses have the duty of creating a work environment in which nurses are made aware of innovation and innovation is encouraged. Regular trainings, scientific activities that will make the process known, make it attractive and guide the way, and role models occupy an important place in activating the innovation process in nursing.

References

1. Yıldırım E. The importance of creativity in the information age and the management of creativity. Selcuk Univ Karaman J Facult Econ Adm Sci. 2007;12(9):109–20.
2. Acıbozlar Ö. Decision making strategies and creativity levels of executive nurses. Master Thesis, Marmara University Institute of Health Sciences, Istanbul; 2006.
3. Denat Y, Memis S. Developing creativity in nursing education. Ege Univ J School Nurs. 2006;22(1):245–52.
4. Feldman LB, Ruthes RM, Cunha IC. Creativity and innovation: competences on nursing management. Rev Bras Enferm. 2008;61(2):239–42.
5. Khorshid L. Creativity and innovation in nursing. 1. Basic nursing care congress book. Izmir, 1–4.18; 2010.
6. Herdman AE, Yazıcı KÖ. Nursing and innovation. J Nurs Educ Res. 2009;6:2–4.
7. Clement O-Brien K, Polit FD, Fitzpatrick JJ. Innovativeness of nurse leaders. J Nurs Manag. 2011;19:431–8.
8. Yamaç K. What is this innovation? J Sci Educ Thought. 2001;1:6–8.
9. Best M, Thurston E. Canadian public health nurses' job satisfaction. Public Health Nurs. 2006;23(3):250–5.
10. Dil S, Uzun M, Aykanat B. Innovation in nursing education. Int J Hum Sci. 2012;9(2):1217–28.
11. Rogers EM. Diffusion of innovations. 4th ed. Simon & Schuster Press: New York; 2003.
12. Todtling F, Trippl M. One size fits all? Towards a differentiated regional innovation policy approach. Res Policy. 2004;34:1203–19.
13. Bradshaw MJ. Fuszard's innovative teaching strategies in nursing. In: Effective learning: what teachers need to know. 3rd ed. New York: Aspen Publishers; 2001. p. 17–26.

14. Ökem G. Innovation in health in Turkey's European Union membership. Istanbul: TUSIAD Publications; 2011.
15. Clair DS. A study of innovation in collegiate business education, graduate school of education and psychology. Doctorate thesis, Pepperdine University; 2008.
16. Kanter RM. Innovation the classic traps. Harv Bus Rev. 2006;11:1–13.
17. Kambarami RA, Chidede O, Kowo DT. Kangaroo care for well low birth infants at Harare central hospital maternity unit – Zimbabwe. Cent Afr J Med. 1999;45:56–9.
18. Karagözoğlu Ş. Individual and professional autonomy in nursing. J Res Dev Nurs. 2008;3:41–50.
19. Yavuz A. National innovation policies and public expenditure: a comparison on various countries. Süleyman Demirel Univ J Econ Adm Sci. 2009;14.
20. Ku YL, Chang CF, Kuo CL, Sheu S. The application of creative thinking in nursing education. Hu Li Za Zhi Chin J Nurs. 2010;57(2):93–8.
21. Cohen S. Don't overlook creative thinking. J Nurs Manag. 2002;33(8):9–10.
22. Ersoy Acıkgoz B, Muter Sengul C. State practices for innovation and EU comparison. In: Management and economy. 2008;15(1):59–74.
23. Kırım A. Recipe for profitable growth: innovation. Sistem Yayıncılık: İstanbul; 2006.
24. Şengün H. Innovation in health care delivery. Med Bull Haseki. 2016;54:194–8.
25. Turanlı R, Sarıdogan E. Science-technology-innovation based economy and society, Istanbul; 2010.

Initiate Change Processes via the Development and Introduction of Leadership Guidelines: A Systemic Approach

4

Ute Grießhaber-Paule and Bernhard Heuvelmann

4.1 Overview of the Facility/Institution

The project described was implemented in a hospital, which is a central care facility with maximum care functions. There are around 2700 employees in the facility. The process covers a period of 18 months. The project involves the development and introduction of leadership guidelines. The primary target group is approximately 200 managers at three board levels.

- Level 1: Hospital's executive board with six members.
- Level 2: Head physicians, nursing managers, department managers administration.
- Level 3: Senior physicians, ward and functional managers of nursing including deputies, team leaders in administration.

To involve the employees is a complementary essential element in the project design.

Current Challenges of the Institution in the Context of Talent Management

Within the last 10 years, the number of beds at the hospital and, correspondingly, the number of employees have increased by a third. In addition, further locations

---

U. Grießhaber-Paule (✉)
Ute Grießhaber-Paule Coaching und Beratung, Fellbach, Germany
e-mail: coaching@griesshaber-paule.de

B. Heuvelmann
Maiconsulting GmbH&Co.KG, Heidelberg, Germany
e-mail: bernhard.heuvelmann@maiconsulting.de

© The Author(s), under exclusive license to Springer Nature Switzerland AG 2022
R. Tewes (ed.), *Innovative Staff Development in Healthcare*,
https://doi.org/10.1007/978-3-030-81986-6_4

have been added. However, the organizational and structural underpinnings could not be readjusted to the same extent. One result was frictional losses with the effect of increased fluctuation. This was exacerbated by the shortage of nursing staff. At the same time, the regulatory framework conditions for hospitals tightened enormously: the changeover to the diagnosis related group system (DRG) led to economic changes. Capping the cost coverage by payers caused the gap between revenues and expenditures to widen. This resulting pressure became noticeable and required a strategic form of control from the hospital management. In the past, the long-standing management had succeeded in turning the hospital into a nationally recognized and very successful enterprise. At the beginning of the project, it did not seem possible to get back on the old track of success, because there was too little connection between the subordinate management levels and the corporate goals. It now became apparent that the managers were acting too much autonomously "on their individual islands" without taking care of the big picture. They thought and lived with the experience: the house was always successful! But that was precisely the rub. To address this problem, hospital leaders wanted to hold executives more accountable for realizing overarching goals. Cascading top-level corporate goals to lower levels of management required a clear understanding of leadership, a clear leadership structure and a helpful set of leadership tools.

What Innovative and Courageous Contribution Does the Project Make to Meeting These Challenges?

The innovative aspect of the chosen approach is that the project design is based on systemic principles. The two project modules Development of Leadership Guidelines (Chap. 3) as well as their introduction (Chap. 4) aimed at using circular communication and interaction processes to involve and irritate all levels of the organization. This was intended to enable a change of perspective. The project deliberately confronted the system of managers—as well as everyone else—with "disruptions" to what was already in place. The communication formats chosen were seen as unusual. The aim was not only to enable change, but to make it tangible, visible, perceptible right from the start. In our understanding, changing an organization always means changing people—their behaviour, attitude, thoughts, their way of communicating, etc. This requires a great deal of personal experience and a lot of communication. This requires a great deal of personal experience and learning on the part of those involved. Experiencing what can work differently, how to talk to each other differently, how to listen differently, how to react differently. Only when people feel that it feels different, i.e. better, will they actually want to do things differently in the future. The project is about broadening the choices of those who act for the sake of togetherness. Each individual just has to do it. Must dare to do it. This was practised and the framework for it was established.

4.2 Leadership Guidelines as a Systemic Instrument of Talent Management

Systems Theory as a Basis for Consideration

One element for the overarching framework for personnel and organizational development in this project are the approaches from the systems theory of the German sociologist Niklas Luhmann. Conversely, it is based on a systemic understanding of an organization, which is nowadays often used as a basis for consulting and development processes [1]. Luhmann assumes that the order of our society is produced by the adaptive performance of the systems within it. Some such systems are, e.g. economy, law, art, politics, education. Our health care system is also one of them. They make sense on their own. Luhmann writes, "An organization is a system that generates itself" [2, p. 45].

Characteristic of the approach are the following premises:

Luhmann's assumptions on system and environment, communication, complexity and meaning

Luhman suggests that social systems provide manageability. "Social systems [...] reduce complexity by mediating between the indeterminate world complexity and the human possibility to process complexity" [3, p. 21]. So the purpose of a system is to reduce complexity. It helps the system to be able to interact with the environment. The exchange of social systems with the environment takes place through communication.

Luhmann understands communication as the individual interactions, actions, symbols, which keep the system "running".

In order for systems to be able to react to changes in the (complex) environment, they themselves must have a certain inherent complexity. Only this will ensure a dynamic further development. The more complex, the more reaction possibilities the system has. Consequently, systems have an inherent complexity.

At the same time, Luhman postulates a world complexity. He refers to the fact that everything is possible that is possible. In Luhman's world there is not only one decision, one variant. There are countless choices available.

Communication/interaction in systems is determined by the particular purpose a system gives itself. It is a circular process that regulates itself as follows: Choices → Purpose → Communication/ Interaction → Current Event → Choices, etc.

It is a system's purposeful self-regulation, which reduces complexity. Systems are continuously engaged in this self-regulation—so they constantly reproduce themselves anew.

In the sense of the aspects mentioned above, hospitals are therefore organizations or systems. They cultivate meaningful self-regulation. They have a very specific communication, which is determined by the purpose the system has given itself. They show a high degree of inherent complexity. Similar to public administrations or authorities, they show themselves to be less willing to change. They are a complex system!

Hospital managers are a subsystem of the hospital system. The levels of management interact with each other as well as their employees through a very specific type of communication. Ideally, it takes place in such a way that individuals are reached and meaning is created for all that "coupling" is possible, as Luhmann would say. Improving this "coupling" through leadership guidelines was the task of the project from a (very abbreviated) systemic perspective.

Systemic Perspective: Constructivism, Wholeness and Circularity

"We perceive reality as we interpret it along our own ideas, conceptions and experiences" [4, p. 36]. Accordingly, we ourselves are part of a construction running in our heads. We ourselves create an image of reality. And this we should always be aware of.

The basic principle of constructivism means in practice to sensitize all participants to the fact that there is no universally valid perception or reality and certainly no universally valid truth. Everyone, individually, is right. At the same time everyone should be open to the perception of others. In the best case, one shows the willingness to change perspective and put on "different glasses". In the long-run, a change of perspective increases choices and brings agility and movement to an organization. It is the beginning of pattern changes in perception, thinking and acting.

A system represents a "wholeness" as described by Steve de Shazer: "A change in one part of the system necessarily affects the whole system" ([5] cited in Schwing/Fryszer [6, p. 24]). However, not in a linear, mechanical way or according to the cause-effect principle, but according to the basic principle of circularity [4, p. 34]. This means that on the way to a goal, there will always be new factors/events, which are taken into consideration, thus influencing the path and the goal. Interactions, communications, etc. can have the goal of "...bringing a dysfunctional system back to an optimally self-controlling function" [4, p. 33]. From a systemic perspective this is due to the fact that systems have the property of always maintaining themselves in a steady state. And you can intentionally make use of it in a change process: a deliberately placed irritation into the system will in turn cause an adjustment reaction there. That way, something new can enter the system. Or old patterns become particularly clear. Both offer the chance to continue working with them.

In systemic terms, in spite of external factors or internal developments, a hospital should thus be able to generate stability—like a balanced mobile. Consequently, the managerial staff are the ones to steer this process for the system, to make adjustment decisions, to prioritize, to reduce relevant environments, etc. At the same time, however, the degree of complexity must be maintained, so that it is consistent with the requirements of the environment. In this respect, managers are of great importance. Leadership guidelines and the preoccupation with what they are supposed to achieve open the view for the connections and the context, in which leadership takes place. They help people to understand to what extent their individual attitude/interaction/communication has a continuous impact on the whole. If leadership does not happen in this comprehensive sense, it will remain ineffective when measured against the requirements.

Systemic Map of Organization and Leadership

The systemic map of organization and leadership [7] ties the above aspects together and shows that we can describe organizations as two triangles facing each other: one focussing on the context of the organization, the other on the context of the person. They each consist of three sub-dimensions. Both triangles need to be considered and worked on together in order to shape the organizational system "hospital". Hospital managers are to succeed in ensuring a harmonious balance between the two triangles as a whole, but also between the inner triangles (Fig. 4.1).

The context of the individual and the context of the organization must fit together. Our project design aims at this.

Our working hypothesis was: the hospital does not yet offer suitable leadership instruments and structures, and neither a leadership culture to manage these adaptation and integration processes in a value-oriented and controlled way. It could therefore be helpful to develop leadership guidelines, giving managers the opportunity to take a look at themselves and their behaviour as well as their effect in the organization. This could aid their subordinate employees in working with the contexts of person and organization harmoniously. It now becomes clear how organizational development and human resource development, in this case management development, are interconnected and yet use different perspectives. While organizational development focuses on the system as a whole, human resource development focuses on the development of managers as a key target group or on other groups of employees. Organizational development deals with those points in the organization's system that trigger pressure to adapt. Management development measures have to be consistently linked to the development of the entire system. As

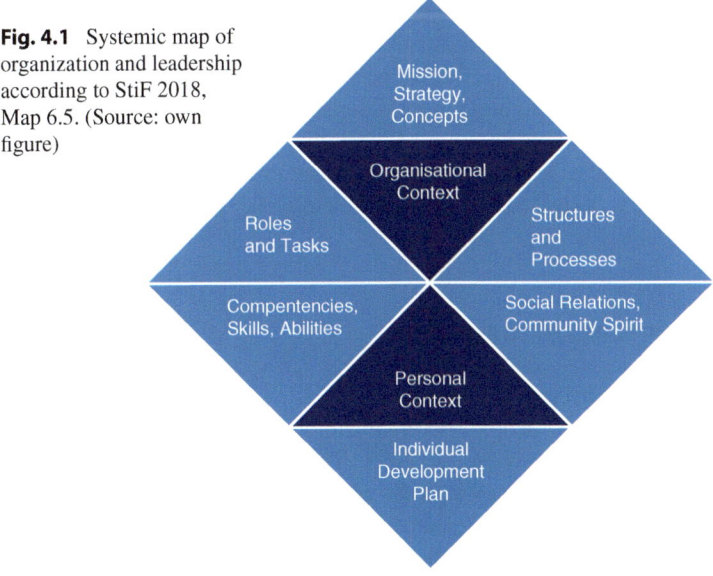

Fig. 4.1 Systemic map of organization and leadership according to StiF 2018, Map 6.5. (Source: own figure)

Königswieser puts it: "Detached individual measures, e.g. an optimization of processes, are not sufficient, if there is no change in the pattern of cooperation...[It is a matter of] understanding and working on the behavioural patterns to be changed and their influence on the processes themselves" [1, p. 120].

Using Systemic Tools

In our project, small and large groups were the most frequently used formats. Systemic questioning techniques were used to trigger reflection processes and changes of perspective: Questions about exceptions, questions about differences, circular questions, hypothetical questions, differentiation questions and the wonder question. Purposefully used, reframing also serves to move away from commonly formulated constructions and attributions. Feedback was practised in both small and large groups.

It proved equally crucial to keep an eye not only on the content but also on the dynamics of the developing process. Where do particular tensions, resistances, coalitions, refusals, cracks, etc. arise? Even in management consulting circles, the realization has arrived: "If change processes follow a pure project logic and disregard psychology, then the process [...] accomplishes nothing. Passagement integrates the psycho-logic into the project logic, so that culture, too, internalizes itself in the change and cultivates the change. [...] Passagement seeks to engage people in change and, in doing so, opens them up to their own development" [8, p. 66 ff]. Passagement describes a concept introduced by Reineck and Anderl as a further development of change management.

Conclusion
Change and development work in organizations means change and development work with the people working in them.

The way an organization communicates, acts, decides, speaks or even remains silent leads to its inherent corporate culture. People can change it, if they become aware that there is a dynamic interaction between their behaviour and the culture, i.e. the micro and the macro level. They have a choice to behave differently. There is an impact. Movement is created. Expanding choices is the sustainable potential of good change processes.

Innovative approaches of the project

Programmed Uncertainty!
Change processes accompany people and organizations on their way to a new situation compared to the one they were in before. The saying "No future without a past" is certainly true, if one relates it to the skills that people and organizations have acquired to date. Nevertheless, it is inherent in a change process that it is characterized by uncertainty—precisely because it is future-oriented:

No one can really say what will happen, still everyone is to get going already.

If the new is to come into the world, we are unlikely to achieve it by constantly repeating the old. The new forces us to endure a certain amount of uncertainty and to go into the uncertainty. Only then can we look around, see what it takes and develop the appropriate skills to be able to shape the future.

In this respect, an innovative change process moves people out of their comfort zone and into uncertainty. Not out of principle, but in the service of the future. It questions assumptions, expectations and experiences in order to find out, which of them will be helpful in the future. It questions behaviour, structures and hierarchies so that people can become creators in and for themselves. It does not accept demarcations, but looks for new and unusual commonalities—which initially only have in common that they are suitable for the future.

But the process does not stop at programmed uncertainty. It invites us to shape the uncertainty. To make something out of it. Such an approach provides the appropriate questions and suitable models—but not the solutions! Although endowed with all this, still the process will not leave us alone. It stays on until something useful is found. In many small and large places and topics, it makes it possible to physically experience what it means to develop the new.

At the end of such a process, pride beckons—in the fact that the people themselves, of their own accord and out of themselves, have created the new.

A reward worth any uncertainty!

The Way Shows the Goal!

A change process is in itself an example of what it seeks to achieve.

When it comes to cultural change, the desired attitude of the target culture already becomes visible in the actions during the change process. This may range from questioning the hierarchy to the claim of "equal speaking time for all" and the likes.

When it comes to structural changes, a change process already sees the described target state as a fact and orients itself to its conditions.

When it comes to innovation, a change process does not accept anything as a given, but always asks for the new, the different, the further development. It does not stand still....

Hence, the future goal also dictates the choice of methodologies, models and interventions:

- dialogical elements
- the attitude that the good solution already exists and just hasn't made it into reality yet
- to be inquiring and curious in search of the best (and not the first) solution
- the attitude that leadership is only as smart (or dumb) as everyone else—and vice versa!
- the question of what all this specifically has to do (!!) with our everyday activities

- the idea that there is certainly room for improvement: the communication, our openness, the transparency, the use of group knowledge, etc.
- the certainty that effectively nothing can happen to me
- ....

All the previously mentioned claims and elements require that there already is a picture of how it will/should be before and during the process. Here this point joins forces with the previous section: if the path shows the goal, then that becomes visible through the leadership. The top(st) leaders have already agreed on such a picture and drawn the conclusions for themselves. However rough that may (still) be....

Participation Does Not Mean Grassroots Democracy!

It is certainly an old rag in organizational development how good organizations could be, "if only the organization knew what the organization knows".

It is true that people in an organization have good ideas for their organization, for example, if they leave behind the hierarchy, departmental thinking and related constrictions. One way for organizations to get from wriggling-along to wriggling out of their peculiarities is honest participation.

Participation here means to listen to people, to ask them serious questions and process their answers. It also means to initially accept the whining and complaining (or whatever the initial cultural reflex to questions is) and yet remain inquiringly curious about the matter.

Interestingly enough, the most common fear of decision-makers is that they would have to implement everything that people have said in the course of participation processes. Just like in grassroots democracy. But in the vast majority of cases these expectations do not exist. It is a scepticism on the part of the decision-makers—but not a fact.

A change process that is transparent in its planning and process is not in danger of raising false expectations.

And if it does, it clears them.

To put it succinctly, participation is meant here as the opposite of "no one asked me".

This may take time and attention.

So what?

Leadership Mikado: He, Who Moves First, Wins!

All the aspects mentioned above apply in particular to the leaders of an organization. But that's not all: leading change is to change leaders!

Managers (and indeed: all managers) are in a sense doubly affected by change processes: they are the ones who are moved in the course of a change. And at the same time they are the ones who are supposed to move other people in the change.

Like it or not, executives' behaviour is microscopically observed, and for some reason, a disproportionate amount of assumptions and attributions are negotiated about it. Executives are, in a sense, the subject of conversation qua office more often than they probably would like. This circumstance is often bothersome and awkward.

But for change management, it's worth its weight in gold.

Change management makes use of the special (in)formal visibility of executives, as it regards executives as role models and multipliers for change at the same time.

A change process therefore pays particular attention to ensuring that managers can be credible role models for the change as early as possible. It ensures that managers make the necessary deductions from the change project and formulate messages from it, which are consistent throughout the management team and can be heard again and again in the same language.

During such a process, the managers examine the consequences of the change for their personal everyday life. From this they develop their personal fields of development:

- for dealing with their employees,
- for their own way of communicating,
- their way of pursuing and demanding goals,
- delegating,
- learning from colleagues,
- for their own claim,
- for the ability to give and take criticism
- and, and, and.....

The process provides appropriate times and places for leaders to actually develop into these fields.

So they can try out and reflect.

So everyone can see it then.

And talk about it—as always!

Conclusion

The focus is on the process—not the result. This is exhausting and demanding and takes time. It triggers uncertainty.

Therefore: a lot of feedback into the system, a lot of dialogue!

Dialogue is meant here as systemic questioning and as a conversation about further development. As an opportunity to try out new things and as an aid for all participants to reflect on and become aware of their own patterns of behaviour and thinking.

4.3 The Process of Developing the Management Guidelines

Basic Considerations for the Project Structure

The concept for the development of the Leadership Guidelines (LGL) and their rollout within the hospital covered a project period of 18 months in total. About 4 months before the start of the project, the procedure for the development was determined.

The project was accompanied by the employee, who was responsible for it internally, and an external consultant, both authors of this chapter. Other external consultants from the network of advisors joined in as needed.

In developing the approach, hypotheses were made applying the experiences from a similar predecessor project in the organization (Process of a Guiding Principles Update, 2013–2015):

- Leaders do not adopt leadership guidelines when they come "from the top".
- If the executive board "proves" that the management guidelines also apply to them, acceptance is higher.
- The executives are critical of the executive board. The executive board sees the executives critically. Both have experiences with each other that led them to this attitude.
- Managers are afraid that the tool will be used to build more pressure and control.
- Long-time executives think, "It's not going to do any good anyway".
- Leaders don't really say what they think, because they fear "punishment".

During the design of the development concept of the management guidelines, the broad participation of staff was of enormous importance. All methods were selected with a view to working in dialogue. In essence, this means that the discussion (no matter how controversial it may be) will determine the outcome. The broader this basis for discussion is laid out from the beginning, the easier it will be later, to roll out certain formats and modules. Because their dialogical form of work is already known and familiar.

The following overview shows the elements of the concept and the loops and feedbacks with the different stakeholders (Fig. 4.2):

Of the 200 managers (including approx. 50 deputies), 40 were brought together in the so-called resonance groups with a maximum of eight people per group,

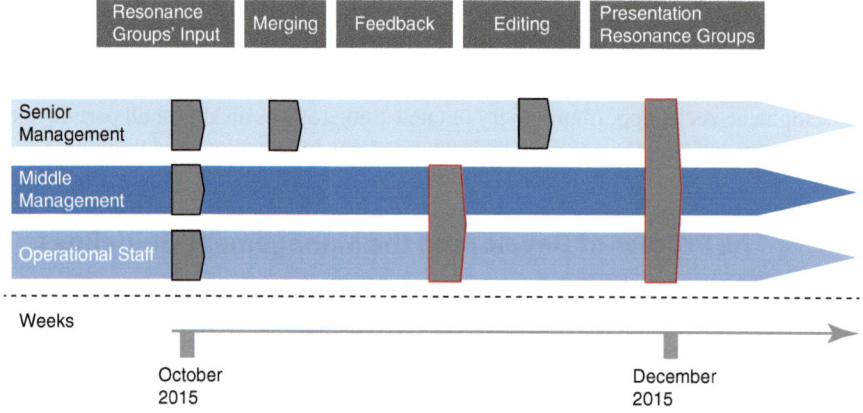

Fig. 4.2 Concept for the development of the leadership guidelines: Formats and participants. (Source: own figure)

applying a good mix (age, professional group, length of service). Eight employees without management responsibility as well as the six-member executive board went through the same programme. The aim of each group was to spend half a day finding out what was important about the topic—to the managers themselves, but also to the employees. We implicitly wanted to explore what could hinder a successful handling of the topic and what we had to pay attention to in the further process. We wanted more information for hypotheses. We wanted to listen and observe from the point of view that every manager is a symptom bearer of the system.

This is how the groups developing the leadership guidelines worked:

Resonance Groups

Purpose and Function
Resonance groups serve to "keep an ear to the ground".

- What are the everyday experiences, pictures and anecdotes about leadership?
- What's going well?
- What is the demand on leadership?
- What would it ideally look like?
- …

Besides the content, these groups represent serious interest in people's impressions. Resonance group participants begin to trust the process. They get to know each other a little better and understand themselves as part of a common whole. They move a little closer together. And they experience that their opinion and their impressions are important and helpful and that there is no "right" or "wrong", but only perceptions "which are different from my impression". My own being different gets space and is accepted.

Methods and Their Effect
Welcome: Introduce the background and the intention of the meeting ("We would like to hear from you what you associate with good leadership and what content you think belongs in the leadership guidelines".). Description of the process flow. Pointing out that the hospital's executive board is also "just" one sounding group among many. Reassuring participants of the confidentiality of the spoken word. Explain that potentially unfamiliar methods will be used and invite people to get involved.

Intended effect: Provide security so that people open up.

Create an understanding that the time is well spent, that it is important for people to participate and that their opinions matter.

Pairing up/warming up: Interview in teams of two; exchange about one's own personality (professional and private). In the group, the participants then introduce their interview partner.

Intended effect: Create a sense of community: We may not know each other, but we work in the same place. Build trust in each other. Discover commonalities. Perceive the other. Feeling perceived yourself. Courage to ask what feels like "personal" questions to a rather unknown person.

Break out group part 1: "Do you remember an experience/situation with leadership that was particularly positive or particularly negative? Please collect them on the flip chart".

Intended effect: Entering the topic through personal experiences. Conscious reflection on leadership. Naming feelings. Important is the exchange: sharing my thoughts and sharing with others. This creates a lively exchange. The group participants discover commonalities. They ask questions, they are interested in the others' experiences.

Break out group part 2: "If you could look at this situation with a film camera, what would the camera record? What exactly is happening? Describe it in words, please".

Here we zoom in and describe the behaviour and the attitude behind it. The participants deal intensively with certain situations. The interesting thing now is that they discover patterns, repetitions or deviations: "It is the same with me" or "I experience it quite differently". This makes the exchange more intense. It brings different "sets of glasses" into the observation.

Break out group part 3: "What would you say now, which leadership behaviour is important to you and should be part of good leadership? Please specify".

The different views are listened to and reconciled with each other. Processes of understanding and comprehension are underway. It becomes clear that the guidelines can apply not only to one's own area of responsibility, but to the entire company.

Present results to the whole group:

Intended effect: Astonishment that some things are the same, while others are different. Recognition of the others' work. Pointing out the diversity. Broadening horizons. Comparing reality and the ideal. Realizing that this is partly far away from the present reality.

Conclusion and feedback session: "How did you do this afternoon? What do you take away?"

Intended effect: Taking the participants seriously. Practising to express one's opinion. Practising to show oneself in the group. Listening to what I can do better. Listening to what might go into the company as feedback. Collecting hints for the next steps.

Observation and Reflection

Interestingly, the results of the six resonance groups did not really differ from each other in terms of content. There were differences between the groups in terms of the degree of openness and casualness. The hypotheses helped to focus the observations. A confirmation was found of the hypothesis that distrust and reservations on both sides are huge. This "construction" is based on the previous experience that countless meaningful projects have already remained fruitless. For middle managers, the scepticism also has to do with their sandwich position. They receive instructions from above, which do not correspond to their own ideas, but they have to represent and enforce these vis-à-vis their teams. It became clear in the exchange that they do not always do this. And over time some refused to do so. Whining and complaining, blaming each other—especially the executive board—and a kind of withdrawal are "normal" for a large number of the participants in all groups. Caution: Problem Trance! Few hold against it, are positive, compare with other houses, "where things are no better", see the basic conditions. They want to make the best of what is available, despite everything. The executive board, on the other hand, sees a lack of willingness to lead on the part of the managers as the sole cause of many problems. They speak pejoratively about people. They do not see themselves in any way as part of the leadership deficit described.

Still, the willingness to get involved was palpable. As well as the pride in and attachment to the hospital and its historical background.

So what does this mean for the next steps? Build trust. Allow trust to be experienced. The stereotypical constructions about "what the other person is like"—who is to blame for everything—should be dismantled. A change of perspective could be helpful. This requires an extreme amount of communication. These findings should be taken into account for the roll-out phase.

From Resonance to the Core—Next Steps of the Elaboration

Working in resonance groups sometimes triggers great expectations among those who participate in the resonance groups. In order to remain credible in the process, it is therefore important to strike a good balance between the individual feedback (and the expectations associated with it by the sender) and the generally valid, further usable content for the entire system.

In addition, the variety of impressions often results in a very heterogeneous picture which, with all its individual aspects, would be very difficult to sustain in the subsequent process, if one were to remain at the level of the individual aspects. It is therefore advisable to aggregate summary theses or thematic fields or fields of action, within which the individual perspectives can be found again. On the one hand, this ensures controllability for subsequent parts of the process, while at the same time all aspects can be found again (also in detail, if required).

For the process of drawing up leadership guidelines, this meant in concrete terms that the first step was to condense the results from the resonance groups.

Condense:	What is the common ground?
	What does the "central thread" look like?
	What's it all about?
	What is the topic behind the topic?

All resonance groups were moderated by an external consultant. At the same time, the internal facilitator was present at all groups as an observer. The facilitator duo (internal and external) now brought the contents together. The contents were clustered and brought together. This process led to topic areas (called "dimensions" in the process). The result of the condensation, i.e. the content-related feedback as well as the dimensions, was presented to the executive board as the first concentrate of the management guidelines. From their side, there were only minor changes.

- Feedback to the groups:
- Together the external consultant and the internal facilitator presented this first concentrate to the members of the resonance groups. The latter were given the opportunity to give feedback under the guiding question: Is this what you wanted to express? Did we understand it correctly? Do you find yourself in it?
- Editorial:
  There was not much feedback, but the feedback given at this point in time served to sharpen the content. Therefore, the facilitator duo did the final editing and presented this version to the executive board with the question: "Are these now the leadership guidelines, which you as the board feel are appropriate for the organization? And are they the guidelines which you will represent in the house?"
- Presentation:
- The then final version was presented to the resonance group participants in a 2-h session by members of the board, who were later open to feedback and questions.

Without going into the details of these phases, two things should be pointed out: the wordings that emerged in the groups were taken over unchanged, even if they did not sound so interesting linguistically. This is a signal of trust: nothing is added or changed afterwards. A fragile trust, however, which became clear again when the participants in the groups expressed the wish: "Can we see the final version before it is presented to selected executives at the strategy retreat?" (strategy retreat is a two-day meeting of management levels 1 and 2 in december 2015) We responded to it by scheduling the above-mentioned "presentation" date, which had not originally been planned. It turned out to be a double signal of trust, as the leadership guidelines were presented by the executive board itself, which was available to answer questions afterwards. The intervention achieved its goal, as confirmed by the feedback: both sides experienced credibility and goodwill, which now confronted the constructed stereotype of "rejection and confrontation" as a new experience.

Hooray, we had a difference!

Result: Five Leadership Guidelines

By both clustering the content into dimensions and formulating detailed descriptions during the summarization process, the structure of the leadership guidelines almost automatically resulted in five dimensions (the clusters, which were sufficiently formulated. The dimensions were: Appreciation, Dialogue, Clarity, Vision and Enthusiasm).

As an example, the text for the dimension of appreciation is presented here:
Appreciation
We actively promote constructive exchange
of knowledge, experience and opinions.
We listen and give feedback.
We pay attention to a fair and
respectful interaction.
This is how we show our genuine interest in
the people we work with.
This creates a trusting relationship.

The internal publication of the management guidelines in paper was designed in a kind of "fan" form and supported by a special graphic concept. The illustrator deliberately worked with a representation of before-and-after situations typical of the organization. The aim was to provide managers with an easy way to identify with what is new (Fig. 4.3).

Now it was important to change direction! The development of the content had largely been bottom-up and with great participation.

So far, so good!

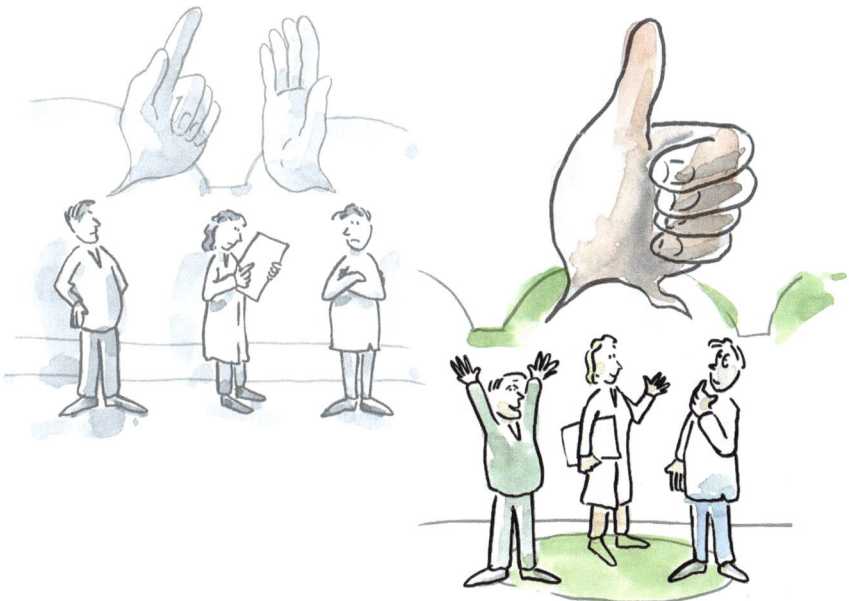

Fig. 4.3 Example illustration of the leadership guideline "Appreciation". It shows the before and after. Graphic design © Christian Ridder. (Source: Graphic design © Christian Ridder)

Rolling it out into the organization now meant introducing those responsible for the organization (i.e. the management team) to the newly developed leadership dimensions. They were to derive the associated requirements for their own leadership actions from the dimensions and their descriptions:

What does that mean for me in concrete terms?

And what does that mean for my work in the system, i.e. for my

work with the people I lead?

The management guidelines were presented to the participants of a strategy meeting (management levels 1 and 2), discussed there and also adopted there.

We now make a big time jump of about 3 months in the process and get back into the next chapter at a later stage, the roll-out phase of the leadership guidelines. You have to imagine that a lot of preparations have been made for this: graphic design of the printed leadership guidelines in the form of the fan to give to all managers, organization of several all-day large group events with 100 participants each, staffing of 16 reflection groups for a total of 200 participants, scheduling of all reflection groups, so that after the first large group event (the kick-off) the reflection groups can start promptly, coordination loops with hospital board, staffing of the external consultant team for the groups, creation and staffing of internal coordination and communication positions, marketing and self-promotion for the process and so on.

Conclusion

Leadership affects everyone: some exert it, others experience it.

So you have to ask people what leadership means.

If you don't ask, it's well-intentioned but poorly done.

Therefore, broad participation from the bottom-up with a lot of dialogue is needed.

Dialogue here understood as the means of listening and understanding.

4.4 Roll-Out Process for the Implementation of the Management Guidelines

In this phase, the new leadership guidelines were made known to all managers. The translation into everyday life was to be encouraged and supported.

In this way, initial changes in the leadership culture were to be achieved and, above all, these changes should be experienced by the organization in a timely manner.

Duration: 12 months.

Event formats during roll-out (see chart below for overview):

- Major events: Kick-off, stopover and closing events for all 200 managers. The external and internal consultant facilitate these all-day events together.
- Reflection groups: 8–10 managers from one hierarchical level meet three times during a defined period. The groups are constantly accompanied by an external consultant and spend a whole day working on questions about their leadership role.

4 Initiate Change Processes via the Development and Introduction of Leadership…

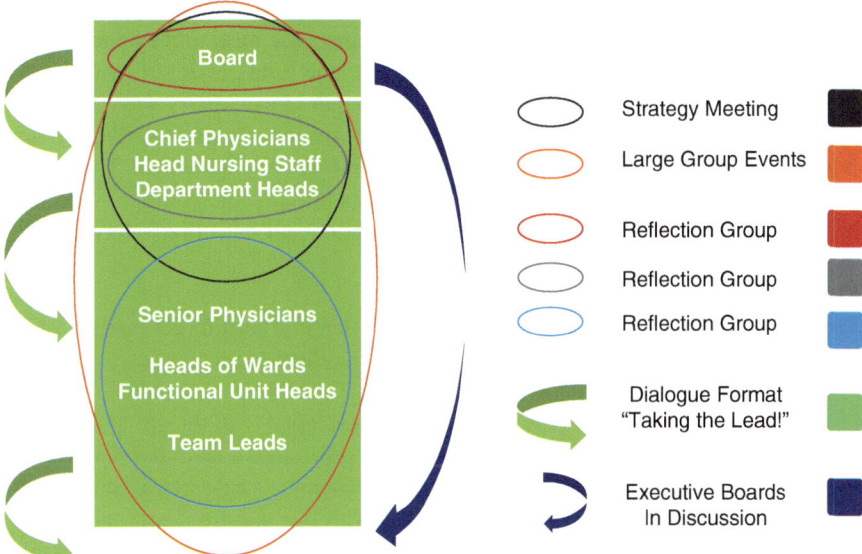

Fig. 4.4 Hierarchical levels (in green box) and their participation in the various event formats (coloured circles and arrows) during the roll-out process. Event formats (coloured circles and arrows). (Source: own figure)

- "Taking the lead": This format supports the practical implementation of the contents of the leadership guidelines on site, directly in the teams. Leaders enter into dialogue with their employees and teams and work on the question, which contents of the guidelines are relevant or interesting for them and how these can then be implemented or achieved in the team as a whole. To prepare for this dialogue in the team, the managers can make use of coaching.
- Executive board in discussion: The hospital management invites all employees (especially those without management responsibility) to twelve 3-h meetings, in which they have the opportunity to discuss the topic of management culture with the executive board (Fig. 4.4).

Large Group Events

What was the goal of large group events? Large group events were designed to bring all stakeholders together. They were scheduled for the beginning of the roll-out, around the middle and at the end of the rollout process. Each of the three large group events was doubled so that 100 of the 200 executives could be present while the other half ensured that clinic operations continued. This allowed all 200 executives to be reached. At each major event (i.e. six times in total), the six-member executive board was present. The events were (as always) dialogue-based, i.e. the aim was to exchange views on the leadership guidelines. Similar to the resonance groups described above, this creates a sense of community among the management team—also and especially because they never otherwise meet and exchange ideas in such a composition. An idea emerges of what "the joint project of management guidelines" is and what its goal is. It can be shown in an exemplary way, what open communication between executives and the executive board can look like and how it is possible to understand the other person better by asking questions. The participants achieve a change of perspective, in which an initially alien point of view later becomes a common point of view (see "Observation and reflection" above).

Fishbowl

This method of conversation is very suitable for large groups to get into conversation with each other and to learn more about each other.

Preparation:

At the beginning of the event, questions are developed with the group of participants. Everyone is to write a question about the project on a card and place it face down in the middle of the large circle of chairs. Then the cards are redistributed by each participant drawing a card from the pile. With this question card, they set out to find someone who has a similar question on their card, then they look for a third and then a fourth. The groups of four are then asked to formulate a question that best expresses the essence of all four questions. The communication demand of the exercise on the participants is high, but it intensifies the exchange on the topic enormously. The evaluation of the questions during the lunch break by the external facilitator clearly brought out one theme (among many others):

"No response from hospital management to executive suggestions!"

Conducting a fishbowl discussion

In the room are two circles; one is an inner circle with ten chairs.

The following were asked to join the inner circle: the nursing director, the managing director, the medical director and one representative each from the medical profession, nursing, administration and service. One seat was for the moderator. One chair remained empty.

The 90 or so other participants sat in the outer circle.

One has to keep in mind that the entire plenum was in the outer circle and listened to the conversation in the inner circle. Talking was only allowed in the inner circle.

If someone from the outer circle wanted to join in, they sat down on the free chair in the inner circle. If all chairs in the inner circle were occupied, and I wanted to contribute from the outer circle, I had to tap someone in the inner circle, who was not speaking at that moment. The person then had to stand up. And I could sit down on that now free chair and participate in the conversation.

Here's an example from the fishbowl:

Facilitator (from collection of cards) to executive board members: "You have heard dissatisfaction expressed about the pace of some decisions. Can you imagine delegating decision-making powers?"

Mr. B. (Managing Director): "There are high demands on quality in our company. I want to make the right decisions".

Moderator: "So you want to think things over thoroughly. I can understand that. How do you feel about waiting for an answer and not hearing anything for a long time?"

Mr. B.: "Sure, I can see that it occasionally takes too long. But our energy is also limited".

Moderator: "You're right about that. How many hours a week do you work, approximately?"

Mr B: "If I don't count the weekend, then it's already around 70 hours. And then still during the weekend".

Moderator: "That sounds exhausting. What do the others think about speed?"

Mr S. (Medical Director): "In the medical field, the delegation of tasks works, it is even clearly regulated".

Mr P. (representative of the medical profession): "But it is still the case that we do not know enough about what is decided. That is really unsatisfactory. Couldn't we be informed regularly?"

Mr S. (Medical Director): "We have committees that work. What I could do is invite the S.C. to some kind of office hours. I honestly just don't know when I should do that as well".

Moderator: "But then it would be a relief to your calendar, if everyone could be informed with one meeting".

Mr. S. (Medical Director): "Mmh..., let's see".

Mrs. D.: (nursing representative): "I see the problem from our side that we actually have a relatively good flow of information in nursing through the nursing conferences, the centre meetings and so on. It is sometimes stupid when we have the impression that the doctors don't know anything, are not informed. But sometimes we also lack the feedback "from above".

A manager from the outer circle spontaneously sits down on the free chair in the inner circle: "Couldn't a decision be made by one member of the executive board alone? Then we wouldn't have the frustration that proposals coming from the bottom stay put forever".

Mrs. M. (nursing director): "Yes, maybe we should define more clearly how the decision-making steps for requests are handled. Maybe you should be able to see where it's jammed, what the status is. Generally, I actually also think that we need less hierarchical decisions. […]"

Observation and reflection

The people in the outer circle listened attentively. The topic concerned everyone. Just by listening, everyone learned from each other how the other person was doing.

This created a change of perspective.

Just the setting of having members of the hospital board sitting in a circle with other leaders in front of everyone sent signals that "We are some of you!" "We are approachable!" "You can talk to us!"

One "outer circle-er" even showed the courage to ask the managing director to leave the inner circle. That was an exciting moment, especially as it was the first time that chairs had been swapped. The fishbowl method sets a personal, but also a collective process of perception and thinking in motion, which can be followed up: one individual can be a model for others. There were reactions like: "Aha, he was able to speak his mind a bit and was not criticized right away. Maybe I'll dare to do the same next time". Surely there is also the expression, "It's always the same... it's no use".

As process-oriented change facilitators, however, we know that the truth is not negotiated in the workshop room—but in the coffee break or over dinner! For us, it is enough to know that these things happened. Then they will already (continue to) have an effect. What individual people think will be exchanged in conversations afterwards or on the side-lines of the events. And they report it to their colleagues. That way, the new impulses (e.g. from the fishbowl) have their impact on the organization.

Reflecting Team

At our first large group event (the kick-off for the roll-out), there were a lot of reservations in the room. Some of them were also articulated on the question cards. At the end of the workshop day, the external consultants reflected their impressions and questions back to the group. To do so, they sat in front of the group and talked about the group without the group being able to intervene. The guideline for the contents of the Reflecting Team was the previously worked hypotheses.

The following topics were addressed:

The topic of persistence: "What is on people's minds here? Our impression is that everyone feels that change is necessary. But 'the others' are to start, before I do something. How about if people here—instead of doubting and pigeonholing themselves or pointing to bad experiences—just acted differently where they can act differently themselves?"

Theme of trust: "We wonder what it would be like, if leaders and people in the hospital could have encounters based on the confidence that the other person cares about a good solution and about the subject matter. No more, but also no less!"

Theme of fear: "We wonder what it would be like, if people could be honest about where they stand and what they are thinking, knowing they are part of a team that backs them up?"

Observation and reflection

This mirroring using the Reflecting Team resulted in positive feedback. It was rather unusual for the leaders to have someone hold a mirror up to them. And it was even more uncertain, whether everyone would be willing to look into that mirror. As a process-oriented passagement consultant, it was enough to know that these things happened. Those who felt addressed would let it continue to work within them. So that the pattern of "it's all the top management's fault", or the blockage of "as long as the others don't do anything, I'll stay the same" could become clearer and be worked on. In smaller discussion groups the aspects mentioned above were taken up—and this would have its effect.

Coaching of the Executive Board

The idea that employees without management responsibility should also be on board was a given for us from the very beginning. The way in which this was to be done was a new idea for the hospital: the executive board was to offer a total of at least twelve open meetings during the project period (in two stages), in which they would listen and ask what the employees thought about the leadership culture at the hospital, how they experienced leadership and whether they had already heard or experienced anything new in relation to the leadership guidelines?

It seemed necessary to encourage not only the 200 managers to deal with the topic, but also all employees. The direct communication loops between employees and top management were also a means to motivate the managers to stay involved. That way, the topical input would reach the entire organization.

These 3-h (!!) meetings were designed for a maximum of 15–20 participants each. They were moderated. The preparation of the executive board for these meetings shows effects of a programmed uncertainty (see above).

The consulting duo had previously exchanged hypotheses about this:

- The members of the executive board are not aware that the employees are afraid of them.
- Getting to know each other and talking to each other helps to perceive each other more sympathetically ("They are not that stupid" or "Now I understand").
- The executive board is afraid of criticism and attacks from the employees.
- The executive board has no practical experience with open, unplanned conversations. They are entering new territory here and are as nervous as could be expected.
- Hospital management wants to send their message and keep the pressure on ("We need to do even better!").
- Employees want to place their questions and concerns at the top.

Mr. B. (Managing Director) to the moderator: "You will still tell us what we are supposed to present?"

Moderator: "You don't have to present anything. We are at the meeting without slides and projector. We sit in a circle of chairs, all of us. It's supposed to be a conversation between you and the staff".

Mrs. N. (Nursing director): "But we don't need three hours for that".

Mr. B.: "...otherwise they'll just start complaining again and blacken everything".

Facilitator: "We need maybe half an hour, three quarters of an hour at the beginning to get to know each other briefly. And then we really want there to be time for the participants' questions". […]

Mr. S. (Medical Director): "Do you actually believe that anyone will come at all?"

Moderator: "Absolutely. After all, the employees never get a chance to talk to you otherwise. Many don't even know what you look like."

Ms G. (HR Director): "What kind of questions should we expect?"

Moderator: "What do you think employees might ask?"

Mr. B.: "Why we built a new building but there is no money for more staff positions..."

Mr. S: "... or that they don't understand what the whole project is actually about".

Moderator: "So, what would these questions be like for you? What would you answer?"

Mr B.: "I could already say something about it. But I would also like to say that the way things are going at the moment is not enough. Everybody has to pull together. Also the employees".

Moderator: "I understand you and I know that this is your concern. But now imagine the employees and how such a statement would be received by them".

Mr. B.: "But that's how it is. It has to be said".

Moderator: "How would you feel, if you were doing your job and putting in effort every day and then you hear from someone that everything is getting worse that what you're doing isn't good enough. How would that come across to you?"

Mr S.: "That's nothing new. I think they realise that already. But it does not help".

Moderator: "How come it doesn't help?"

Mrs. M. (Director of Nursing): "They don't understand the context, they're struggling enough with their situation on the ward or wherever... that's of higher priority".

Moderator: "You think it's not because of a lack of interest, but because employees have a lot on their plate in their daily lives? Did I understand that correctly?"

Mr. B.: "Yes, we are also under pressure".

Moderation: "Aha, but the employees probably don't see that. Maybe you could explain to the employees why it is necessary to get better again".

Mr. S.: "I wonder if they want to hear that".

Facilitator: "Just try it. I imagine it will go down well, if you explain yourself and your stance and show that the pressure isn't being put on you over nothing".

Mrs. M.: "Maybe it won't be so bad".

Moderator: "By the way, we make sure that many get to speak and that a good conversation ensues. You'll see, it'll be worth it".

Observation and reflection

The board's anxiety about this meeting was palpable. It was a very unusual format to go into a 3-h meeting so openly and without any agenda. It had already been so difficult to schedule the meeting that it became clear to us, how great the internal resistance was. So it was all the more important that we did not yield.

The preparatory interview makes it clear that there was still the goal to communicate the economic situation. It was difficult to imagine what the employees' reasons might be for not doing exactly what the management thought was necessary. It was less about listening. As the conversation progressed, different opinions within the executive board become visible. It became clear that there was a division of roles, which made an honest exchange difficult. The managing director and the medical director were the spokespersons. They brought scepticism into the process and ventilated it a lot. The others remained silent or attempted cautious steps. In the follow-up to this discussion and the dialogues with the employees, the executive board began to work further on constructive cooperation. This process was accompanied externally.

Surprisingly, the events themselves had the character of real conversations. Few employees showed up (8–12), but they had brought a lot of questions. And surprisingly, the members of the executive board were able to engage well with them. The accompanying duo even got the impression that they really enjoyed it. Despite the fact that really critical topics were also discussed.

During these and other meetings, the inner process, in which the executive board members found themselves, became tangible. The employees registered positively when a member of the board expressed his/her learnings from the change process. The following final question to the board in the meeting was helpful: "What would you say, what have you already learned in the course of the project and in your reflection group?" The board members' answers ranged from "I have tried and intentionally praised my staff", to "I take it upon myself to listen better. I have noticed that most of the time I already think I know what the person I am talking to wants to tell me. I want to learn to listen well", to "It was good to have an open exchange. Especially in the circle of colleagues [here: executive board]. I thought it was good that we gave each other feedback".

The second run of six more such events was not implemented—scheduling difficulties were given as the official reason.

The final major events and even more reflection groups for the managers were held according to plan.

Conclusion
It's about experiencing.
Not explaining.
By experiencing, people get an impression of what would be different "if...". And they can try it out.
At best, good examples lead the way.
That takes guts.
But it works.

4.5 Learning Experiences from the Project

Like every project, this project, too, stands in the light of the question, what was pursued and what (of it) was actually achieved?

The first goal was to create and formulate leadership guidelines for the organization and to make them known. Leadership in general was to be addressed at all levels of the organization, with the aim of making people aware of the phenomena as well as the demands on leadership. Leadership behaviour was to be adapted in line with the new guidelines. In a nutshell, after the end of the project, leadership in the organization was to be perceived differently than before.

The result is that the guidelines have been formulated and transported to the different levels via various dialogue formats. In the course of this, the management team was able to get to know each other across professions and build up an inner closeness.

The content-related and personal work on the topic was carried out via reflection groups and exchange formats. This incidentally created (personal) connections, which still provide an opportunity for exchange to this day.

The topic of leadership could be (re)set in the organization and there was and is—in the form of a newly established leadership academy—a specific qualification on leadership-relevant topics in the organization.

The long-term, visible change in the management culture at the hospital was not achieved. The topic is being continued thematically and there is support for organization-wide measures at selected points. At the same time, the top management continues to demonstrate leadership in a way that is different from the way it is formulated in the guidelines. And since this is a hierarchical system by nature, non-conforming (i.e. hierarchy-reducing) behaviour has got a hard time here.

What are the reasons for this?

There were and are behaviours in prominent places that were or are unacceptable—if you relate them to the leadership guidelines. They rather represent a repetition of patterns and certainly not an interruption of patterns. The process did not succeed in making these the subject of deeper consideration and processing.

One reason for this is surely that reflection on such behaviour would have represented an extreme personal challenge. In this respect, resistance to it was and is understandable.

Speculatively, one could say that perhaps there was too much to lose ("How does that kind of behaviour fit in with my position? That would make me untrustworthy!"). Another aspect could be that the advisory relationship was not (yet) strong enough. In projects of this kind it often happens that the nature of the relationship with external people changes—and has to change—from "consultant" to "coach" or "companion". Especially when it comes to leadership, it is true that the professional is to a large extent personal. This means that questioning a person will inevitably arise at some point and should also be answered. At the beginning of such a process many clients are not aware of this. And many facilitators fail to make this aspect clear from the outset. In the end the fact remains that on the home stretch—when it is no longer about the first visible changes, but about substantial, personally more strenuous, self-questioning issues—there is no actual change in attitude or behaviour. And so the visible figureheads (and clients) of change are no longer experienced as such.

In retrospect, one possible approach to avoiding such a situation seems to be that the cooperation in the management could have been scrutinized earlier and more intensively. In the course of this, the (critical) shares of each member of the executive board would have been addressed. This concern was presented as the next step. However, agreed project dates were cancelled due to scheduling problems or because of overriding issues so that the connection to the management became increasingly weaker and the project ultimately came to an end.

Point out all consequences right from the beginning

The lessons learned from the project are that right at the beginning of the project, it is essential to point out expected developments—based on the experiences from similar, previous projects: that frictions will arise that there will be conflicts. It must be made clear from the outset, how difficulties are to be dealt with. Do the clients then want to gloss over such critical issues and "sweep them under the carpet"? Or do you want them to continue to be dealt with? And how openly can this be done? Addressing this clearly and agreeing on a common line is important. We, as the people responsible for the project, should show what support change management or process support can offer here. In the end, the commitment for the project order/contracting also provides clarity. This should be phrased in a very differentiated way, because it also creates awareness of the dimension of such a change project. It is advisable to explicitly address the work that the top management bodies will have to do: it should be made clear how intensive and personally challenging the process will be or can be for them. After all, a willingness to self-reflect is a component of systemic working. And for many in a professional context this is foreign and sometimes exhausting. It therefore helps to ask in advance: what do you think this plan/project will entail for you personally? What can we do as project managers to support you in this? This willingness to "get involved" is as binding as possible and allows the consultants to refer to it and take it up during the course of the project. In doing so, the clients always remain co-responsible for the process. It should be clearly stated that there will be no lasting change or impact on the organization without a sustained visible change in the behaviour of senior leaders. And that the consultants—in the sense of a successful process—have the task of addressing old patterns and not allowing any taboo topics. In this context, it is not without a certain paradox that, as a facilitator, one has to conduct a conversation of such openness and clarity at the time of contracting. From our point of view there is no alternative. If we as facilitators do not make it clear what is in store for the participants, they have every right to drop out of the process. If such processes are to succeed, radical transparency is needed right from the start—even if the relationship between facilitators and participants/clients is by no means as strong at this stage as it will be later.

Make the Time Requirements Clear

Especially when short-term success is targeted by the client, it is important to emphasize the long-term nature of an approach such as ours. This means that everyone needs to be willing to invest time in the project. And to be allowed time for the project. Leaders need time, but so does the top management. Because one thing is certain: change does not happen by the way. It needs the space and time to emerge. The most effective way is for the facilitators to outline the time budget by taking a concrete look at the clients' calendars and making it clear, which amounts of time will be required in what time spans. Certainly there are short-term successes, but the real benefit of such change work lies in the sustainable and long-term change of attitudes and behaviour. This is how things truly change! So it is good that this is clear to everyone at the beginning!

Point Out Risk of Cancellation

In this context, it is equally important to point out the danger of premature project termination. If such a process is allowed to expire or is aborted, it gambles exponentially more credibility than it could gain. In other words, it leads to lasting mistrust and damage.

Create Time and Space for Reflection and Feedback on the System

It helps those who responsible for the project, to reflect at certain intervals (determined according to the duration of the project) at the meta-level, whether the path still fits the goal, what has been achieved, what is next and whether the long-term perspective is still being maintained? And what then needs to be done. The result of these considerations should be fed back to the client. After all, they are part of the system. And systems stabilize themselves through patterns. Reflection at the meta-level touches on questions like: Do we recognize a pattern? What might it be? Is this pattern helpful now? Or dysfunctional, because it is detrimental to the change goal? What might it mean, for example that other issues are now being prioritized higher and there is no time for the conversations or events originally planned? What does this say about the system? What might it mean for the process going forward, if leaders realize that the project is not moving forward as planned? These kinds of questions belong in the regular exchange between the client and the project managers/consultants as defined in the contract.

In Short

When clients are at the beginning of a change process, they have usually thought it through well in advance and, in their own way, already have an idea of it. For example, about how the project should proceed, what should happen, etc. The mood may lie somewhere between enthusiasm, inevitability or determination. This is always associated with expectations of the process facilitators.

If now, in this mood, the companions—even before things really get going—point out the possible demands of a project, if they warn against abandonment and speak of reflection, then they may be experienced as killjoys, naysayers or self-promoters or, or.... In extreme cases, they may even be asked, "Do you want to be the facilitator or not?"

But it does not help: at the beginning, the companions should name everything that may arise in the course of the process. Not in order to have known better. But because it is part of it. That is only fair. It creates a sense of reality. And respect for the process. It facilitates the discussions which will occur as the project progresses. Because then the facilitators can refer to what they shared and talked about with the client at the beginning of the process. Then, the feedback from the facilitators and their reflection on (critical) developments in the process can be classified together with the client. The exchange enables the client—with the helpful outside perspective of the consultants—to look at the developments. This in turn sharpens the understanding of what is happening in the organization.

And that gives the process a chance to move forward.

And that's what counts. So? Would we do it again? Yes, of course!

But why?

Because it's about "get going!"

It's about seeing what happens.

And to ask yourself if what you're seeing is helpful.

In doing so, one must not make oneself a slave to the goal.

Too much happens along the way anyway for it to turn out the way you initially thought it to be.

So, once again, it's a case of "Continue to fail ahead successfully!"

References

1. Königswieser R, Hillebrand M. Einführung in die systemische Organisationsberatung. 8th ed. Heidelberg: Carl-Auer-Verlag; 2015.
2. Luhmann N. Organisation and decision. Wiesbaden: Westdeutscher Verlag; 2000.
3. Schuldt C. Systems theory. Hamburg: Europäische Verlagsanstalt; 2003.
4. Bamberger G. Lösungsorientierte Beratung, Praxishandbuch. 5th ed. Weinheim: Beltz-Verlag; 2015.
5. de Shazer S. Ways of successful short-term therapy, Stuttgart; 1989.
6. Schwing R, Fryszer A. Systemisches Handwerk, Werkzeug für die Praxis. 7th ed. Göttingen: Vandenhoek & Ruprecht; 2015.
7. StIF : Zettelkasten. Stuttgart Institute for Systemic Therapy, Consulting, Supervision and Systemic Coaching, Stuttgart; 2018.
8. Reineck U, Anderl M. Mythos change. Verändern verändern. Weinheim: Beltz-Verlag; 2015.

Further Reading

Boos F, Mitterer G. Einführung in das systemische management. Heidelberg: Carl-Auer-Verlag; 2014.

Frauenknecht X, Winkler M. You up there! Upward appraisal as a contribution to changing leadership culture in health care companies. KU Health Management; 8/2016. p. 43–9.

Garbsch M. Systemische Führungsentwicklung. Linking leadership and organisational development using the example of a hospital. Heidelberg: Carl-Auer-Verlag; 2012.

Heinze R. No fear of change. Managing change processes successfully. Heidelberg: Carl-Auer-Verlag; 2004.

Janas J. Doomed to fail? KU Health Management; 9/2015. p. 68–70.

König E, Volmer G. Handbuch Systemisches Coaching, Für Coaches und Führungskräfte, Berater und Trainer. 2nd ed. Weinheim: Beltz Verlag; 2012.

Luhmann N. Trust. Ein Mechanismus der Reduktion sozialer Komplexität. Stuttgart: Enke-Verlag; 1973.

Pearls of Wisdom: The Evolution of a Healing Healthcare Model

5

Emily Nowak and Valerie Lincoln

5.1 Introduction

Healthcare in the United States (US) continues to evolve at paces unprecedented historically. Over the past 20 years, the use of complementary and alternative medicine (CAM), also known as integrative services (IS), within the acute care setting has exploded. Increased attention to IS is largely driven by consumer desire for additional options for approaching their personal well-being and, systems desire to increase revenue streams. The most recent statistics by the National Center for Health Statistics (NCHS) reports that nearly 40% of all Americans use some form of CAM, spending 33.9 billion dollars annually in doing so [1].

The phenomenon of hospital based IS is seen across all regions of the country and in all cross sections of the acute care hospital industry including community based and academic institutions and for profit and not-for-profit organizations. Hospitals that offer integrative services do so for various reasons such as consumer preference, market factors, and differentiation strategies. An emphasis on patient satisfaction as a legitimate outcome of care, organizational mission, resource availability, and other service expansion approaches are also contributors. Mann et al. [2] identified seven models of integrative care, two of which focus on inpatient acute care models: hospital based integration and integrative medicine in academic medical centers. Integrative models of care have several aims. These include the desire to improve patient and family experiences of health care in an inpatient setting; a desire to honor the commitment to providing integrated care; expanding patient care

---

E. Nowak (✉)
Department of Nursing, Henrietta Schmoll School of Health, St. Catherine University, St. Paul, MN, USA
e-mail: ewnowak@stkate.edu

V. Lincoln
Integrative Nurse Consultant, Lake Ann, MI, USA

options; improving communication and relationships between patients and caregivers; reducing dependency on pharmaceutical and technological interventions; providing greater attention to wellness, disease prevention, and self-care; enhance the reputation of the hospital, and other potential benefits such as nursing and service staff retention [3].

The integration of IS into the acute care setting requires attention to assuring the place, the people, and the processes are synergistically aligned. In this chapter, the authors describe one small community hospital's development, implementation, and evaluation of a holistic model of care in the acute care setting and the evolution of the holistic model across the larger system. The chapter concludes with suggested opportunities for increased integration of concepts of holistic care into academic programs to assure adequate preparation of new healthcare professionals with the foundational skills and knowledge to meet the growing demand for these services.

5.2 The Place: Woodwinds Health Campus

Woodwinds Health Campus (WHC) is a small 86 bed community hospital in the Twin Cities metropolitan area of Minnesota. WHC opened in August of 2000 to serve the southeast metro using integrative approaches to health care. At its birth, WHC was one of three hospitals within a smaller system uniquely positioned to provide care in this innovative way. Now a part of Fairview network, a large non-profit organization with 12 hospitals and 56 clinics across the state, the hospital remains unique in both the design and delivery of the care provided as demonstrated through the patient experience [4]. In addition to the acute care beds, WHC houses an outpatient cancer center, emergency care center, and several independent primary and specialty care clinics. Attention to environmental influence on health is notable in each design feature. Inviting public spaces like the Town Center entice patients, visitors, hospital staff, and volunteers through live piano performances, access to the healing gardens and labyrinth, a three-season patio and a fireplace to warm up by in the winter months. Private individual spaces like patient rooms provide outdoor views, spacious accommodations, a variety of lighting options, and a place for family members to rest and provide support to loved ones.

Publically reported outcomes such as the HCAHPS (Hospital Consumer Assessment of Health Plan Survey) and the Leapfrog Hospital Safety Grade demonstrate the quality of the unique care that WHC provides for those it serves. WHC was awarded a 4-star rating in the 2019 Centers for Medicare and Medicaid "Hospital Compare" HCAHPS survey placing the health campus in the top 30% of hospitals in the country and was graded "A" overall by The Leapfrog Group [5]. Data from HCAHPS reflects the patient perceptions of hospitalization including communication with doctors and nurses about medicine, responsiveness of hospital staff, pain management, quality of discharge instructions, cleanliness of the hospital environment, and the quietness of the hospital environment. Leapfrog data represents overall safety measures such as number of infections, problems with surgery, practices to prevent errors, safety problems, and qualities of doctors, nurses, and staff. These qualities are in line with the concept of an Optimal Healing Environment (OHE) and Holistic Nursing (HN).

Optimal Healing Environments

Although WHC was created and operational before the concept of an optimal healing environment (OHE) was published by the Samueli Institute, the efforts of WHC are supported by the seamless integration of the overall healing environment as later presented by Jonas and Chez [6]. Jonas and Chez's seminal work provides a comprehensive review of the factors affecting the inner environment of the persons in relationship (developing healing and intention, experiencing personal wholeness, and cultivating healing relationships), as well as the outer environmental factors (applying collaborative medicine creating healing organizations and building healing spaces). The bridge between the two realms of the inner and outer environment is represented by practicing healthy lifestyles, which is seen as both an inner and outer process.

OHEs are defined as systems that "surround the individual with elements that support the innate healing process" [7]. These elements include healing intention, personal wholeness, healing relationships, healing organizations, healthy lifestyles, integrative care, healing spaces, and ecological sustainability. OHEs support healing and the achievement of wholeness which uniquely includes a focus on self-care, the conscious development of intuition and focusing on the inner states of awareness by embracing intentions of healing, love, and compassion. The integration and assimilation of principles of OHE include balancing financial values, patient-centered leadership, community involvement, and the mind–body connection within different models of integrated care [6].

Recognizing the unique opportunity to create a healing environment from the bottom up, WHC took a multidisciplinary approach to the principles and pillars of this model [8]. The overarching WHC culture recognized and focused upon these six P's of the WHC Healing Healthcare Model: people, philosophy, place, process, policies, and practice. The design was comprehensive and integrated. The interior halls are curved to eliminate a straight rectilinear, institutional feel. Every patient room is private and is large enough to accommodate support persons and caregiver needs. All rooms look out unto a large campus imbued with nature. The healing power of nature is supported by outdoor spaces, a healing garden and a large labyrinth which is also visible from within the hospital. Two gazebos are available for both patient and staff renewal. The vast majority of the extensive artwork is inspired by nature. In addition, the Chapel embraces the visual support of earth, wind, fire, and water to embody the desire for a spiritually inclusive environment. Local Ojibwa elders assisted in the blessings of the healing space and healing gardens. The classical elements are also emphasized throughout the campus; some departments have aquariums to invoke the water of the land, and multiple fireplaces provide warmth and light in most patient and family sitting areas. The overall design calls forth the iconic Northwood's cabin of Minnesota (Figs. 5.1, 5.2, and 5.3).

Fig. 5.1 Entrance of the hospital

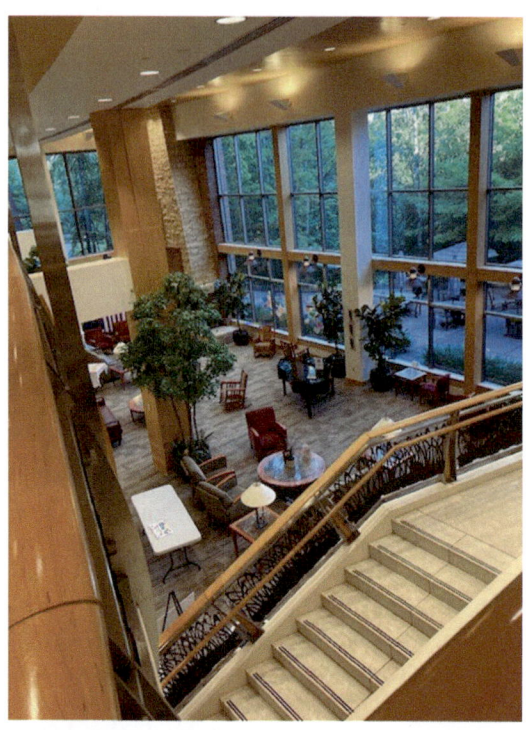

Fig. 5.2 Curved interior halls

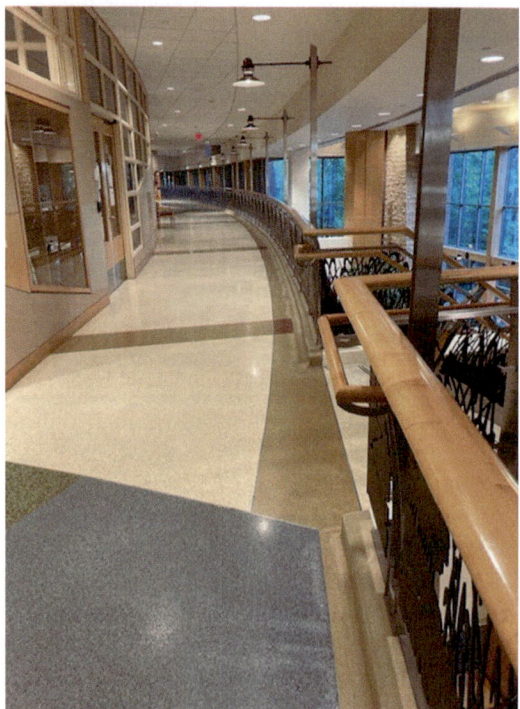

Fig. 5.3 Healing garden

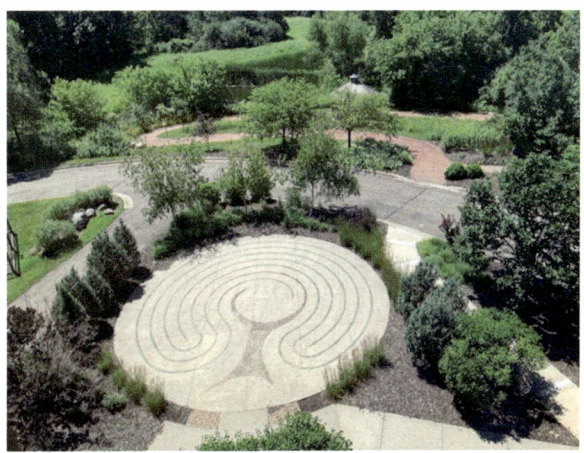

Holistic Nursing

HN is synergistically in alignment with the concept of an OHE. Holistic Nursing Models (HNM) are rapidly emerging as salient models in nursing education and practice. Nursing theories and philosophies underpin holistic nursing models and are further supported via the integrated use of healing art therapies (HAT) such as essential oils, guided imagery, healing music, and energy based healing (Healing Touch, Reiki and Therapeutic Touch). HATs compassionately support care of both the nurse and the patient in addition to expanding the therapeutic strategies that nurses can use to provide holistic care.

The HNM recognizes and honors that each clinical shift brings with it challenges to the delivery of compassionate, holistic care. Like all fast-paced acute care nursing divisions, WHC is similarly experiencing increased acuity, quick patient volume turnover alongside challenging clinical circumstances. The HNM encourages nursing staff to access healing presence and consciousness as a facilitator to the healing moment and to set the intention to be of service to others, including their co-workers and to remember the moment.

5.3 The Process: Woodwinds Health Campus Healing Healthcare Model

The founding vision of Woodwinds' Healing Healthcare Model (HHM) was to be an innovative, unique, and preferred resource for health for the local community. The purpose of the HHM was to promote health and healing of body, mind, and spirit, through relationships, choices, and learning. The founding values and guiding principles of WHC described an organization that was committed to integrative, innovative, collaborative, responsive, and compassionate service to the community [9]. This was represented in the core values and standards of the Woodwinds Health Campus' organizational mission which foundationally supported the integration of the practice of holistic nursing. Both the organizational philosophy of servant leadership and the use of the HNM were considered innovations within the healthcare system at the time. To translate the vision of the HHM into practice took years of commitment and leadership (Fig. 5.4).

Step One: Identification of the Issue

The Integrative Service Department at WHC is a support department which is integrated into the budget process as a highly valued service to the care model and is part

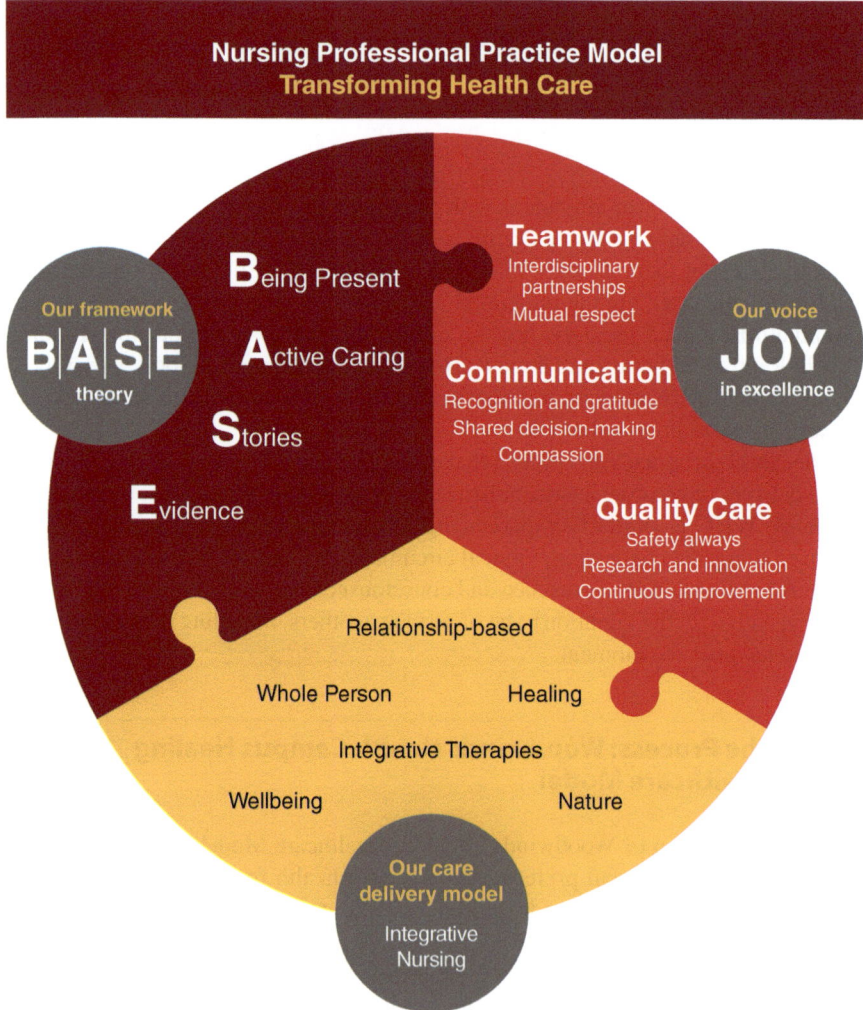

Fig. 5.4 Nursing professional practice model. (Source: M Health Fairview (2019))

of the operations budget currently without philanthropic support. The department is led by a clinical leader to champion the grassroots initiatives and lead the education, practice, clinical research, and clinical outcome evaluation of these services.

During a period of nursing shortages in Minnesota, the Minnesota Organization for Leaders in Nursing (MOLN), a statewide organization found in most states, sought to identify reasons for job satisfaction and tenure as a means in which to retain current workforce. Through their work, MOLN identified that the work environment of acute care hospitals was a potent influencer of nursing shortages in key segments within the State of Minnesota. In response to this new knowledge, MOLN selected six Minnesota hospitals to participate in the development and implementation of projects to improve the acute care work environments and subsequently, job satisfaction and tenure. WHC was chosen for their interest as well as to represent a smaller community based hospital within the metropolitan area of Minneapolis and St. Paul, Minnesota.

Representatives from each of these six hospitals met under the leadership of the MOLN. The projects varied widely. Staff nurse members involved in designing the project at WHC deferred to announce their focus for their project electing instead to first survey all staff nurses for their opinion on the best project to address. Although many ideas emerged, the one identified as the most important to staff members to improve their work environment was "to implement a holistic nursing model." Following the identification of the project, a Holistic Practice Council (HPC) was established to lead the charge. The HPC included representation from each department within nursing. Together they worked to establish goals, identify problems, and develop strategies to support the education, practice, and evidence based processes to support the HNM. The overarching goal for the HPC was to: care well for self and soul and to support a sustainable healing environment for patients, families, practitioners, staff, and community [10].

The leadership of the HPC was shared by the Director for Integrative Services and a staff member. Membership included nursing personnel from each unit, nursing leaders, patient care associates, and representatives from other disciplines and departments. The HPC was responsible for facilitating the holistic nursing professional model with a specific focus on education, practice, clinical evaluation, and research. The HPC partnered to develop holistic nursing educational and practice competencies, procedures related to select Healing Arts Therapies (HAT), educational programming such as annual education and competency validation, the annual WHC Healing Healthcare Conference, and larger house wide initiatives such as the Prayer Shawl Ministry and the Pause for Prayer process. The Prayer Shawl Ministry was facilitated by a HPC leader, in partnership with the Director of Spiritual Care, and consisted of both volunteer staff and volunteer community members who wished to create prayer shawls. Members of the Prayer Shawl Ministry came together one evening per month to knit or crochet together. The shawls created during these evenings were donated to the hospital as a spiritual offering for patients, families, and employees going through challenging times including but not limited to terminal diagnoses or unexpected loss. These gifts could be initiated by any member of the healthcare team. The Pause for Prayer initiative serves patient, staff, or family members who request the spiritual support of other's healing intention. A few seconds of healing flute music is heard overhead to call the spirit of healing to individual's consciousness. This is done for both patients and staff who are facing deep challenges. Additionally, like many organizations, a few moments of a lullaby are played overhead to announce the emergence of a child into our larger community.

Step Two: Creating the HNM

The philosophy, core beliefs, and standards for the HNM at WHC were deeply informed by the American Holistic Nursing Association (AHNA) scope and standards for practice [11]. The nursing division at Woodwinds adopted the HNM to guide patient-centered care in all nursing departments. The HNM was intentionally created as a fluid entity that evolved as the hospital and the people changed over time. After a decade of use, the foundational aspects of holistic nursing practice, education, and research via the HNM were deepened to include concepts from Watson's Caring Science [12] and Koerner's Healing Presence [13]. Concepts from Watson and Koerner incorporate a sensitive balance between art and science, intuitive and analytical skills, and the use of the healing capacity of the body, mind, and spirit. The HNM intentionally called nurses to commit personally and professionally to the principles of holistic care with a special emphasis on self-care and healing presence.

Step Three: Support for the HNM

The nursing division made the decision to adopt a HNM with the integrated use of HAT to supplement their practice. The team identified the following HAT interventions for use: energy based healing (Healing Touch, and later Reiki and Therapeutic Touch), essential oils, healing music, acupressure, massage, and guided imagery. A comprehensive literature review ensued to evaluate the acute care hospital use of these modalities. Literature of high quality was cataloged leading to the establishment of a HAT Journal Database. This was done to allow quick reference to the literature by patient type, clinical presentation, modality, or holistic nursing category. The database became a comprehensive repository of pertinent literature that can augment contemporary literature searches.

Within the first year of operations, a Healing Arts Therapy Volunteer Program (HATV) was also established to lead and supervise the delivery of select HAT to augment the care of the direct caregivers [14]. The volunteers' care included delivery of Healing Touch, Reiki, massage, guided imagery, use of essential oils, and healing music. Integrative services offered by specialty certified or licensed professionals such as Certified Music Practitioners (CMP), Certified Massage Therapy (CMT) or Acupuncture (LAC) have also been robustly offered. Acupuncture is offered in all of the inpatient units from medical-surgical, to maternity care, and in outpatient units such as the emergency department and the cancer care clinic. Most patients receive essential oils, healing music, or guided imagery, while 25–35% of patients receive energy based healing or acupuncture treatments during their hospital stay.

Step Four: Forming Partnerships

Forming strategic partnerships with Medical and Practitioner Staff, Nursing Leaders, community members was necessary to support the integration of the HNM. Advanced practitioners in medicine and other specialties recognized that a HNM is the professional realm of nursing, however, partnering closely with key medical practitioner staff to enhance their awareness and keep them well informed serves to improve the experience of patient as a whole. The use of HAT is a component of the HNM and as such medical orders are not necessary as this is viewed as nursing practice. Additional key partnerships included nursing leadership within the individual units as their support was critical to achieving the degree of success desired.

Step Five: Intentional Communication

At the beginning of the project, members of the HPC and nurse leaders acknowledged the difficult task of keeping staff informed of the process. In response, several communication vehicles were created. The first was the creation of a resource box. In this box staff could find key supportive resources such as practice standards, patient education brochures, and brochures related to special holistic classes. The second was a newsletter specific to the holistic model. These vehicles have now been moved to the online intranet environment and are easily accessed during working hours or after hours via the individuals home internet services. This was initially mailed to the homes of staff but is now located on the electronic intranet. In addition to avenues for communicating with staff, vehicles for communicating with community members were also necessary. A community class "Supporting Your Healing Process" was established and was well attended for many years.

Step Six: Assuring Educational Equity

Identifying the educational needs of the staff to develop the educational curriculum largely drove this step in the process. The original house wide RN survey served as a rich source of staff identified educational needs. From these results the HPC developed a required 2 day long seminar related to the holistic model. This content, although focused on the nursing staff, was also available to other interdisciplinary professionals. Clinical competencies were identified related to the safe use of the HAT and were seamlessly integrated as a part of the general clinical orientation as well as unit specific orientation. Mandatory online modules were a required part of staff education each year to assure up to date knowledge and use of both the model and HATs.

Step Seven: Establishing Protocols and Procedures

Establishing protocols, procedures, and practice documentation standards was necessary to support this important work. The standard of "every patient, every shift" created an easy reminder for the expectations of nursing staff. At the onset, the decision was made to purposefully view the use of HAT as a standard of care in line with the HNM that would not require special procedures. To that end, only the use of essential oils and acupressure has a specific procedure. The other HATs including are delivered and documented as any other nursing intervention. Initially all documentation was facilitated by the use of a paper form. Documentation of the clinical use of HAT then became an integrated part of the routine electronic medical record (EMR).

Step Eight: Evaluation

Recognizing the unique opportunity to contribute to the advancement of nursing practice as well as to improve patient care services for future patients, establishing a HAT registry supported by the institutional review board (IRB) became a priority. All patients who were admitted to the acute care setting were asked for their consent to enable the organization to retrospectively analyze the clinical use of any HAT received. This registry served as a rich repository for data for many years and enabled the analysis of clinical research related to the use of HAT. Currently there are over 20,000 study registrants in this HAT Registry; however, the registry itself is no longer active. Data storage and retrievals are now available via the EMR.

As a whole the collective HATs are most commonly used to promote relaxation and general well-being and to reduce nausea, vomiting, anxiety, pain, and urinary retention. Two notable studies have demonstrated the effectiveness of the HNM and the HAT combined. The first study by Lincoln et al. [14] used retrospective data from the HAT Registry to examine the concomitant use of two HAT modalities, Healing Harp (HH) and Healing Touch (HT) as a means of reducing pain, anxiety, and nausea in the post-operative patient. The results demonstrated the effectiveness of using concomitant HT and HH to significantly reduce moderate to severe pain ($p < 0.0001$) and anxiety ($p < 0.03$) in this patient population compared to just HT or HH alone (Fig. 5.5).

The second study examined the patient perception of care at WHC [15]. Using the Caring Factor Survey [16] and narrative inquiry, patients described the caring behaviors they experienced in four themes: the attitudes and attributes of the nurses, the actions the nurses took to make the patient feel cared for, honoring the patients' spirituality, and receiving care within an optimal healing environment. Qualitative

Healing Touch and Harp				Healing Touch or Reiki alone	
Pain level	N	Pain Reduction	p-value	N	Pain Reduction
Severe (7-10 on 10-pt scale)	22	87% *	<0.001	662	53%
Moderate (4-6 on 10-pt scale)	21	90% *	< 0.001	971	61%
Mild (1-3 on 10-pt scale)	38	not statistically significant		698	-------

Research Results: Reducing pain level by Healing Touch and Harp or Reiki

Fig. 5.5 Research results of pain reduction by healing touch and Reiki

findings included four overarching themes. Themes included Attitudes and Attributes (of patient caregivers), *"They listen to me; and react..."*; Actions, *"People always ask, 'Is there anything else I can do for you?'"*, *"...a pat on the arm after helping getting lifted into position or something like that, those are the kinds of things that I'm always seeing and always appreciating..."*; Honoring Spirituality, *"Everybody that I know of that knows my faith has strongly upheld it or upheld me, and, therefore, I feel honored, cared for..."*; and Environment which had three sub-themes, Personnel *"They all seemed to kind of interconnect and work together..."*, Physical Space *"This is the best hospital I've ever been in..."* and Healing Art Therapies, *"It (healing touch) made me feel special; I was just taken aback that someone would come in and do that, and that the nurse would see that as something I could benefit from...I think people here see or connect to how a person might be feeling – it's nice..."* The findings from this study stress the importance of relationship and presence.

Currently, the use of HATs is considered a standard of care. Each care provider must offer at least two HATs to each patient each shift. While there is ample data now available in the EMR to evaluate patient outcomes associated with the use of HATs, current limitations only serve to provide audits of use rather than associated outcomes.

5.4 The People

Steps that supported the accountability of both the nursing staff and the nurse manager to seamlessly integrate the HNM philosophy into practice were fundamental to the success of the HHM at WHC. Accountability begins with the hiring process. Expectations for embracing the culture are embedded into each nursing division job description. These "Holistic Nurse Professional Expectations" make clear the expectations that are indicative of a dedication to the HNM, including self-care and clinical excellence in the nurse's specialty area. As nursing staff advance thru the orientation process, they are assessed on their performance of allopathic nursing skills as well as their performance and literacy related to the HNM. Unit Educators and Clinical Preceptors have been key nursing leaders to support the advancement of the HNM for all new and current unit staff.

The process for new employees included meeting with their nursing leader at 1 month, 3 months, and 9 months and then annually. At this annual evaluation the leader would review the HNM competencies, and the staff nurse would complete a Holistic Resilience Reflection. The reflection required the staff nurse to provide at least one holistic personal and professional goal they wished to accomplish. For example, the staff nurse may state they wish to attend a Healing Touch class to learn how to serve future patients (professional) and to set a goal of supporting a daily meditation practice (personal). In the spirit of encouraging familiarity with aspects of nursing inquiry and personal reflection, the staff nurse was also asked to submit a short reflective summary of a holistic patient encounter from which they learned more deeply about a caring moment or which demonstrates understanding of practice-in-action related to healing presence.

Interdisciplinary Evolution and Assimilation

The HNM has had an overall influence on the culture at WHC. It is evident in that several non-nursing units are also offering HAT to their patients, specifically healing music, guided imagery, and in many cases, offering essential oils to reduce pain, stress, or nausea. Radiology was the first non-nursing department to ask to be educated about the safe use of these therapies to improve the patient experience. For example, in Breast Care Services when a woman is asked to change into a patient gown to get ready for the mammography procedure, they are asked to remove any deodorant as a procedural necessity. Instead of offering a cold alcohol wipe(s), the staff offers oshibori with lavender oil. This is prepared using warm washcloths with lavender oil. Not only does the oshibori aid in removing deodorant, but also delivers lavender essential oil with the expressed clinical purpose to reduce anxiety often associated with medical testing.

5.5 The HHM Today

Over the past 6 years WHC and the Healtheast System as a whole have undergone significant changes in both leadership and subsequently structure. In 2012, a new president for Healtheast sought to align the hospital systems into one care model and prepare the system for integration with Fairview, a larger more financially robust system in the Twin Cities. During this time, new leadership in IS re-established the commitment and energy needed to uphold the HNM as systems level changes occurred. Holistic nurse clinicians were assigned to each of the three Healtheast sites as champions doing *with* the nursing staff rather *to* the nursing staff through revised education and a focus on staff self-care. In just over 3 years the IS team trained over 2000 nurses and saw marked improvements in audits scores which have been sustained over time. Formal and informal survey results showed an improvement in engagement of nurses and improved results in meeting the standard of care [17].

In 2017 the merger of Healtheast and Fairview into one system began a new path for establishing a holistic nursing model that would represent the two organizations as one whole. Over the course of the last 2 years, each layer of the two systems has slowly merged. The nursing division remains segregated with legacy protocols and procedures informing nursing practice at each site. As such, nursing and auxiliary staff at WHC largely continued to practice under the former HNM with continued success as demonstrated by the awards and accolades mentioned previously.

With nursing services nearing their own merger, the HNM as it was formerly known has sunset, but core aspects remain including a newly revised Nursing Professional Practice Model (PPM; Fig. 5.4). The PPM has three elements or puzzle pieces that create the whole. These include the framework for nursing practice, JOY within the organization and, the care delivery model. The first puzzle piece is Potter's BASE of nursing theory [18] which serves as the framework for nursing practice. BASE represents four domains unique to nursing, being present (B), active caring (A), stories/narratives (S), and evidence from science (E). The second puzzle piece represents the voice of the nurses within the organization. This piece captures what has been learned about how to create joy in the workplace through gathering feedback from voices across the organization through intentional rounding. Components identified for supporting JOY in the work environment include excellence and professionalism with concepts of teamwork, communication, and quality care as key contributors. The third and final piece of the puzzle is the care delivery model, Integrative Nursing. The care delivery model highlights the way in which care for the whole person within the whole system is facilitated.

The core values and standards of the Fairview system support and uphold the practice of the holistic nursing including a call to dignity, integrity, service, compassion, and innovation [19]; however, the work to educate and roll out of the new model is just beginning. With 12 hospitals, 56 clinics, and a number of long-term care facilities to integrate, leadership anticipates the process taking several years to implement. With lessons in hand from the development, implementation, and evaluation of the former HNM, the process for implementation of the new NPPM will largely follow suit with an expressed focus on presence as the core attribute to transforming health care and doing *with* rather than *to* being foundational to getting buy-in.

5.6 Lessons Learned

The world continues to evolve and change at paces unseen before our time, including but not limited to the rapid technological and economic influences. Like all organizations undergoing massive structural and cultural change, our habits of working, thinking, and of acting are all subject to scrutiny and challenge. These challenges to all that we have known can feel stressful and uncomfortable leaving us yearning for the "old ways" but if we look closely, and think broadly, we also find that this scrutiny has opened the door for questioning much that was once taken for granted. As Eisler and Potter [18] note, this questioning is part of a much larger movement for change: the global partnership movement toward more democratic and egalitarian relations in both the so-called private and public spheres and the possibilities for what this means in our health care and educational systems are limitless.

Change is full of chaos and contradictions; the Newtonian approach to organizational design is no longer viable. To understand and respond fluidly to the quickly changing world around us, we must leave behind the reductionist perspective of A plus B always equals or leads to C, and instead understand that there is much more complexity to achieving any desired outcome. Every single individual, and every component of that which surrounds us, in turn influences how life is experienced, perceived, and manifested. Change therefore must be viewed as a process, not a singular event. Organizational change does not happen instantaneously because there was an announcement that this was the desired outcome. Fortunately or unfortunately, individuals do not change simply because they received word that they were expected to do so. When we experience change, we move from what we have known and done through our own lived experiences, through a period of transition where we eventually arrive at a desired new way of behaving and doing.

5.7 Expanding Consciousness

The expansion of IS to the acute care delivery model is evident in the disciplines of both medicine and nursing. Concepts of IS are now included in curricula in medical residencies and fellowships and are evident in all levels of professional nursing education including doctorate in nursing practice programs. Other professional international organizations continue to follow. At the heart of the profession of nursing is the intention to attend holistically to all individuals through the extension of competent relationship centered care. The changing face of healthcare over the last several decades, including reliance on technology and increased patient acuity, has overshadowed *being* (a nurse) with *doing* (nursing tasks). Academic nursing programs necessarily prepare students to become proficient at clinical reasoning, relying heavily on empirical knowing to prepare students for practice. However, as individuals, families, and communities call for healthcare to meet more than just their physical needs, nursing must re-focus on both the being and the doing essential to holistic care. Of the 966 baccalaureate nursing programs in the US, the American Holistic Nursing Credentialing Corporation (AHNCC) endorses only 14 [20]. The rapid evolution of healthcare requires academia to follow suit. Responding energetically with innovative curricula to prepare the nurses of tomorrow for a future yet to be defined is necessary.

5.8 Conclusion/What Others Can Learn from Us

The evolution of the healing healthcare model at WHC is one example of how organizations and systems can begin to approach the integration of IS into the acute care setting. Key learnings that can improve the opportunity for success include assuring the place, the people, and the processes are synergistically aligned. Starting small by establishing a cultural intention to be present to those being served and to be of service to those who are serving is imperative. Without intention to serve it will not matter how many tools or modalities providers are given to use, their potential impact will be limited. Once the cultural shift has occurred, begin slowly. Do *with* the healthcare provider instead of *to* the healthcare provider. Each system or organization will have its unique strengths and weaknesses. Knowing in advance how to maximize the strengths and minimize the weaknesses as the integration of IS occurs can provide a more seamless integration.

In conclusion, leaders, aspiring leaders, clinical educators, and development staff within the healthcare organizations have the opportunity to change the experience of giving care and receiving care using a healing healthcare model. Assessing the needs and desires of those using the services and delivering the services is a crucial first step. The approach to change thereafter will be unique to each organization; however, the experience at WHC can serve as one example of success.

References

1. Nahin R, Barnes P, Stussman B, Bloom B. Costs of Complementary and Alternative Medicine (CAM) and frequency of visits to CAM practitioners: United States, 2007. National health statistics reports 18. 2009. https://nccih.nih.gov/sites/nccam.nih.gov/files/nhsrn18.pdf.
2. Mann D, Gaylord S, Norton SK. The convergence of complementary, alternative and conventional health care: educational resources for health professionals. University of North Carolina at Chapel Hill, Program on Integrative Medicine; 2004.
3. Gannota RJ, Zoller J, Brantley J, White A. Perceptions of medical directors and hospital executives regarding the value of inpatient integrative medicine programs. Wake County Med Soc J. 2009;1:1–7.
4. Fairview. Woodwinds health campus. 2019. https://www.fairview.org/locations/woodwinds-health-campus.
5. The Leapfrog Group. Hospital safety grade: woodwinds health campus. 2019. https://www.hospitalsafetygrade.org/h/woodwinds-health-campus?findBy=zip&zip_code=55125&radius=50&rPos=316&rSort=distance.
6. Jonas W, Chez R. Toward optimal healing environments in health care. J Altern Complement Med. 2004;10:1–6.
7. Samueli Institute. Optimal healing environments. 2016. http://www.samueliinstitute.org/research-areas/optimal-healing-environments/ohe-framework.html.
8. Lincoln V. Nontraditional healthcare: emerging into integrative healthcare. In: Condon M, editor. Women's health: an integrated approach to wellness and illness. Upper Saddle River: Prentice-Hall Health; 2000. p. 182–94.
9. Lincoln V, Johnson M. Staff nurse perceptions of a healing environment. Holist Nurs Pract. 2009;23(3):183–90.
10. Lincoln V. Creating an integrated hospital: woodwinds health campus. Integr Nurs. 2003;2(1):12–3.

11. American Nurses Association. American holistic nursing association - holistic nursing: scope and standards of practice. Silver Spring: American Nurses Association; 2013.
12. Watson J. The philosophy and science of caring. Denver: University Press of Colorado; 2008.
13. Koerner J. Healing presence: the essence of nursing. New York: Springer; 2012.
14. Lincoln V, Nowak E, Briggs T, Wax G. Impact of healing touch with healing harp on inpatient acute care pain: a retrospective analysis. Holist Nurs Pract. 2014;28(3):164–70.
15. Nowak & Lincoln. The patient perception of caring: preliminary findings. Perceptions of healing. 2014. https://www.healingbeyondborders.org/images/Newsletter/2014-2ndQuarterNewsletter.pdf.
16. Nelson J, DiNapoli P, Turkel M. Concepts of caring as construct of caritas. In: Nelson J, Watson J, editors. Measuring caring: a compilation of international research on caritas as healing intervention. New York: Springer; 2011.
17. Verner T. Personal Communication, 12 June 2019.
18. Eisler R, Potter T. Transforming Interprofessional partnerships: a new framework for nursing and partnership-based health care. Indianapolis: Sigma Theta Tau International Honor Society of Nursing; 2014.
19. Fairview. Mission, vision, values. 2019. https://www.fairview.org/about/who-we-are/mission-vision-values.
20. American Holistic Nurses Credentialing Corporation. Current endorsed nursing programs. 2019. https://www.ahncc.org/school-endorsement-program/current-endorsed-nursing-programs/.

A Strategically Engaged Programme of Person-Centred Culture Development in Health Services: The Courage of the Irish!

Brendan McCormack, Lorna Peelo-Kilroe, Margaret Codd, and Debbie Baldie

6.1 Background

The Health Service Executive (HSE) is responsible for providing all public health services in hospitals and communities across Ireland. The vision for the HSE is 'a healthier Ireland with a high quality health service valued by all' [1, 2]. To this end a number of structures and initiatives were put in place to improve quality, enhance the experiences of people who use the service, achieve greater efficiencies and control rising costs. Recent high profile examples of poor practices have created debate about the extent to which 'training' can address deeper issues relating to cultures of care and practice and the impact that it has on quality of care, care experiences and staff well-being. It also raised questions about what it means to be person-centred and how we evaluate it. What became obvious from this debate was the variety of interpretations and understandings of person-centredness and person-centred care in the Irish context. It was widely assumed that person-centredness was the business only of some staff, mainly those who worked in the delivery of services to patients.

This chapter will outline the courageous journey that the HSE has taken to enable a culture of person-centredness that includes and involves everyone in the organisation irrespective of discipline or grade and whether in direct care, administration or corporate settings. It can be seen from our story that although nurses are involved in this programme and indeed have been the forerunners of a similar but smaller scale national programme within older persons residential services [3], our focus and story will encompass all the disciplines and services taking part in this work. We will start by giving a brief overview of the Irish health service and population trends. After that, we will describe the journey of the programme, the work involved, including methodology and methods, and the preliminary outcomes from the evaluation so far.

6.2 The Irish Health Service

Ireland has a comprehensive, taxation funded public healthcare system. A person living in Ireland for at least 1 year is considered by the HSE to be 'ordinarily resident' and is entitled to either full eligibility (Category 1) or limited eligibility (Category 2) for health services. Approximately 30% of the population are in Category 1 which means that they receive a wide range of services and medicines free of charge. The largest numbers of people in this category are people aged 70 years and over. The remainder 70% can avail of services and medicines either free of charge or at a reduced cost, usually supported through personally purchased healthcare insurance.

The public health service is the largest employer in the country employing 131,926 staff, comprising a mixture of clinical and non-clinical grades [4]. Nurses account for almost one-third of that figure at 31.9%. Like many other countries, the Irish health service is experiencing difficulty in the area of staff recruitment and retention with a turnover rate estimated to be 6%. This problem, if not reversed, can only increase as the average number of employees aged over 55 has increased from 13% in 2007 to 21% in 2017.

In 2007, the Department of Health introduced an independent health and social care monitoring and licencing authority, Health Information and Quality Authority (HIQA), whose role is to develop standards, inspect and review health and social care services and support informed decisions on how services are delivered.

6.3 Population Changing

Figures from the Irish Department of Health [5] indicate that the population has been growing steadily year by year over recent decades. In 1968 the population of Ireland was three million and had increased to 4.7 million by 2016. The number is expected to increase by a further 8% by 2026 with a 23% increase in people aged over 60 and an associated increase in life expectancy and persons living with chronic disease and co-morbidity. Irish women are currently expected to live

83 years, which is in line with the EU average, and Irish men expected to live in excess of 79 years, approximately 1 year longer than the EU average. This changing population will have significant implications for health service availability. The Department of Health proposes that the addition of each chronic condition leads to an associated increase in primary care consultations, hospital out-patient visits, hospital admissions and ultimately to the total healthcare costs.

6.4 The Catalyst for Our Person-Centred Journey

A small number of complaints about care practices and systems failures that fell below acceptable standards received a high profile in the Irish media. Particular issues in intellectual disability services were identified as they underwent specific scrutiny and evolution from institutional settings to small home settings. The National Patient Experience Survey [6] and Employee Engagement Surveys [7] indicated dissatisfaction with how staff engage in decisions about them and about the level of involvement by both people who use the service and those providing it. The HSE Corporate Plan [1, 2] has centre-staged the organisation's values and beliefs of care, compassion, trust and learning and the challenge for everyone is to make them a lived experience.

Several pilot, short and longer term initiatives were introduced into the system that broadly addressed areas of values, behaviours, leadership and practice. National initiatives such as Values in Action, [8], Caring Behaviours Assurance System—Ireland [9] and Health Services Change Guide [10] to name but a few were introduced, all with a common goal of service improvement. It was an opportunity to review other successful initiatives that took place over previous years so that capacity developed within the system could be used to drive change from inside the service rather than always looking outside for expertise that may already exist.

6.5 Learning from Previous Experience

In 2007, the HSE sponsored a 2 year national practice development (PD) programme in older persons' residential services to introduce a model of person-centred practice. That programme was the first of its kind to use an emancipatory practice development approach (ePD) to empower staff to lead their own change. This approach is a particular method of practice development that supports healthcare teams to develop their knowledge and skills and to transform the culture and context of care. It is enabled and supported by facilitators committed to systematic, rigorous continuous processes of emancipatory change that reflect the perspectives of service users. It draws on knowledge and experience from a variety of sources to holistically inform facilitation of practice, taking account of knowledge of self; learning styles; the individual and their context; interpersonal processes; group theory and processes; systems, organisations and power; and change theory and processes [11]. The programme was nurse lead and involved nursing and support staff along with residents in 18 hospital and residential units across the country engaged in a national facilitated programme. It was also the first time that a specific framework, The Person-centred Nursing Framework [12], was used to guide and evaluate person-centred changes in practice. Findings from that programme identified positive outcomes for residents, staff and organisations and a report was developed outlining achievements and the key recommendations for future development [3]. The approach used in the programme positively influenced other international programmes and provided a basis for a similar programme focused on end of life care in acute hospitals from 2010 to 2012 [13, 14]. This work went largely unnoticed within the overall system and this was a key learning because without senior managers supporting and championing this work it does not 'stick'. The work was slow and did not 'fix' structure and process issues in the system; therefore, the impact was not immediately noticeable. However on HIQA inspections, sites that engaged in this programme consistently fared better in reports. Feedback from staff indicated that person-centred practice endured and some sites progressed their practice beyond that achieved on the programme, all this largely without the support of senior managers and corporate leaders. This raised the question of whether or not there was a need to look at enabling a supporting culture first before embarking on developing care practices. It also raised big questions about who needs to be person-centred in the organisation. Is it just the business of staff providing care to patients or should everyone be involved? Therefore it was decided to adopt a whole-systems approach involving everyone regardless of role, position or service.

6.6 Promoting the Idea

The National Framework for Improving Quality [15] was developed by the HSE National Quality Improvement Team (National QI Team) to support quality improvement throughout the Irish health service. Central to the framework is *'a culture of person-centred quality care that continually improves'*. This opened the way for a proposal to establish a national programme to enable cultures of person-centredness to be led by the National QI Team and supported by the National Office of Nursing and Midwifery (ONMSD). The strategic approach meant the programme was aligned with national organisational goals, and building on previous experience, it meant we had tangible evidence to support the culture development approach and the skills within the system to take ownership.

Courageous Step 1

The National Director of the National QI Team and the Director of the ONMSD both demonstrated courage in standing behind the proposed programme and giving it their full support. By backing something that had never been achieved in any other health service, a whole system approach to culture change, their credibility as leaders was in the spotlight nationally. Also, as they were not familiar with the approach or the detail of the programme it required a leap of faith to trust those who did to take the lead.

Courageous Step 2

Corporate leaders within the HSE listened to what was being proposed, pondered, sought further clarity and in time gave the programme permission to proceed. They recognised that even if services were resourced with sufficient training and better care environments this would not necessarily equate to good care experiences and good relational care. They showed courage by taking the risk to support a proposal that uses a very different philosophy and approach to learning and development, especially at this time when demonstrating value for money was paramount. They knew that failure had the potential to reach the national media and perhaps beyond but they were brave enough to support person-centredness as their way to assuring the development and sustainability of person-centred practice and care. This is commensurate with the growing evidence that staff must experience person-centredness consistently in order to provide more than person-centred moments to those they provide care to and that for this to be realised practitioners need to be supported in a culture of person-centredness [12, 16].

6.7 Partnering and Planning

At the time in Ireland, there were a small number of people who had the skills to provide this programme. However, undertaking the development and provision of a programme of this magnitude was too much for this number of people to provide without help and expertise. It was decided to partner with external experts to support the planning and implementation phase of the programme and provide accreditation and support with research and evaluation. Following a tendering process, Queen Margaret University (QMU), Edinburgh, UK was selected as the partner of choice for the first 3 years of the programme. In total, a team of four facilitators, two from the HSE's National Quality Improvement Team and two from QMU came together to co-design and deliver the programme. As lead facilitators, each had advanced knowledge, skills and experience in person-centred facilitation and large scale programmes of change within health services. As a collaborative team we needed to learn to work together and share individual and collective expertise, insider organisational knowledge and international perspectives, as well as expertise to plan and shape the new programme.

6.8 Programme Description

Following a year of negotiation and planning, the *National Programme to Enable Cultures of Person-centredness* began in 2017 with 70 participants from a range of settings and services across the country. The overall aim of this year long programme is to embed cultures of person-centredness within services systematically and incrementally by:

- Developing multi-professional facilitators who would lead person-centred culture change within their own services.
- Provide a means for services to embed person-centred ways of working as the norm for how they do their business.

The programme offers learning and development in person-centred facilitation, knowledge and skills but with an emphasis on being reflective, critically creative and using creative practices. The programme is focused on person-centredness for everyone—staff as well as persons using the service and their families. Time and patience are required to unlearn traditional assumptions and for a culture of person-centredness to become a reality.

Two programmes were established in year 1, one for participants from intellectual disability services and one for all other services and this was repeated in year 2. Nominees from all disciplines who had the authority and ability to lead change within their work area were invited to undertake the 12 month programme. The curriculum is built around six broad themes. Each theme is linked with specific person-centred activities that enable it to be facilitated and operationalised in practice. The themes are:

1. Helping teams to know and develop shared values and beliefs about person-centred practice.
2. Facilitating the development of a shared vision for person-centred practice.
3. Developing teams and building an effective culture of person-centredness.
4. Introduction to evaluation and engaging in participatory evaluation method.
5. Facilitating learning in the workplace.
6. Action planning.

The time commitment of the programme is as follows:

- 5 day introduction to person-centredness spread over 2 months
- 10 one day modules to develop skills in facilitating person-centredness in practices.

Each participant works with a group of their colleagues for the duration of the programme to practice their facilitation skills and share their learning. With their colleagues they develop shared values about person-centredness and work together to evaluate and improve their team's culture and practices in systematic and rigorous ways. The size of the working groups varies depending on the size of the organisation, ranging from four to five members in small organisations and up to ten in larger ones. The collaborative, inclusive and participative processes used provide a means of involving everyone on the team in decision-making and planning, resulting in a wider spread of engagement. The approach is not about 'telling' but collaborating, not 'training' but learning and development so that a culture of person-centredness and engagement with the wider setting is incrementally enabled and embedded. So too, the competencies and confidence of participants as facilitators are enabled.

To date 133 participants from 85 sites have participated in five programmes. Unsurprisingly, nurses make up approximately 65% of those. It is expected that by the end of year 3 at least 160 staff members will have engaged in the programme directly and approximately 1500 other staff will have been involved in developing cultures of person-centredness in their services. Programme participants have the opportunity to apply for academic accreditation at masters' level through Queen Margaret University, Edinburgh, Scotland. Accreditation meets with European standards and depends on attendance at programme days and submission of a written assignment based on reflective learning chosen from a specific topic guide.

6.9 Methodology and Methods

The programme is underpinned by the philosophy of person-centredness focusing on the right of every person to flourish. Knowing how to provide the conditions for human flourishing to take place is crucial to achieving this philosophy and in turn to transform thinking, practice and culture. The programme recognises that Healthcare organisations have different cultures at different levels, departments and teams [17] and this programme focuses on workplace as opposed to organisational culture as this is the level that has most impact on people and influences the way they behave and talk [18]. It looks at the embedded patterns about how things are done [19] and unpicks the deeper levels of assumption, values and beliefs that lie beneath [20]. Participants are facilitated to engage with cognitive and creative methods to uncover the realities and possibilities for their workplaces. An adult learning approach called Active Learning [21] is used to enable that transformation process to take place. By using facilitation approaches, participants engage their colleagues in work-based learning instead of traditional classroom learning.

An integral element of the programme is ongoing evaluation that is both formative and summative. In keeping with the philosophy of person-centredness we use diverse and creative approaches to collect and analyse data so that it can be owned and used by all involved to tailor and contextualise learning and actions in various contexts. The approaches to evaluation used include the following:

- Participants' self-evaluation through personal reflection on their personal values, ways of being and development as a facilitator.
- Group reflection exercises that helped people seek and provide feedback that was aimed at enhancing personal growth of self and others.

- Group evaluations both from programme days and from local working group sessions that taught groups to evaluate how they work together and to continually improve so that they become increasingly person-centred, effective, collaborative, inclusive and participative.
- Records of meetings with working groups; observations of practice, environmental walkabouts and stories from people who provide and use services.
- Claims, concerns and issues helped reflect on progress, uncover embedded patterns within the workplace and critically explore particular issues impacting the programme.
- Focus groups and critical creativity work to uncover learning and development.
- Individual interviews at midway and end of programme to understand people's learning on the programme and how that is used in practice.
- We tested the use of a culture assessment index to explore if it could be used to quantitatively assess change in culture over time. We found however that it was not well suited to our evaluation at this time as many participants worked across a number of sites, the focus on care provision posed difficult for those not working in direct care roles and there was confusion initially over the instrument as a tool for service evaluation versus research.

6.10 Key Learning from the Work to Date

At the end of year 1, a formal evaluation was undertaken to ascertain participants' perceptions of the benefits of the programme; how it had influenced them as a person, their facilitation practice and the health care culture they worked in. A collaborative data analysis approach called critical creative hermeneutic analysis [12] was used to synthesise the data and agree the key themes that were emerging. Five themes were identified as well as data related to the person-centred outcome of the existence of a healthful culture. The five themes include: consciousness raising; transformation of self; development of facilitation knowledge, skills and expertise; sharing responsibility for person-centredness; learning and doing. When considered in combination with our overall experience, there is significant learning available about the things that have worked well in relation to the programme in the Irish context and what needs further attention.

Learning for Participants

For many participants this was the first time they had participated in a programme that provided a structured methodology to raise their consciousness and knowledge of self, articulate their own values and facilitate others to do this too. From the outset, participants' entrenched assumptions arising from a narrow interpretation of person-centredness needed to be challenged. By bringing to life embodied knowing of what it might feel like to experience person-centredness and human flourishing, many participants started to transform their thinking about person-centredness and how it related to them. They reflected on their way of being and how they engaged with others. They questioned existing decision-making and problem-solving structures and started to embrace more collaborative, inclusive and participatory approaches with colleagues. In some cases this was echoed in the way they interacted with persons using the service too. This provided opportunities for collective shared responsibility for person-centredness and workplace culture so that changes could be informed from and in practice together rather than this being imposed on them.

Trusting and using person-centred processes took time and required a willingness to let go of traditional ways of thinking about learning and facilitation. For many, the focus on critical creativity as a means of exploring and enabling new ways of working and being was challenging and took time to appreciate. The temptation to apply quick fixes to complex problems was challenging for most. Having time and space to unpick old ideas and assumptions using creative as well as cognitive methods provided the opportunity to dig much deeper into the assumptions and patterns in practice that drive decisions and behaviours.

Holding Back the Tide

Another area that quickly needed to be addressed was the misperception that the programme would affect a rapid change in workplace culture. Many participants felt under pressure by managers and colleagues to bring about changes before they had completed their learning as facilitators and for some, interest started to lessen when this did not happen quickly. It needed to be constantly emphasised that it takes a year of consistent focus and practice to develop the facilitation skills needed to begin changes in culture. The complexity of person-centredness and workplace culture took time to appreciate and letting go of long held beliefs required time and patience.

Consistent, Visible Support from Managers

Participants identified early on that an important factor determining success and sustainability of the person-centred work they doing was managerial buy-in. While assurances were given at the outset, the reality in terms of support for both participants and their working groups in some cases fell short of what was required. Support by managers could be the difference between success and failure. Participants who met regularly with their line managers and secured the time and resources needed to establish and facilitate local working groups progressed significantly better than those who did not. Consistent, visible support enabled participants to feel more confident to implement what they were learning. In doing so, they strengthened positive relationships within their teams and were enabled to consider and challenge norms that compromised person-centred ways of being and doing in the workplace. Conversely, for those who did not experience the same levels of support, progress as facilitators and influencers of change was hindered. They often felt they were swimming against the tide, trying to get time to prepare for working group meetings and trying to get colleagues released to attend. For them, it was difficult to convince people of more effective ways of working, reduce hierarchical decision-making and introduce more person-centred, shared decision-making that could benefit them and the people with whom they engaged. All of this highlighted the need for robust structures for monthly engagement between participants and managers to ensure a shared understanding of the work, ideas for change and the support needed. As this is a knowledge and skills development programme, structures to embed these new ways of working and ways of being must be considered from the outset. For future programmes it has also led to a change in the application process with commitment and supporting structures more clearly outlined.

Overall much courage was demonstrated by participants in going back to their workplaces to behave in ways that were completely against anything they had ever learned about facilitating change or leading meetings. But for the majority of people, they held firm to the principles of person-centredness and holistic facilitation when for many, it would often have been much easier to let go.

Clarifying and Simplifying

As programme facilitators, we have developed and refined the programme as we have actively learned with and from participants. We quickly realised that we needed to constantly clarify and simplify our message and the processes we use on the programme so that they could be understood and useable in different work contexts. As part of that clarification, a new HSE new position statement about person-centredness emerged (Fig. 6.1).

Getting the balance right between enabling, learning and providing direction was a challenge. For many it was frustrating having to figure out together what person-centredness meant for them and their contexts through collective learning with their working groups rather than simply being told. As lead facilitators we had to listen carefully to what the groups were telling us as well as to our inner wisdom and craft knowledge so that we could get it right.

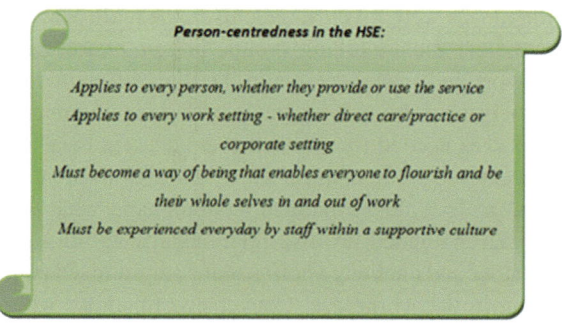

Fig. 6.1 Person-centredness in the HSE

Excitingly, the experience of implementing this innovative, programmatic, whole system approach across the range of Irish Health Services has led to the emergence of new knowledge, tools and processes that can be used in this work. They include the articulation of PIP (purpose, intended outcomes and processes) as a means of clarifying the processes and exercises used when facilitating this work. In response to participant feedback, a *Facilitator Debrief Document* was developed to enhance learning from the experience of running person-centred culture change groups. The document is a checklist that provides a structure for facilitators to use as they reflect on each of their group sessions. It prompts them to consider the links between the person-centred facilitation theory, the methods they are learning and their practice. It can be used individually or jointly by co-facilitators or groups. It draws attention to areas such as:

- Clarity of PIP (purpose, intended outcomes and processes).
- Elements that worked best/least might be done differently.
- The use of creativity.
- How CIP principles (collaboration, inclusion, participation) and agreed ways of working are 'lived' by the group.
- Supportive challenge and feedback.
- Types and effectiveness of facilitator interventions.
- Active learning processes.
- Managing story-telling and rescuing.
- Ideas for further sessions.

As part of the programme, lead facilitators offer to visit participants in their workplaces as they facilitate their person-centred culture change groups. Within our health system currently there is a proclivity of external reviews for the purpose of assessing and critiquing performance. The site visits offered by the programme are different in that they focus on the learning and development needs of participants. Using creative processes, guiding principles for supportive site visits were developed (Table 6.1). Finally, creative approaches have resulted in the use of puppetry

Table 6.1 Guiding principles for supportive site visits

1	Create foundations	This work is generative and flexible but the methods and process we use are solid, well tested and provide robust foundations
2	Recognise the curious	Being alert and aware of the 'curious' individuals and opening pathways for them to connect and engage
3	Enable movement	Being reflexive and responsive in order to facilitate a movement or shift in individuals thinking, heart or mind—i.e. their landscape
4	Going with the chaos	Accepting and working with the chaos that exists in every person and every workplace when it happens
5	Cherish the fertility	Seek out and cherish the expertise and opportunities that are available and unique to each site
6	Help to change the landscape	Each site visit should positivitely change the practice setting in some way

© HSE National Programme to enable cultures of person-centredness and the development of a bespoke Person Centred Framework game to bring core concepts such as CIP (collaboration, inclusion and participation) and the Person Centred Framework to life.

6.11 What Is Happening Now?

In the third year of the programme in Ireland the landscape in terms of commitment and support for this systematic approach to enabling cultures of person-centredness changed. Person-centredness is now embedded as the central driver of the National Quality Improvement framework [15] and the programme is identified as a strategic goal in the National Service Plan 2019 [22]. A new board was appointed to the Irish HSE in early 2019 for whom a focus on patient safety, quality, culture and values are early agenda items. Interest in the programme has increased substantially since year 1 as evidenced by the applications received, and interestingly, 50% of new participants are from organisations already engaged in the programme. In response to need, the programme has evolved to incorporate a suite of different implementation models including a whole hospital approach sponsored by the National Human Resource Division, a 1 day foundation programme in person-centredness and a 6 days over 6 month programme for corporate leaders to develop person-centred ways of working. Work to develop a network of participants through which skills and knowledge in person-centred facilitation can be furthered is ongoing.

6.12 Conclusion

This chapter outlines the courageous journey undertaken by the HSE to enable a culture of person-centredness for everyone irrespective of discipline or grade and whether in direct care, administration or corporate settings. It recounts the success and challenges experienced in implementing a National Programme using this innovative, programmatic, whole system approach across the range of Irish Health Services. It points to some of the new knowledge, tools and processes that have emerged during the first 2 years of implementation. It is still early days, but the progress in terms of commitment and support for this systematic approach to enabling cultures of person-centredness is exciting.

Tips for people thinking of implementing a person-centred facilitator programme
- Take time to cultivate support at strategic level before you begin, be that at organisational or national level
- Clarify the PIP (purpose, intended outcomes and processes) for your programme
- Culture change takes time. The focus during the programme year needs to be on making sure participants have the time and support they need to develop as facilitators. It takes courage to resist the urge to show organisational or system level changes rather than smaller workplace changes or personal development

- Be clear about your selection criteria for participants. They need to have enough seniority, interpersonal and critical thinking skills and influence to be able to lead and facilitate others
- Managerial support can be the difference between success and failure. Build in regular meetings with managers to keep them informed and on-side about what is happening. This helps to build their support for both the programme participants and members of the local culture change groups
- Remember that person-centredness includes everyone. Membership of the local culture change groups should be open to staff from all grades and disciplines, as well as service users if that is appropriate for your service
- Invite service managers and directors to join the local person-centred culture change groups. Often they are unaware that they could or should be part of the groups. Their involvement gives a clear message of support and enhances relationships within the workplace team
- Be faithful and diligent about how you use the person-centred methods and processes. Do not short-cut

Trust the person-centred groups to co-create the changes they want to make that will bring their shared values to life. Rally support for them to put the changes they want in place. This approach to sustainable culture change is not about implementing projects that have been identified or desired by others

- Stay focused and have fun

References

1. Health Service Executive. Building a high quality health service for a healthier Ireland: Health Service Executive corporate plan 2015–2017. Dublin: HSE; 2015.
2. Health Service Executive. Building a high quality service for a healthier Ireland – Health Service Executive Corporate Plan 2015–2017. 2015. https://www.hse.ie/eng/services/publications/corporate/corporateplan15-17.pdf. Accessed 15 June 2019.
3. McCormack B, Dewing J, Breslin L, Coyne-Nevin A, Kennedy K, Manning M, Peelo-Kilroe L, Tobin C, Slater P. Developing person-centred practice: nursing outcomes arising from changes to the care environment in residential settings for older people. Int J Older People Nurs. 2010;5(2):93–107.
4. Department of Health. Employment in the Public Health Service. 2018. https://health.gov.ie/publications-research/statistics/statistics-by-topic/employment-in-the-public-health-service/. Accessed 12 June 2019.
5. Department of Health, Ireland. Working together for health a National Strategic Framework for health workforce planning. Dublin: Department of Health; 2017.
6. Health Service Executive. National patient experience survey. 2017. https://www.hse.ie/eng/services/list/3/acutehospitals/natpatientexperiencesurveyprogramme/. Accessed 12 June 2019.
7. Health Service Executive. Employee engagement survey. 2015. https://www.hse.ie/eng/services/list/3/acutehospitals/natpatientexperiencesurveyprogramme/. Accessed 13 June 2019.
8. Health Service Executive. Values in action. 2017. https://www.hse.ie/eng/services/publications/corporate/corporateplan15-17.pdf. Accessed 19 June 2019.
9. Health Service Executive. Listening, responding and improving. The HSE response to the findings of the National Patient Experience Survey 2017. 2017. https://www.patientexperience.ie/app/uploads/2017/12/HSE_QualityImprovementPlan_2017.pdf. Accessed 12 June 2019.
10. Health Service Executive. People's needs defining change. Health services change guide. 2018. https://www.hse.ie/eng/staff/resources/changeguide/resources/change-guide.pdf. Accessed 12 June 2019.
11. McCormack B, Garbett R. The characteristics, qualities and skills of practice developers. J Clin Nurs. 2003;12(3):317–25.

12. McCormack B, McCance T. Person-centred nursing: theory and practice. Oxford: Wiley-Blackwell; 2010.
13. Irish Hospice Foundation. National Practice Development Programme: end of life care in major acute hospitals in Ireland. Dublin: IHF; 2013.
14. Shannon M, McCormack B. Practice development – ein Konzept zur Entwicklung der beruflichen Pflegepraxis in Irland. In: Tewes, Stockinger, editors. Personalentwicklung in Pflege- und Gesundheitseinrichtungen. Berlin: Springer; 2014. p. 165–78.
15. Health Service Executive. Framework for improving quality. 2016. https://www.hse.ie/eng/about/who/qid/framework-for-quality-improvement/framework-for-improving-quality-2016.pdf. Accessed 12 June 2019.
16. McCormack B, McCance T. Person-centred Nursing and Health Care – Theory and Practice. Oxford: Wiley Publishing; 2017.
17. Manley K, O'Keefe H, Jackson C, Pearce J, Smith S. A shared purpose framework to deliver person-centred, safe and effective care: organisational transformation using practice development methodology. 2013. https://www.fons.org/Resources/Documents/Journal/Vol4No1/IPDJ_0401_02.pdf. Accessed 19 June 2019.
18. Manley K. Workplace culture: is your workplace effective? How would you know? Nurs Crit Care. 2004;9(1):1–3.
19. Plsek P. The challenge of complexity in health care. Br Med J. 2001;323:625.
20. Schein EH. Organizational culture and leadership. 3rd ed. San Francisco: Jossey-Bass; 2004.
21. Dewing J. Being and becoming active learners and creating active learning workplaces; the value of active learning. Chapter 15. In: McCormack B, Manley K, Wilson V, editors. International practice development in nursing and healthcare. Oxford, Blackwell Publishing; 2008.
22. Health Service Executive. National Service Plan 2019. 2019. https://www.hse.ie/eng/services/publications/serviceplans/national-service-plan-2019.pdf. Accessed 09 May 2021.

Developing Practice Together with the University: Changing Health Care to Be Evidence-Based and Person-Centred

Renate Tewes, Irén Horváth, and Lydia Ulrich

7.1 Introduction

With the increasing academisation of the health professions, the networks of universities with their practice partners are growing. The cross-fertilisation in research, teaching and practice development has so far been unsystematic in Germany and is dependent on the interests of the individual networks and their sponsors. Although change processes are part of everyday life in the health care sector and the need for knowledge on effective and efficient change management is enormous, no change managers have been qualified for this at university level to date. In order to close this gap, the first course of study on practice development in the healthcare sector was established at the Evangelische Hochschule Dresden (ehs). Practice development with a focus on person-centredness are concepts developed by Brendan McCormack and Tanya McCance [1] and researched internationally. Their success for healthcare practice has been demonstrated in many studies: in rehabilitation [2, 3], in the care of people with dementia [4], long-term care [5, 6], acute care [7] or in psychiatric care [8].

The study programme takes up the concepts of practice development and person-centred care [1] and provides part-time students with the necessary scientific foundations and practical skills to become active as future change managers in the healthcare sector. This includes the teaching of evidence-based, nursing science expertise as well as knowledge of organisational development and conflict management and in-depth communication and reflection skills. Students are enabled to

---

R. Tewes (✉)
Crown Coaching International, Dresden, Saxonia, Germany

Department of Practice Development, Evangelische Hochschule (ehs), Dresden, Germany
e-mail: tewes@crown-coaching.de

I. Horváth · L. Ulrich
Department of Practice Development, Evangelische Hochschule (ehs), Dresden, Germany
e-mail: Iren.horvath@ehs-dresden.de; Lydia.ulrich@ehs-dresden.de

© The Author(s), under exclusive license to Springer Nature Switzerland AG 2022
R. Tewes (ed.), *Innovative Staff Development in Healthcare*,
https://doi.org/10.1007/978-3-030-81986-6_7

implement scientific evidence in person-centred care practice and to accompany their colleagues and teams in organisational development processes.

For this article, we have chosen Duchscher and Windey's [9] transition model as the theoretical framework in accordance to describe the implementation of the practice development course. Originally, the transition model describes the common phases of professional entry for nurses after their training, or studies. These three phases of doing, being and knowing also provide a good explanatory basis for our study programme development. They are described in the following.

After training/study, new entrants to the profession grow into their roles and go through three phases within the first year. Research on this shows that these phases of transition are often experienced in practice as a shock that needs to be overcome [9]. The shock is associated with doubt, disorientation, confusion and loss. Duschcher's [10] transition model describes three salutary process phases to overcome.

The structured and relatively predictable procedure during training/study is now followed by a phase of new expectations and responsibilities, which initially triggers an intense experience of uncertainty. In order to do the right thing (doing), performance, learning, adaptation and understanding must be aligned accordingly.

The second phase is characterised by great progress in thinking, knowledge and skill development. Nevertheless, they reach limits with their knowledge and experience frustration, disappointment, devaluation and feel incompetent. At this stage, it is no longer about what I do, but who I am (being). To overcome the disappointment, the usual procedure is now questioned, doubted, examined and uncovered.

The third phase is about finding one's own path, which is different from those of other colleagues. Personal knowledge (knowing) reaches a deeper level, which can also be accompanied by feelings of instability of one's own identity. This phase is characterised by separating oneself, exploring, criticising and accepting.

Following these stages of development, this chapter first describes what our students do (doing), how the university enables practice development to come to life (being) and finally how this knowledge flows into practice (knowing).

7.2 Enabling Professional Action Through Interactive Learning (Doing)

In order for students to become successful practice developers in the healthcare sector after graduation, they need a wide range of knowledge and skills that serve as a secure basis for their future professional activities. In addition to imparting knowledge and training skills, it is important to anticipate possible uncertainties during the transition to the new field of activity and to develop coping strategies together with the students during their studies.

To this end, we have been relying on interactive teaching methods for years. Therefore we offer a wide range of activities, like regular reflection on practice in all modules of the study programme, carrying out a nursing research project, working with acting patients from theatre and learning in the simulation laboratory.

Reflecting on one's own professional practice is the starting point for further developing nursing practice. Without becoming aware of one's own professional actions in dealing with patients and relatives as well as colleagues or in the interprofessional team, the need for change will not become apparent. This requires a critically reflective view from a meta-perspective. To this end, students learn about approaches to reflection and practice reflecting on their professional actions themselves [11, 12]. Each reflection begins with a description of a situation or event (Who? Where? When? What? How? With whom?) that did not go well and led to negative feelings for the student. This is followed by an analysis of their own feelings within the situation and what influence these feelings had on their actions. A first evaluation of the situation is the next step (What went well? What did not go well? What did I want to achieve? Did I achieve it?). The particularly problematic aspects of the situation are then considered in more depth with the help of further reflection questions [11, 12]:

- What consequences did my behaviour have for the patient, colleagues or for me?
- What triggered my behaviour, thoughts and feelings?
- What knowledge and skills were available to me? What knowledge and skills would have helped me?
- To what extent was I able to act in the best possible way and in accordance with my values/the values of the organisation?
- How could I impact the situation different so that I act more professionally in the future?
- What factors might prevent me from behaving differently the next time I am in that or a similar situation?
- Do I feel able to realise different behaviour in a comparable situation? What knowledge or skills do I need for this? How can I acquire this?
- What are the next steps I need to take to make this happen?

The knowledge of a multitude of reflection questions and the practised reflection enable the graduates of the course to guide and accompany colleagues in reflection.

Successful practice developers not only need very good reflection skills, but also versatile communication and counselling skills. Our students learn and train these skills by working with acting patients and in the simulation laboratory. The persons trained for this purpose by experienced teachers, actual actors or selected laypersons simulate patients in various demanding and complex care situations (e.g. a man with incipient dementia, a mother of a deceased baby, a man in a palliative stage). The students, initially under the guidance of teachers, then independently, conduct professional conversations with the acting patients. The conversation or counselling goals developed for the respective situations are communicated with the students in advance so that they can prepare themselves well. In addition to the feedback from the student group, it has been shown that the feedback from the acting patients after the exercise sequences is irreplaceable, as important aspects are addressed that cannot be perceived in this way from the external perspective of the teachers. Learning in the simulation laboratory also offers the advantage that students can not only practice communication skills in a protected setting, but can also try out nursing actions on controllable manikins. Manikins represent people who need to be cared for, where, e.g. heart and lung sounds, movements, bleeding but also verbal interaction are controlled by the teachers using computer technology [13]. In addition to interaction situations, specific nursing actions, examinations or emergency situations can also be practised. The learning environment in the simulation lab is characterised by interactivity, trust and a learner-centredness [14], which is appreciated by students and can give a sense of security when they are in practice.

In order to further develop the practice of health care towards a person-centred care practice, practice developers need skills to make use of scientific evidence for their own professional actions. They need to understand how scientific evidence is generated, interpreted and evaluated. This is best taught by having students generate their own scientific evidence in their own small research projects under the guidance of teachers, presenting it both orally and in writing and addressing its limitations. Students develop scientific questions that they bring with them from their professional practice and investigate these by means of written or oral surveys or in the form of observations in a selected target group (e.g. a specific patient group or their own colleagues). The topics are diverse and range from the perception of the profession of nursing in society to the impact of work in the COVID-19 pandemic to fundamental questions of nursing care for patients.

In two respects, the study programme thus provides good starting conditions for future practice developers and the subsequent transition phases described by Duchscher and Windey [9]. The acquired specialist knowledge as well as the communication and reflection skills enables the practice developers not only to shape development processes in their organisations, but also to realise their own personal development, so that upcoming challenges during the transition into practice can be mastered well.

7.3 Enabling the Role of Practice Development (Being)

The second transition phase is primarily about the question of who we are. In order to find out, the boundaries are explored, the meaning of contents and procedures are questioned, methods are doubted and the uncomfortable is uncovered. In the process, we push the limits of our knowledge, which can lead to feelings of incompetence and frustration. In the struggle for our values and the clarification of what is really important for a successful person-oriented course of studies, we create spaces in which we can "be". We need to find an attitude with which we can teach, research and lead authentically. In the following, we will explore the question of how it is possible to actively take on the role of a role model and adopt a person-centred attitude in teaching and research.

How Do We Become Role Models for Person-Centred Interaction?

In order to support students in their future role as person-centred practice developers, teachers need to be role models for exactly this. This is easier said than done. Person-centredness is about being in relationship, being in the social world, being in the room and being with oneself [1:17]. This needs a high level of awareness of self and others, as well as the spatial and social environment. How do teachers generate this awareness? The only honest answer to this is lifelong learning and continuous self-reflection.

Now, universities are generally good places for learning, at least for students. Self-critically questioning one's own competencies is not necessarily one of the strengths of university lecturers [15]. An important task of university lecturers is to assess students' performance. In a study by CHE Consult on the quality of teaching at universities, Christoph Berthold confirms in an interview with DIE ZEIT that professors show little self-criticism and mostly look for the reasons for declining student performance only at the students themselves [16]. According to a review by Mohammadi et al. [17], critical self-reflection proves to be an important methodological building block for clinical instructors in order to be a good role model for students.

And it is this competency, of knowing self, that plays an important role in person-centredness. Defined as the way in which a person experiences one's own knowing, being and becoming as meaningful through self-reflection, self-awareness and engagement with others [18:34].

At our Protestant University of Applied Science, Dresden we use various possibilities to develop the reflection of one's own competence. All courses are evaluated anonymously by the students at the end. The results are discussed verbally with the students at the beginning of the new semester. Here the lecturers ask specifically what they can improve in the future. Entering into dialogue via feedback and thus deepening cooperation has become an important instrument.

Helpful questions for self-reflection are provided by the core values of person-centred practice [19:15].

- Am I respectful of the values of others when I make decisions?
- Am I being authentic and facilitating meaningful relationships?
- Am I developing trusting relationships and enabling students to make informed decisions?
- Do I show respect for the active engagement of others with their different skills, preferences, lifestyles and goals?
- Do I promote mutual respect and understanding?
- Do I use caring behaviours as an intervention to support positive outcomes?
- Do I take personal responsibility and have a healthy lifestyle?

Since the introduction of the Practice Development course with its focus on person-centredness, we have used these questions regularly in the Department of

Nursing in the various sessions. In team meetings of the lecturers and coordinators of the nursing study programmes, we each take 5–10 min to reflect on one of these above-mentioned questions. Usually a team member has prepared one of the questions and reports on it self-critically from their own experience. When do I succeed in respectfully dealing with the values of others and when do I find it difficult. After this personal statement, the other colleagues join in and report on their experience. It is important for us not to judge what is said, but to listen and thus open up a space in which we can honestly communicate. In this way, we create small places of reflection in our everyday professional lives. These moments are often experienced as a gift, as they promote both mutual trust and the courage to admit mistakes.

How Does a Person-Centred Approach Succeed in Teaching and Research?

Lecturers at universities also have leadership responsibilities in addition to teaching and research activities. The supervision of students, if taken seriously, has the character of personnel development. This means that teaching also becomes a leadership task.

The preconditions for person-centred teaching and research are professional competence, interpersonal skills, commitment to the profession, clarity of one's own beliefs and values and knowledge of one's own self. Working on one's own attitude is essential grounding for person-centredness. Tom Eide and Shaun Cardiff [20] describe this stance of both researchers and leaders as a dance with colleagues and staff. As in a tango, the steps of togetherness are subject to their own dynamics that emerge in the dance, creating something new in the movement that would not have been possible alone. This approaching each other, daring to turn, enabling a new perspective at a distance and engaging in a connection again describes not only the tango, but also the dance of teaching and research. Eide and Cardiff studied this dance among leaders. In doing so, they were able to identify five concepts that describe person-centred leadership can easily be related to teaching and research. These are *presencing, communing, contextualising, sensing and balancing*. These concepts describe being and engaging in the encounter; creating a space for shared communication that can shape the future from the now; sensing and reflecting on possibilities and balancing needs and expectations in dialogue.

We have chosen two approaches for the transfer of these concepts into everyday university life. First, we discuss the concepts and their personal meaning for us in our team meetings. At the end of a meeting, one person agrees to prepare one of the concepts for the next meeting. It is about a 5–10 min input on it. This can be scientifically derived or the meaning is described in their own words. The person giving the input always reports on an everyday situation in which this concept was used.

Conversely, we bring these concepts into teaching and discuss them with the students. Students and lecturers talk together about how it can be personally successful to get involved, to be completely there, to actively seek the conversation, to use the space of togetherness, to strengthen the ability to perceive and to find balance. Often this engagement ends with a statement, such as, "I will not use my smart phone for personal purposes during the course and will engage fully with the content and the togetherness". It is important here that each course finds its own statements and that we as lecturers exchange ideas about them.

The most important principle of person-centred research is the ability to connect with other network partners and research colleagues. Cooperation rather than competition thus becomes an essential foundation. Jacobs and her colleagues (2017) have described three principles of person-centred research. These are (1) *attentiveness and dialogue,* (2) *empowerment and participation and* (3) *critical reflexivity.*

In our research centre apfe at the Protestant University of Applied Science in Dresden we have started to reflect our research interests more critically than before. Thus, before applying for research projects, we ask ourselves the question of power: who benefits from our research results? Do we apply fairness and keep socially marginalised groups in mind? We pay attention to gender-appropriate language and enable students to accompany larger research projects with their questions.

Since our university has been politically active for the disadvantaged since its foundation, this part is not difficult for us, it is just made more conscious. The challenge is rather to maintain the dialogue between the many research projects. So far, we have presented the ongoing projects to each other twice a year. More synergies could be found here if we could report to each other more frequently. However, since all researchers have to cope with a large teaching load at the same time, time is always a criterion here. We are currently discussing additional dates for the fruitful exchange.

The Next Step

The shared goal of our Department for Nursing is to make the entire university flourish and to infuse our reflective processes throughout the university enterprise. But before we take this next step, we first want to complete the first course of students together and evaluate our teaching and learning experiences (Fig. 7.1).

7.4 Bringing Person-Centred Care from the University into Practice

According to Duchschner's transition model [10], the stage of knowing begins for graduates of nursing education and/or nursing studies with a separation, in the sense of an inner distancing from existing conditions, work processes and colleagues in nursing practice. Ideally, it ends with acceptance—an inner attachment to the profession of nursing in a larger community of professional nurses ([10:447], see also above). Following this, we as a team of nurse educators are currently realigning our professional stance by expanding our profile. The expansion consists, on the one hand, in the fact that we want to carry the approach of person-centred from university to the meso level of care institutions. On the other hand, we want to promote person-centred practice and research on an international level in networking with universities in other countries.

The cooperation of the nurse educator team at the Protestant University of Applied Science Dresden (ehs) with practice partners is not new. It has already been

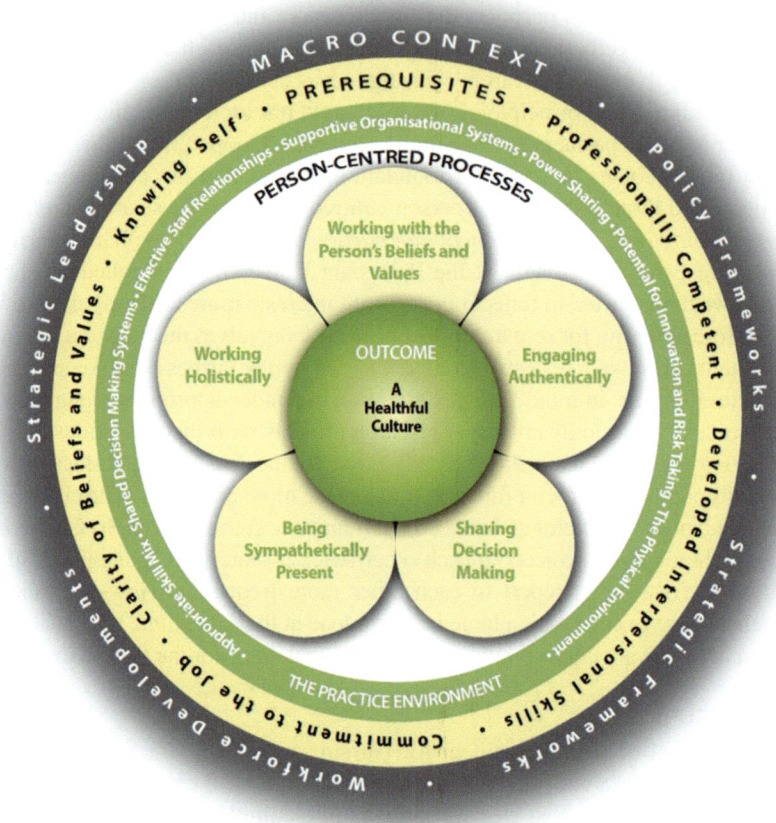

Fig. 7.1 Framework of person-centred care [1]. (Reproduced with permission of the author)

taking place for many years, e.g. in the course of undergraduate nursing education (B.Sc.), political commitment and in the implementation of research projects[1] in nursing facilities.

What is new is our intention to have a direct impact on practice conditions. The shared decision to embody, live, communicate and establish person-centred care in the practical field of our students affects and changes our professional identity.

As with the transition from the Doing stage to the Beeing stage, we did not plan the move to the Knowing stage. Rather, it developed out of an initial dissatisfaction. It arose from the obstacles that our students faced as soon as they wanted to provide person-centred care to people with care needs in their workplaces. Frequently, in-service students reported how they were only able to implement a fraction of the

---

[1] For example, a project on the social inclusion of older people in community living arrangements and a project on Double Duty Carers, the double burden of carers who provide both professional and personal care. Involvement of older people in shared housing.

skills they had acquired during their studies due to working conditions and the culture of care. As soon as it came to the concrete implementation of person-centred care under real practice conditions, resistance, blockage and limitation dominated the perception of both the students and us. In practice development we identify this resistance as a normal period in change.

Let's have a look into the Person-centred Care framework [1].

Of the four domains—represented by four circles from the outside to the inside—we have already addressed the first. This is the outer circle, the personal prerequisites that a nurse must have in order to provide person-centred care. We have written these competencies into the curriculum. And since the course started in spring 2020, we have aligned our teaching and exam performance to them. It is a starting point, but only a beginning, and it does not yet do justice to the holistic approach of the model. Based on this insight, it was necessary to extend our work to the other three domains of the person-centred care model, the care environment, the person-centred care process and expected outcomes [1]. And our arguments about the way in which we would like to integrate the model in its entirety into our work ran for several months and continues into the present. The way to an answer is to plan concrete steps and prioritise them.

Since our students study part-time, the practical shock described by Duchscher is reduced at the end of their studies. This is because they already introduce change projects into their practice during their studies and are accompanied by the lecturers. Possible resistances in the professional everyday life can be analysed and reflected at the university, in order to prepare arguments for the practice. After graduation, the university offers a network for the practice developers through conferences and working groups.

This leads to the second domain—represented by the second circle from the outside in the person-centred care framework model—the care environment [1]. This is where the management of our students' organisations plays a major role. In order for practice development to be person-centred, leadership must be brought on board. Our goal is not only to provide person-centred moments for our students, but for all care to be person-centred [1].

Since leaders are the key to the success of person-centred practice development, we will offer workshops for them. The following topics will be covered:

- How can a care facility benefit from the use of academically qualified practice developers?
- What roles can the academic practice developers play in the healthcare organisation?
- How can managers support the academic practice developers in their role identification and activities?

How Can a Care Facility Benefit from the Use of Academically Qualified Practice Developers?

The focus here is on the benefits for the companies. For this purpose, study results are presented, best practice examples from international network partners are presented and the advantages of person-centred practice development are elaborated.

The positive influence on the quality of care and the cooperation in the teams will be discussed as well as the importance of systematic practice development for the image and the economic success of the company.

What Roles Can Academic Practice Developers Play in the Healthcare Organisation?

The possible roles and fields of activity of practice developers are manifold. They can develop evidence-based standards and guidelines and check the quality of existing ones. They act as facilitators for change processes and thus engage in active change management. Their dual perspective, that of the practitioner and that of an evidence-based trained person, predestines them for this role in a special way [21:258 ff]. In doing so, they critically question existing structures and processes and motivate colleagues to do the same. Another typical role of graduates is to manage the nursing process for patients with complex health problems and care needs [22:15 ff].

In collaboration with managers, practice developers function as consultants and experts for nursing clinical expertise. They cannot be assigned to a hierarchical level; rather, their role is "across" the entire organisation. This makes them an important resource for both middle and top management, and the investment in their studies pays off.

How Can Managers Support Academic Practice Developers in Their Role Identification and Activities?

The field of activity of practice developers is new and has yet to be consolidated in job descriptions. The range of tasks should be defined as well as the organisation of the support of change processes. It is advisable to assume the role of practice developers in teams other than one's own. Ideally, another academic nurse (M.Sc.) accompanies the process [21, 22:15 ff].

In order to integrate the person-centred care process into our work, the third domain in the person-centred care framework model, we will develop a curriculum for continuing education in person-centred care at the university level. The target audience for the continuing education is nurses who have a bachelor's degree. These may or may not be managers. The person-centred care process is to be at the centre of the further training. With the PRAWIMA project,[2] our nursing department has already successfully carried out[3] three further training courses at Master's level, so that we can build on the experience gained. The conception of further training is our medium-term goal in the further development of person-centred care.

---

[2] PraxisWissenschaftsMaster: Project for the development of master's degree courses in nursing and childhood education.

[3] Evidence-based Nursing, Pain Management, Change Management.

The category of expected outcomes, the fourth domain according to the person-centred care framework model [1], comes into play in the expansion of our regional network of practice partners, which we plan as a long-term project. We pursue the goal of accompanying and evaluating the implementation of person-centred care in practice facilities. In addition, we would like to elicit clinically relevant research questions in cooperation with practice facilities. In the further course, some of the research questions will be investigated in research projects. In order to realise these projects, we have already applied for project funding.

In summary and in retrospect, we have gone through three decisive turning points in our development as a person-centred team: the decision to design a study programme with a focus on practice development; the decision to live person-centred care also in the cooperation of the teachers and the decision to implement person-centred care in practice fields. In retrospect, the development seems like a sequence of logically predictable steps. In concrete situations, it sometimes seemed more like a cautious approach with occasional setbacks. Moreover, according to Duchschner [10], the transition process is just as non-linear as the implementation of person-centred care into practice. Developing a person-centred culture requires sustained dedication through collaboration, inclusion and participation [1]. However, both of these models provide a framework and structure for our work and that of the students on the Nursing Practice Development (B.Sc.) programme. In this way, we want to make a contribution against a fragmentation of nursing science, management and practice and instead promote collaboration and networking.

References

1. McCormack B, McCance T, editors. Person-centred practice in nursing and health care: theory and practice. 2nd ed. West Sussex: Wiley Blackwell; 2017.
2. Davidson L, Bellamy C, Flanagan E, Guy K, O'Connell M. A participatory approach to person-centred research: maximising opportunities for recovery. In: Person-centred healthcare research. Oxford: Wiley Blackwell; 2017. p. 69–83.
3. Gracey J, McMillan A. Person-centred rehabilitation. In: McCormack B, McCance T, Bulley C, Brown D, McMillan A, Martin S, editors. Fundamentals of person-centred healthcare practice. Oxford: Wiley, Blackwell; 2021. p. 179–88.
4. Skovdahl K, Dewing J. Co-creating flourishing research practices through person-centred research: a focus on persons living with dementia. In: Person-centred healthcare research. Oxford: Wiley Blackwell; 2017.
5. Buckley C. A narrative approach to person-centredness with older people in residential long-term care. In: Person-centred practices an nursing and health care theory and practice. Oxford: Wiley Blackwell; 2017. p. 183–92.
6. Moore K, Kelly F. Experiencing person-centredness in long-term care. In: Dewing J, McCormack B, Tischen A, editors. Fundamentals of person-centred healthcare practice. Oxford: Wiley Blackwell; 2013. p. 199–208.
7. Boomer C, McCance T. Meeting the challenges of person-centeredness in acute care. In: McCormack B, McCance T, editors. Person-centred practice in nursing and health care theory and practice. Oxford: Wiley Blackwell; 2017. p. 205–14.
8. Borg M, Karlson B. Meeting the challenges of person-centredness in acute care. In: McCormack B, McCance T, editors. Person-centred practices in nursing and health care theory and practice. Oxford: Wiley Blackwell; 2017. p. 205–14.

9. Duchscher JB, Windey M. Stages of transition and transition shock. J Nurses Prof Dev. 2018;34(4):228–32.
10. Duchscher JB. A process of becoming: the stages of new nursing graduate professional role transition. J Contin Educ Nurs. 2008;39(10):441–50.
11. Bulmann C, Schutz S. Reflecting practice in nursing. Oxford: Wiley; 2013.
12. Oelofsen N. Developing reflective practice: a guide for health and social care students and practitioners. Banbury: Lantern Publishing; 2012.
13. Lopreiatro JO. How does health care simulation affect patient care? [Internet]. 2021. Verfügbar unter. https://psnet.ahrq.gov/perspective/how-does-health-care-simulation-affect-patient-care.
14. Jeffries PR, Rodgers B, Adamson K. NLN Jeffries simulation theory: brief narrative description. Nurs Educ Perspect. 2015;36(5):292–3.
15. Coskun L. Is the teacher self-critical? In: 16th international conference on social sciences, Paris; 24 Nov 2018.
16. Wiarda JM. The professors' fallacy. A survey shows: University professors have misconceptions of the typical student. Die ZEIT [Internet]. 22. 2011;39. Verfügbar unter. https://www.zeit.de/2011/39/C-Studentenirrtum.
17. Mohammadi E, Shahsavari H, Mirzazadeh A, Sohrabpur A, Henri S. Improving role modeling in clinical teachers. A narrative literature review. J Adv Med Educ Prof. 2020;8(1):1–9.
18. Brown D, Tropea S. Knowing self. In: McCormack B, McCance T, Bulley C, Brown D, McMillan A, Martin S, editors. Fundamental of person-centred healthcare practice. Oxford, Wiley Blackwell; 2021. p. 33–40.
19. McCormack B, McCance T, Martin S. What is person-centeredness? In: McCormack B, McCance T, Bulley C, et al., editors. Fundamentals of person-centre healthcare practice. Oxford: Wiley Blackwell; 2021. p. 13–22.
20. Eide T, Cardiff S. Leadership research: a person-centred agenda. In: McCormack B, van Dulmen S, Eide H, editors. Person-centre healthcare research. West Sussex: Wiley Blackwell; 2017. p. 95–115.
21. Behrens J, Langer G. Evidence-based nursing and caring: Methoden und Ethik der Pflegepraxis und Versorgungsforschung. 3., überarb. und erg. Aufl. Bern: Huber; 2010. 379. (Pflegeforschung, Pflegepraxis).
22. Eberhardt D. Practice development as a strategic framework for implementation academic nursing roles. Clin Nurs Res. 2017;3:15–27.

Part II

We Are Bold: Emotional Intelligence Pays Off

empCARE: An Empathy-Based Relief of Strain Training for Carers

Ludwig Thiry and Vera Lux

8.1 What Is empCARE?

"That I am allowed to have my own feelings and needs," says one participant when asked what important insight she gained in the empCARE training. This statement exemplifies that it is not natural for carers to be in touch with their own feelings and needs in emotionally challenging situations. The loss of contact with oneself is one of the sources of exhaustion and loss of professional motivation. EmpCARE reduces the stress experienced by nurses because they learn to perceive their feelings and needs and to integrate them into their nursing work. Thus, the training aims at professional motivation and (re)awakens the joy of the most beautiful aspect of the nursing profession: the encounter with people.

EmpCARE is the abridged version of "Care for Nurses: Development and anchoring of an empathy-based relief concept in care work." empCARE was funded as a research project from November 2015 to April 2019 by the Federal Ministry of Education and Research. Within the program "Preventive measures for the safe and healthy work of tomorrow." Prof. Marcus Roth from the Institute of Psychology at the University of Duisburg-Essen was responsible for the scientific coordination and management. The University Hospitals of Cologne and Bonn and the intensive care service Aaron from Cologne participated as joint partners. The project consisted of the development of a training measure, its implementation and the scientific evaluation of its effects. Almost 300 employees of the partners took part in the

L. Thiry (✉)
Uniklinik Köln, Köln, Germany
e-mail: ludwig.thiry@uk-koeln.de

V. Lux
Geschäftsführung Pflege, Medizinische Hochschule Hannover, Hannover, Germany
e-mail: Lux.Vera@MH-Hannover.de

training and the accompanying study. All three face the typical challenge of acquiring and retaining personnel but had different tasks within the project.

At the University Hospital Cologne, the trainings were offered as open seminars for nurses of inpatient nursing. Some of the wards involved sent larger groups, others sent individual persons. At the University Hospital of Bonn, the extent to which the concept can be carried into the departments by mentors was tested. There, two persons from each of the participating wards were trained, and they were given the task of additionally developing a dissemination concept for their nursing team. The participants of Aaron Intensive Care took part in the standard trainings. The aim here was to evaluate the effect of the training on employees in outpatient intensive care some of whom care for their clients in their home environment for up to 12 h a day over a period of years [1].

For the University Hospitals of Cologne and Bonn and the Aaron nursing service, it was a great effort to release the large number of nurses for a total of 25 training sessions, coaching sessions and, last but not least, the surveys during the planning period of 6 months. The motivation for taking this risk came from the conviction and the will to leave the well-trodden paths of stress seminars, back schools and other established forms of health-promoting measures. Instead, the partners agreed on a concept that unfolds its relief effect in an area that is constitutive for nursing, namely the interaction with the people who are being cared for. In empCARE training, caregivers learn to perceive their own and other people's feelings and needs, to integrate them into the interaction and to remain in contact with themselves and the people they care for.

8.2 How Are Empathic Working and the Health of Carers Related?

How does it happen that carers neglect their feelings and needs? There are answers to this question from the sociology of work. F. W. Nerdinger explains that part of the role expectation of nurses is that they get patients to allow actions that a person would normally refuse because they are associated with pain, shame or other unpleasant consequences. In order to get patient cooperation, nurses outwardly display different feelings than those they feel inside, whether they are embarrassed, disgusted, frightened, or simply stressing themselves out for other reasons. Nerdinger, referring to A. Hochschild, defines this as "emotional dissonance"and sees it as one of the main stress factors for nursing professions [2].

An extension of this explanatory model is offered by Böhle, Stöger, and Weihrich, who have intensively researched interaction work in service occupations [3]. They describe four factors of interaction work: cooperation work, subjectifying work action, sentimental work, and emotional labor (see Fig. 8.1).

Nurses enter into a cooperative relationship with their patients. The cooperation of the person receiving care is necessary for him or her to carry out an activity or to allow another person to act. The cooperative relationship must be established again and again because the reaction of a person receiving care cannot be predetermined

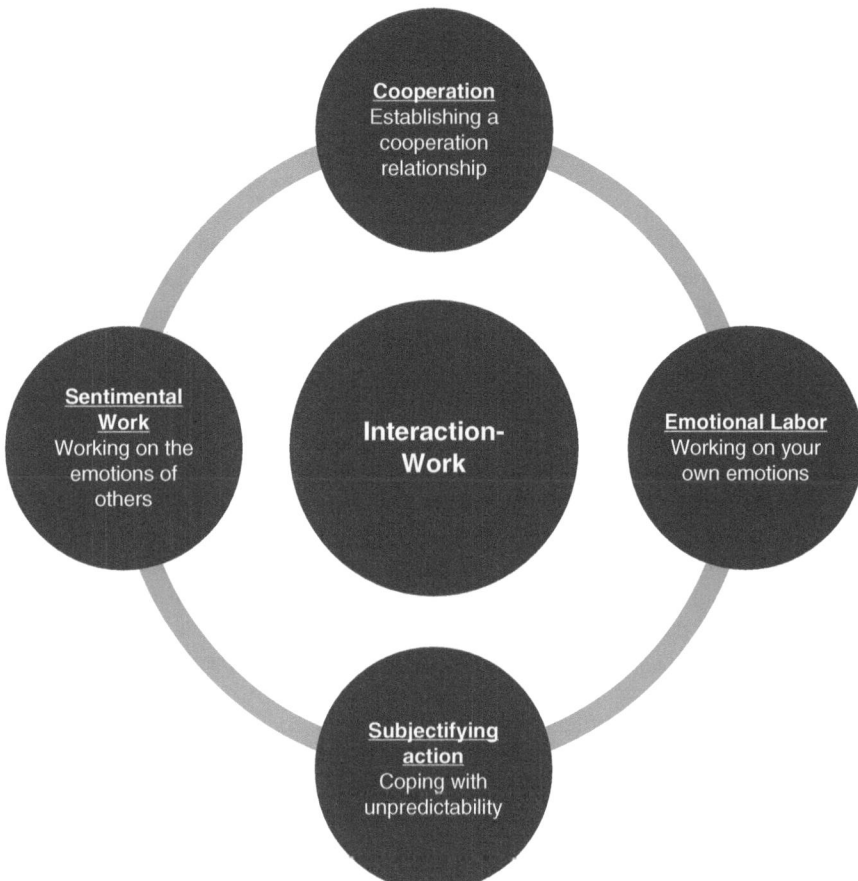

Fig. 8.1 Interaction work according to Böhle, Stöger, Weihrich. (Source: own illustration)

once and for all. Anyone who has experienced people in the existential situation of a serious illness knows that they do not behave consistently, but often act ambivalently. Therefore, carers have to adjust themselves again and again and find the best possible reaction in each situation. Care thus corresponds to a subjective work action that cannot be predetermined by algorithms.

The progressive economization of care is putting subjectivizing work under increasing pressure. Attempts to develop economic measurement criteria for nursing work and digitization in nursing require the definition of standardized work units, which contradict the creative requirements of a subjectivizing way of working [4]. The economic pressure exerted by political decisions on hospitals and on providers of outpatient and inpatient care should not worsen the quality of outcomes. Therefore, economic hospitals are flanked by quality assurance requirements that lead to further standardization of nursing activities. On the one hand, quality development holds the chance that the evidence-based, best way of providing care will prevail, but on the other hand, there is also the danger that the specifics of each case will be disregarded. These are all reasons why nurses are confronted with ever greater formalization which narrows the scope for subjectivizing action [5].

Through these developments, the two other components of interaction work, sentimental work and emotional labor, fall behind. Cooperation work and subjectifying action depend on sentimental work. In this context, carers must correctly recognize, respect and respond to the emotions of the person they are caring for [3]. Emotional labor, in turn, depends on carers being able to regulate their own emotions [3]. If emotional labor cannot be performed adequately, this leads to psychological stress, stress symptoms, a reduction in professional motivation and, in the case of many, to an exodus from the profession.

8.3 How Can Interaction Work Be Designed to Promote Health?

At the policy level and within organizations, structural measures are needed that provide sufficient space for successful interactional work. At the team level and within departments, nurses need a culture that allows the individual to do extensive interaction work. One of the findings of the empCARE project is certainly how dependent the relationship building between carers and the people they care for is on the team culture. And finally, on the interpersonal level of the relationship with the patients, the individual nurse needs concrete tools with which to improve the interaction work. This is exactly where empCARE comes in. The focus is on the question of how sentimental work and emotional labor can succeed in the long term without the nurses either becoming emotionally exhausted or distancing themselves and turning away from the people they care for.

8.4 The Empathic Short Circuit as a Means of Short-Term Emotion Regulation

In everyday life, many carers use a mechanism for working with emotions and feelings for which the empathy researcher Tobias Altmann has found the term "empathic short circuit" [6]. In the empathic short circuit, the perception of an event is followed immediately and without further reflection by the interpretation (what is going on here?), the emotional resonance (how does the other person feel?), and then a reaction (what is best now?) (see Fig. 8.2).

The empathic short circuit is an instrument with which carers can quickly regulate their own feelings in a challenging situation. Reflected sentimental work and emotional labor are inadequately replaced by seemingly empathic reactions such as appeasement, quick solutions, or lecturing. Emotion and feeling work remain ineffective [7, 8]. Here is an example:

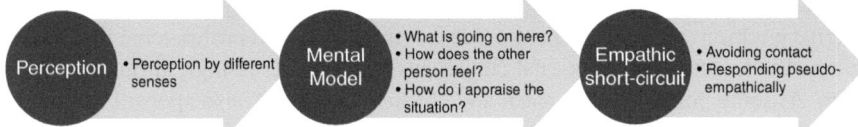

Fig. 8.2 Empathic short circuit according to Altmann. (Source: own illustration)

▶ A nurse enters the room of a patient with a newly placed ileostoma from which the stool bag has detached. The stool has spilled into the bed. The patient is sitting in bed and crying, gesturing with their hands up and trying not to touch the stool. The nurse says, "It's not that bad. I'll clean it up quickly." After the nurse leaves, the patient thinks, "How gross, what's this going to be like when I get home?" and the nurse thinks, "What kind of job am I doing here? Come on, it's part of the job. What was I going to do next?".

This short sequence shows how empathic short circuits work. The nurse comes into the room, interprets the patient's behavior as restless and hectic, responds with appeasement and quickly has a solution ready. There is no further reflection on the situation. Both are dissatisfied afterwards. The empathic short circuit allows the nurse to escape the situation without coming across as obviously rude, unfriendly or, indeed, non-empathic. They must, after all, move on briskly elsewhere. However, a real confrontation with the patient's feelings or the topic that is currently occupying him or her takes place just as little as the realization and processing of one's own feelings. In order to remain able to work in the concrete situation, they push aside their own feelings and those of others. It is obvious that these nevertheless continue to have an effect.

Patients in hospital, residents in a retirement home or clients of an outpatient care service need support to get to know their own feelings better, to find a productive way of dealing with grief, despair, fear or shame and to cope better with an illness or the frailty caused by their age. When this support is lacking, downright vicious circles can develop. The person receiving care feels unseen and unheard, unable to deal constructively with their illness, their dependency, their frailty. It need not be surprising that the cared for exhibits behaviors that are interpreted by those around them as regressed. These people call the nursing staff more often, are confused more quickly, are more likely to have nausea, are more likely to be unhappy or even aggressive. They show a variety of manifestations, which Hildegard Peplau described long ago as "unexplained discomfort" [9]. Since this essay is primarily about the carers, we will not pursue these thoughts further for the time being and look at what effects empathically short-sighted acting has on carers in the long run.

In a discussion within the empCARE project group, Tobias Altmann once compared the long-term consequences with transferring a patient from bed to a transport couch. Because it has to be done quickly, everyone "grabs hold" and manages the transfer without moving in a way that is easy on the back. None of the people involved will immediately have back pain or permanent back damage. These only occur after carers have acted in this way for years. Similarly, if caregivers use empathic short circuits for a long time and almost exclusively, that is, they do ineffective emotion work. A creeping process sets in, in which professional motivation gradually declines and emotional challenges become increasingly difficult to cope with. At some point, psychological and physical symptoms also appear [7].

For some, empathic short circuits no longer work at some point to regulate their own feelings, at least in the short term. The transitions to non-empathic, degrading, even aggressive reactions are then fluid. It can come to the devaluation of the people whom one actually wanted to be close to, whom one wanted to care for. Frightening comments from carers can be: "Some relatives are simply stupid" or "I don't need such training. I've been at it for so long, I'm hardened."

8.5 What Are the Mechanisms at Work in empCARE?

EmpCARE counteracts such hardenings which inevitably have an impact on the quality of interactions with patients but also on the health of the nurses. Participants in the trainings can learn how to replace empathically short-sighted behavior with reflective empathic behavior. This reflection involves working through a causal chain of unsatisfied need, the negative emotion triggered by it and the resulting behavior (Fig. 8.3), which Marshall Rosenberg described in the context of non-violent communication [10] and which requires closer examination.

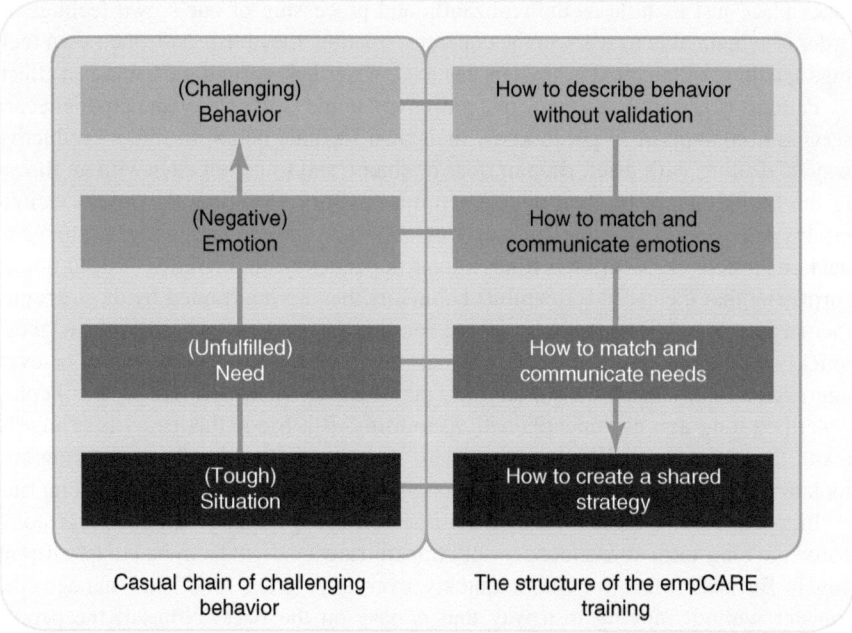

Fig. 8.3 Causal chain structure: Derivation of the training structure from the experience of the interactions partners. (Source: own illustration)

8.6 The Central Importance of Needs

Needs often remain unconsciously hidden behind perceptible behavior and compassionate feelings [10]. Needs are basic motives such as food, attention, protection, safety, or autonomy. They cannot be negated or questioned. For example, a patient can be expected not to eat before surgery (behavioral level) but not to be not hungry (need level). The success of an interaction depends largely on whether the needs have been correctly identified. Disruptions in an interpersonal relationship occur at the behavioral level and not at the needs level. Mutual reproaches between patients and nurses refer to behavior: "The nurse is always so short-tempered." or conversely, "I've explained it to them so many times, but the patient just won't go along with it."

At the same time, it is true that a need cannot be satisfied by only one type of behavior. It is precisely the insistence on only one behavioral option that leads to conflict with others or even with oneself [10]. In a partnership, both people may have a strong need for togetherness and yet argue at the behavioral level about whether this should be satisfied by spending an evening watching television together or attending a sporting event. There are almost always other options for need satisfaction. The need for togetherness can also be satisfied by sharing a cup of coffee, going to the cinema or taking a trip together. This creates a scope for negotiation at the behavioral level.

It becomes particularly problematic when behavior and need are confused. If it is said "I need a coffee now," this does not express a need, it can rather be about different needs: Relaxation, companionship, stimulation. Let's look at these connections in our case study.

> ▶ With an empathic short circuit, the nurse defused the situation emotionally and otherwise solved the existing problem purely instrumentally. The nurse has fitted a new ostomy bag and re covered the bed. The patient is left alone with their disgust and insecurity. These continue to have an effect and cause them to call for the nursing staff frequently. They are told to keep checking the stoma so that such a situation does not happen again. The nurses then explain that it was an exceptional case and that the patient should not worry about it at home. Nevertheless, the patient reports more and more frequently and the relationship with the carers deteriorates visibly as a result. At some point, a nurse in the handover says: "The patient's really getting on my nerves with their constant ringing about nothing."

The example is a typical situation that participants often bring to empCARE trainings. Almost all of them have experienced a gradual deterioration of the relationship with a patient. This goes so far that members of the care team avoid contact if possible. "Can you please leave now, I can't take this anymore with the patient" is then said. The deterioration of the relationship takes place because neither the feelings and needs of the patient nor those of the nursing staff have been worked out and expressed. Then, there would have been the possibility to think together about which alternative behaviors could have satisfied the respective needs. Let us assume that the patient's need for security was particularly active. If this had been recognized and expressed, a dialogue could have taken place about how the need for safety could be satisfied other than by frequent reporting.

8.7 The Directions of Action of the Training

The empCARE training is structured in such a way that the participants work their way in reverse to the causal chain described, from the perceptible, external behavior via the clarification of emotions to the ultimately decisive needs (Fig. 8.3).

In doing so, they can gain experience in two directions: the external effect on their relationship with the patients and the internal effect on self-perception and the inner experience of nursing interactions. For a better understanding, the two directions of impact are presented separately here; in the didactic design this separation does not take place in this way. Many of the exercises simultaneously target external and self-perception [11, 12].

8.8 How Does empCARE Affect the Interaction with Patients?

Let us first look at how a better understanding of patients in emotionally tense situations comes about. Nurses learn in several steps to understand a behavior that challenges them as an expression of a need on the patient's side that is not immediately visible, perhaps not even conscious, to enter into conversation with the patient about it and to look for constructive solutions together.

- First of all, they practice reproducing an event in a non-judgmental way. It is not easy to describe only the surface of an event without interpreting it emotionally in some way or even evaluating it morally. The difference between the phrases "They rang the bell three times in the last hour" and "The patient rings all the time" makes it clear what is meant.
- In the second step, the nurses check with the patient whether they have correctly identified their feelings. In this example, is the patient's disgust or insecurity or fear actually in the foreground? In an emotionally challenging interaction it is very important that patients experience that there is nothing wrong with their feelings and that there is an honest interest on the part of the carer to learn about them. The participants practice listening and looking carefully recognizing what feelings the person they are talking to is showing. This is the prerequisite for the next step.
- Recognizing and naming a feeling makes it possible to reduce its immediate, unreflective behavioral impact and to enact conscious elements of behavioral control. In empCARE training, this is done by reflecting on

what unmet need has triggered a patient's strong feelings. The trick is not to try to convince the other person of any of their own interpretations. The patient, represented in the training by another participant, rather receives support only to the extent that they can find out for themselves which unmet need is active in the concrete situation. The exercises lead to active silence rather than to active listening in the classical way. The renunciation of one's own interpretations, the giving of time for reflection, is extremely difficult for many nurses who see themselves as knowledgeable experts.
- Letting things happen and waiting is then also a challenge in the last step. For now it is a question of which productive behaviors could help the patient to satisfy his needs in a different way than through the behavior that the environment has so far assessed as challenging. Once the patient is clear about what is really important to them, they will be able to develop alternatives to the previous behavior.

8.9 What Effect Does empCARE Have on the Inner Experience of the Caregiver?

The improved interaction with patients is in itself a benefit for the nurses. But the effect of empCARE goes beyond that. "Only when I become aware of my feelings and needs can I develop appropriate strategies and inquire about the feelings and needs of my counterpart" and "For me it was important that we learned that our needs are also important" are statements from the formative evaluation of the training. The mere fact of being able to perceive one's own feelings and needs at all, of being able to take them seriously, was a new and relieving experience for some participants. In the training, this experience takes place in several steps [12, 13].

- In a partner exercise, the carers report a situation that was emotionally challenging for them. The partner has the task of identifying the emotional parts of the report in the verbal and non-verbal expressions. The dialogue continues until the feelings are accurately named. Without hearing the content of the conversation, this moment is often recognizable to the training facilitator by a change in posture or facial expression. The person telling the story suddenly straightens up a bit, leans back, eyes widen, a smile comes to the face. Although it is usually a matter of strong negative feelings, it is already possible to experience during the training what a relieving effect it has to become clear to oneself about a feeling and to share it with a counterpart.
- In a further step, the focus is on one's own needs. The participants experience the central importance of needs for their own experience and actions.

> They experience in exercises how negative feelings arise from their lack of satisfaction and clarify which of their own needs were affected in concrete nursing situations in which they felt a negative feeling.
> - And finally, the participants reflect on the behavior through which they satisfy their needs and what alternatives there might be to this. Values and conventions within their work team also play a role here. With which self-image does the team work, which demands are made on the team members, how does this influence their way of working and is reflective empathic work supported by the team?
> - In the end, there is again a negotiation process with the counterpart on how to proceed together so that both sides are satisfied.

8.10 Relief Effect Through Self-Awareness

The relieving effect of empCARE is achieved on the one hand through the improved interactions with patients. The nurses are able to maintain the relationship even in difficult situations and to refrain from distancing themselves through empathic short circuits. It stands to reason that this supports professional motivation. The reflected empathic contact with patients is complemented by empathy towards oneself, self-empathy. empCARE enables nurses to perceive their own feelings, even negative ones, without judging them morally. They learn to understand their own feelings as an expression of an underlying need and to make this clear to themselves. This enables them to find alternative ways of behaving in contact with patients and colleagues, which satisfy the respective need in a constructive way and at the same time maintain contact with others.

The relief effect through self-awareness as it occurs with empCARE has also been proven by other methods and their research. For example, Angelika C. Wagner has developed a method of mental self-regulation and introvision, in which "observing and noticing" plays an important role. In this method, bodily sensations, thoughts, and feelings are perceived attentively, but only in a stating way and not in an evaluating way. Similar to empCARE, this leads to a disconnection from mental models which lead to unreflective and immediate action [14].

Boris Bornemann and Tania Singer describe similar mechanisms of action [15]. As part of the ReSource project, they investigated which brain regions are affected by compassionate action. The semantic distinction made in the ReSource model between empathy and compassion cannot be explained here due to space limitations. Similar to empCARE, the ReSource method is about, among other things, staying in touch with one's own and other people's feelings and thoughts, detaching oneself from automatically running thought and behavioral programs through defusion, and thus achieving greater flexibility in terms of behavior, thoughts, and affective reactions.

8.11 Which Effects of empCARE Can Be Proven?

The empCARE project consisted of the development and implementation of the training and an extensive evaluation and lasted a total of 3 years. The long project period made it possible to conduct a longitudinal study to evaluate the effects of the training, including a control group without training. The evaluation concept included a summative as well as a formative survey in an anonymous form by questionnaire [16].

The summative part of the evaluation was conducted using standardized questionnaires measuring various characteristics such as empathic competence, job satisfaction, stress experience, or psychological well-being. Baseline data were collected before the training and the surveys were repeated in three follow-up measurements at intervals of 4 months. This allows statements to be made about the sustainability of the changes in the participants. The self-assessment of the study participants is completed by surveys of colleagues on the team culture, of patients on the working atmosphere, and on the empathic behavior of the nurses as a whole, as well as by an anonymized external assessment by persons from the personal environment of the participants. The extensive results are comprehensively presented in a separate publication [17]. At this point, initial results are summarized which were presented at the final meeting of the project in October 2018.

The summative survey showed a steady increase in empathic competence in the sense of the model of reflected empathy presented here over the measurement period of 12 months. It can be concluded from this that the participants made the tools learned in the training their own and made steady progress. This is associated with a decrease in burnout symptoms, body symptoms, and depression, particularly in the first few months after training. This effect remains stable or then diminishes slightly in the following months. This suggests that the continuation of the concept makes sense. This is also confirmed by the participants' comments in the formative evaluation. This took place immediately after the end of the training. The participants evaluated the training itself, its contents and the didactic implementation and gave an assessment of its practical relevance and feasibility. Despite some skeptical comments ("difficult, because you often don't have that much time"), the assessment that the concept is relevant and applicable in practice ("I can take a lot back to my everyday work through the practical exercises") predominates. The feasibility is often linked to conditions, such as further practice opportunities or support in the nursing team ("Further support in everyday nursing" or "Good! With courage and support from colleagues") [13, 17].

8.12 Conclusion and Outlook

EmpCARE has a positive effect on individual health promotion. However, it has effects that go beyond this and prompts further reflection. In the course of the project, it became increasingly clear that empCARE stimulates reflection on the culture in nursing teams or in organizations as a whole.

"In our ward, he would get an announcement," is the literal statement of a participant during the training about a patient who, in a difficult situation for him, shows behavior that is challenging for the nurses. A colleague from the same ward sits next to her and nods eagerly. Here, evaluations and values not only of two individuals but of a whole team become apparent. Part of the role of "patient" in this value system is to make an effort, to participate, and not to make too many demands. Nurses can and perhaps should "tell patients off." They are entitled to evaluate and influence patient behavior. EmpCARE challenges such normative ideas. In one team, this changed the way they looked at patients. In coaching, one nurse reported, "We don't necessarily talk differently to patients yet, but differently about them." This shows that individual interaction work must always be viewed systemically. It does not only depend on individual willingness. According to the experiences in the project, the factor team culture is of determining importance. The team culture even seems to be more decisive than the time factor, which is never available in sufficient quantities. The question of the extent to which interaction work is limited not only by a lack of time, but also by existing team and organizational cultures, would be an occasion for further research.

Of course, intensive interaction work and intensive conversation need time. Both are insufficiently taken into account in surveys of nursing intensities and, above all, in the measurement of nursing working hours. Without serious steps in this direction, the performance of nurses for the care of sick and frail people due to old age is not adequately reflected [5]. Conversely, interaction work is always performed during instrumental tasks such as personal hygiene or changing dressings. And last but not least, the time spent to keep a patient with challenging behavior cooperating over and over again with empathic short circuits must be offset against the time spent on an intensive conversation that defuses the situation in the long term.

Organizations that want to work with empCARE benefit more if they embed the trainings in a framework of further development of team and company cultures or in prevention programs. Since empCARE is a scientifically evaluated program, refinancing according to §20 SGB V is possible in Germany and should be examined in individual cases. This is particularly promising if departments in which mental stress is particularly high are identified as part of a risk assessment carried out in accordance with §5 of the Occupational Health and Safety Act. Within the organization, the program should be publicized and marketed in a targeted manner. In order to achieve and maintain a high participation rate in the departments, it is of decisive importance to win over middle management to the approach. A special seminar for ward or division managers, held at the beginning of an empCARE project, makes it possible to dispel concerns from this circle and to win over managers for ongoing support of the project. Central project coordination, which can be located in an education center or a staff unit of the nursing directorate, ensures the coordination and sustainability of the project. This also includes opportunities for continuous practical reflection. The empCARE concept is excellently suited for case discussions, which can be held regularly or as needed. When selecting the training leader, care should therefore be taken to ensure that he or she has experience in the area of collegial counseling. empCARE strengthens the ability to act and self-efficacy of employees and thus individual resources. Positive effects can also be observed in communication with patients, relatives, and colleagues. Nursing management has a decisive role in shaping the necessary framework conditions, be it in securing financial and human resources and prioritization in difficult bottleneck situations or in conflicts [18].

The results of the evaluation encourage the partners to continue and further develop empCARE. The seminars are also offered at the university hospitals in Cologne and Bonn for employees of other institutions, interested trainers can participate in special seminars and will benefit from the publication of the concept and its evaluation in a separate book. There will be further developments of the concept for team and ward managers who want to lead their staff empathetically while remaining healthy themselves. The same applies to practice instructors and their students. The expansion to other occupational groups with patient contact is also desirable. EmpCARE will be available after the end of the project period to other companies in the health care industry that are looking for ways to maintain and increase the professional motivation and health of their employees.

References

1. Kocks A. Projektübersicht empCARE: Förderung, Teilprojekte, Öffentlichkeitsarbeit. In: Thiry L, Schönefeld V, Deckers M, Kocks A, editors. empCARE - Arbeitsbuch zur empathiebasierten Entlastung in Pflege- und Gesundheitsberufen. Berlin: Springer; 2020.
2. Nerdinger FW. Emotionsarbeit und Burnout in der gesundheitsbezogenen Dienstleistung. In: Büssing A, Glaser J, editors. Dienstleistungsqualität und Qualität des Arbeitslebens im Krankenhaus. Göttingen: Hogrefe; 2003. p. 181–97.
3. Böhle F, Stöger U, Weihrich M. Interaktionsarbeit gestalten - Vorschläge und Perspektiven für humane Dienstleistungsarbeit. Berlin: Sigma; 2015.
4. Jungtäubl M, Weihrich M, Kuchenbaur M. Digital forcierte Formalisierung und ihre Auswirkungen auf die Interaktionsarbeit in der stationären Krankenpflege. Arbeits- und Industriesoziologische Studien Heft. 2018;2(October):176–91.
5. Thiry L, Weihrich M. Interaktionsarbeit erhalten - Gesundheit schützen. Pflege Zeitschrift. 2019;5(2019):57–61.
6. Altmann T. Empathie in sozialen und Pflegeberufen. Wiesbaden: Springer; 2015.
7. Altmann T, Roth M. Mit Empathie arbeiten - gewaltfrei kommunizieren. Praxistraining für Pflege, Soziale Arbeit und Erziehung. Stuttgart: Kohlhammer; 2014
8. Schönefeld V. Pseudo-Empathie – Theorieentwicklung und empirische Beiträge. Published dissertation. University Library of the University of Duisburg-Essen, Essen; 2019.
9. Peplau HE. Interpersonal Relations in Nursing: a conceptual frame of reference for psychodynamic nursing. Springer; 1988.
10. Rosenberg M. Nonviolent Communication, A Language of Life, Encinitas CA; 2019.
11. Thiry L. Vierdimensionale Didaktik - eine Einladung zum reflexiven Lernen. In: Thiry L, Schönefeld V, Deckers M, Kocks A, editors. empCARE - Arbeitsbuch zur empathiebasierten Entlastung in Pflege- und Gesundheitsberufen. Berlin: Springer; 2020.
12. Thiry L, Altmann T, Deckers M, Kaschull K, Schönefeld V, Roth M. empCARE - Das Trainings manual. In: Thiry L, Deckers M, Schönefeld V, Kocks A, editors. empCARE - Arbeitsbuch zur empathiebasierten Entlastung in Pflege- und Gesundheitsberufen. Berlin: Springer; 2020.
13. Thiry L, Kaschull K, Deckers M, Kocks A. Reflecting on training leads and evaluating participants - how to improve a training concept. In: Thiry L, Schönefeld V, Deckers M,

Kocks A, editors. empCARE - Arbeitsbuch zur empathiebasierten Entlastung in Pflege- und Gesundheitsberufen. Berlin: Springer; 2020.
14. Wagner AC. Gelassenheit durch Auflösung innerer Konflikte. Mentale Selbstregulation und Introvision. 2nd, fully revised ed. Stuttgart: Kohlhammer; 2011.
15. Bornemann B, Singer T. Das ReSource Modell des Mitgefühls. Eine kognitiv-affektive neurowissenschaftliche Perspektive. In: Singer T, Bolz M, editors. Mitgefühl in Alltag und Forschung. Munich: Max Planck Society; 2013. p. 184–98.
16. Schönefeld V, Deckers M. Maßgeschneiderte Forschung: Das Evaluationskonzept von empCARE. In: Thiry L, Schönefeld V, Deckers M, Kocks A, editors. empCARE - Arbeitsbuch zur empathiebasierten Entlastung in Pflege- und Gesundheitsberufen. Berlin: Springer; 2020.
17. Deckers M, Schönefeld V, Altmann T, Roth M. Forschungsergebnisse zur Wirksamkeit des empCARE-Konzepts. In: Thiry L, Schönefeld V, Deckers M, Kocks A (Hrsg) empCARE - Arbeitsbuch zur empathiebasierten Entlastung in Pflege- und Gesundheitsberufen. Berlin: Springer; 2020.
18. Lux V, Pröbstl A, Schliffer D, Kocks A. Veränderungen und Entwicklungen gestalten - Die Umsetzung von empCARE aus Sicht der Führungsebene. In: Thiry L, Schönefeld V, Deckers M, Kocks A, editors. empCARE - Arbeitsbuch zur empathiebasierten Entlastung in Pflege- und Gesundheitsberufen. Berlin: Springer; 2020.

WellBeing at the Workplace: The Urgency and Opportunity

Mary Jo Kreitzer

9.1 Nursing in the USA

In the USA, as in many countries of the world, nurses are the largest group of health professionals. It is estimated that there are over three million nurses employed across a wide variety of settings including hospitals, clinics, public health, and community-based facilities such as schools and senior care settings. Nurses are also employed as leaders, educators, and scientists and often lead employee health and health and wellness initiatives within the business sector.

Unlike like many other western countries, the USA has not had a national health insurance system that assures citizens access to health care. Federal health care programs have been limited to seniors (Medicare), low income and persons with disabilities (Medicaid), and veterans who are eligible to receive care through systems operated by the Veteran's Administration. While the USA has achieved unparalleled health care advances and has access to very modern facilities and the most advanced technology in the world significant health disparities exist and the USA ranks fairly low among industrialized nations in mortality and morbidity. The recently passed legislation, the Affordable Care Act, that provided broader access to health care is presently under siege politically. This creates enormous anxiety within the US population as people fear that they will lose their health care coverage.

In 2008, The Robert Wood Johnson Foundation (RWJF) in collaboration with the Institute of Medicine (IOM) launched a 2-year initiative on the Future of Nursing.

The impetus for the initiative was the recognition that the nursing profession faced several challenges in fulfilling the promise of a reformed health care system

---

M. J. Kreitzer (✉)
Earl E. Bakken Center for Spirituality & Healing, School of Nursing, University of Minnesota, Minneapolis, MN, USA
e-mail: kreit003@umn.edu

© The Author(s), under exclusive license to Springer Nature Switzerland AG 2022
R. Tewes (ed.), *Innovative Staff Development in Healthcare*,
https://doi.org/10.1007/978-3-030-81986-6_9

and meeting the nation's health needs. The goal of the initiative was to produce a report [1] containing recommendations for an action-oriented blueprint for the future of nursing that would include changes in public and institutional policies at the national, state, and local levels.

During the course of its work on the Future of Nursing, the committee responsible for producing the report developed a vision for a transformed health care system. The future system was described as follows: "A future system makes quality care accessible to the diverse populations of the United States, intentionally promotes wellness and disease prevention, reliably improves health outcomes, and provides compassionate care across the lifespan." In this envisioned future, primary care and prevention are central drivers of the health care system. Inter-professional collaboration and coordination are the norm. Payment for health care services rewards value, not volume of services, and quality care is provided at a price that is affordable for both individuals and society. The rate of growth of health care expenditures slows. In all these areas, the health care system consistently demonstrates that it is responsive to individuals' needs and desires through the delivery of truly patient-centered care.

The recommendations of the report centered around four themes:

1. Nurses should practice to the full extent of their education and training.
2. Nurses should achieve higher levels of education and training through an improved education system that promotes seamless academic progression.
3. Nurses should be full partners, with physicians and other health professionals, in redesigning health care in the USA.
4. Effective workforce planning and policy-making require better data collection and an improved information infrastructure.

9.2 Wellbeing of the Health Care Workforce

Achieving the aspirational vision described above requires a robust health care workforce. Stress and burnout of healthcare providers have become a major healthcare issue that has implications for not only workforce projections, but the cost and quality of patient care and the lives of healthcare providers and their families as well. Burnout, characterized by loss of enthusiasm for work, feelings of cynicism, and a low sense of personal accomplishment [2], is associated with early retirement, alcohol use, and suicidal ideation [3, 4]. A 2014 survey [5] found that 68% of family physicians and 73% of internists would not choose the same specialty if they were to start their careers anew.

A plethora of research has documented the severity of burnout and its impact across the health professions [4, 6–9]. There is evidence that burnout among US physicians is getting worse. A study conducted by Mayo Clinic researchers in partnership with the American Medical Association compared data from 2014 to metrics they collected in 2011 and found that more than half of US physicians were experiencing professional burnout [8]. They note that burnout leads to poor care, physician turnover, and a decline in the overall quality of the healthcare system. In the 2011 survey, 45% of physicians met the burnout criteria, with highest rates occurring in the "front lines"—general internal medicine, family medicine, and emergency medicine. In 2014, 54% of responding physicians had at least one symptom of burnout. Satisfaction with work–life balance also declined. While the rate of burnout in nursing is not as high as in medicine, it is still significant. McHugh et al. [6] found that 34% of hospital nurses and 37% of nursing home nurses report burnout.

As healthcare scrambles to respond to patient needs, fiscal realities, and workforce projections, the concept of the triple aim [10] has been introduced as a way to optimize performance. The focus of the triple aim is on improving the health of the population, improving patient experience, and reducing costs. Bodenheimer and Sinsky [11] have proposed that the triple aim be expanded to a quadruple aim, adding the goal of improving the wellbeing of the care team. The wellbeing of the health care workforce is critical to achieving improved patient care and system performance. The remainder of this chapter will introduce a wellbeing model and focus on a staff development initiative focused on giving leaders and clinicians knowledge and skills to create cultures of wellbeing.

9.3 Why Wellbeing?

Wellbeing is not a particularly new concept, but perhaps an idea whose time has come. In [12], the World Health Organization defined health as a state of complete physical, mental, and social wellbeing and not merely the absence of disease or infirmity. Over 30 years ago, Aaron Antonovsky [13], a professor of sociology, coined the term salutogenesis to describe an approach to care that focuses on factors that support human health and wellbeing, rather than on factors that cause disease.

At a personal level, wellbeing is certainly impacted by health but is also heavily impacted by many other factors illustrated in Fig. 9.1 including our sense of purpose and meaning in life, the quality of our relationships, the vitality of the community in which we live, our environment, and our perception of safety and security. When any of these factors are compromised, our overall wellbeing is affected.

Our role as nurses and leaders is to increase people's *capacity* and *potential* within each area of wellbeing. This requires a whole person, whole systems, integrative perspective.

Health: Health encompasses more than physical health. A whole person approach requires that we consider the inseparability of body, mind, and spirit and be equally attentive to emotional, social, and spiritual health as well as physical health. While health is affected by genetics and social determinants, such as the circumstances in which people are born, grow up, live, work, and age, and the systems put in place to deal with illness, the largest determinants of health are lifestyle behaviors and choices. It is estimated that 90% of people's health [15] has nothing to do with hospitals, healthcare providers, and drugs per se. Rather, the state of our health is influenced much more by the food we eat, how much we exercise, how we manage our stress, and how much we sleep, as well as our social, environmental, and genetic

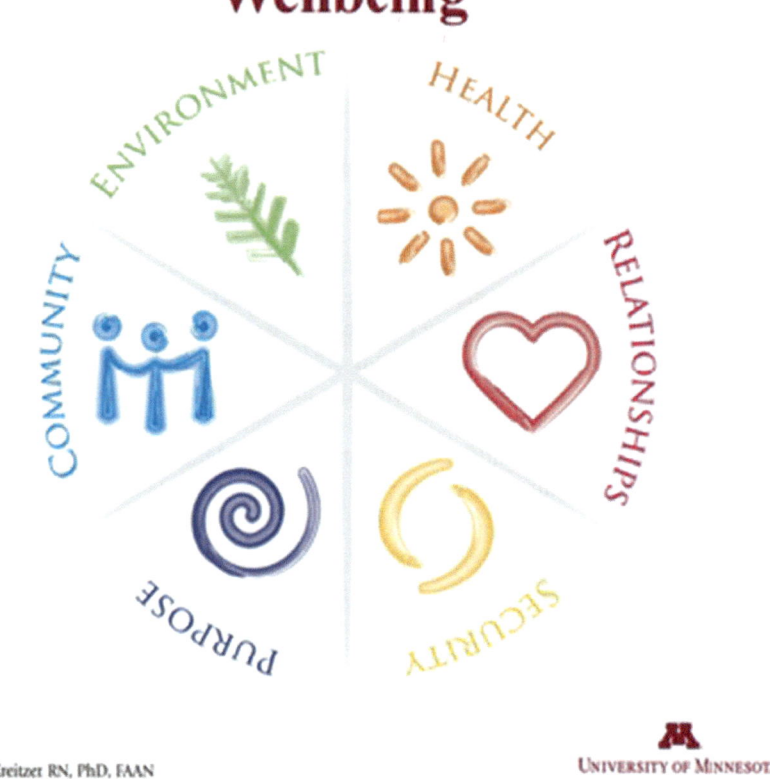

Fig. 9.1 Wellbeing Model [14]. (Source: Mary Jo Kreitzer Earl E. Bakken Center for Spirituality & Healing, University of Minnesota)

influences. Social determinants of health are shaped by a broad set of economic and political forces, as well as social policies that are beyond the control of individuals. Lifestyle choices, however, are very much within our control.

To build personal and system capacity and potential, it is important to convey to employees that in many respects, "health is in their hands." Literally, how healthy people are has far more to do with lifestyle choices and decisions that they make each day than anything that a healthcare system might offer. An example of robust resource to teach people how to take charge of their health can be found at: www.takingcharge.csh.umn.edu.

When people begin to take charge of their own health and wellbeing, it impacts not only their own lives, but also the organizations in which they work and the communities in which they live. Businesses and worksites recognize that the health and wellbeing of their employees affect not only the cost of health care, but also productivity and creativity. It directly impacts the bottom line.

Purpose: Having purpose and meaning is important at every age and stage of life. Purpose guides life decisions, influences behavior, shapes goals, offers a sense of direction, and creates meaning. In her book The Power of Meaning, Emily Esfahani Smith [16] notes that the search for meaning is not a solitary philosophical quest nor is meaning something that we create within ourselves and for ourselves. Rather, she writes, meaning largely lies in others. When we focus on others, we create a sense of belonging for them and for ourselves. In other words, finding purpose and meaning in our lives requires that we reach out, and it is through our discovery of purpose that we find meaning.

Purpose can induce episodes of "flow," an optimal state of being in which one's creative and intellectual limits are challenged but not stretched beyond one's ability [17]. There is abundant evidence that purpose is directly related to both health and happiness, and whether we have clarity about our sense of purpose and live our purpose in our lives will have a major impact on our wellbeing. Purpose is not only associated with better physical and psychological health, but enhanced civic engagement, pro-social behavior, and personal relationships, as well as increased resilience - the ability to overcome life challenges [18, 19].

A significant amount of research on purpose has been conducted in Japan, where the concept of *ikigai*, or a "reason for being," is prevalent in the culture. These studies link strong purpose to long life and a decreased risk for cardiovascular disease [20, 21]. A 2014 study [22] found the same connection between purpose and longevity. Greater purpose in life consistently predicted lower mortality risk across the lifespan, showing the same benefit for younger, middle-age, and older participants. People with a sense of purpose had a 15% lower risk of death, compared with those who said they were aimless.

Purpose is also important at the organizational level. When an organization does not have clarity of purpose, it impacts workflows, productivity, employee engagement and morale and ultimately, the wellbeing of the organization, including the financial bottom line.

Relationships: It has now been well documented that "isolation is fatal." In fact, loneliness and isolation are risk factors for disease that are comparable in impact to obesity and hypertension [23]. Lives devoid of positive relationships have less joy, meaning, and ultimately wellbeing. Recent research suggests that loneliness predicts depression and fatigue in cancer patients [24], high blood pressure [25], and a 50% increased mortality risk [23]. Likewise, strong relationships provide support that can act as a buffer against the negative effects of stress, leading to a longer, healthier life. Research on healthy communities around the world, called Blue Zones, estimates that committing to a life partner can add 3 years to one's life expectancy [26].

The quality and nature of relationships is also important at an organizational level. If there are poor relationships among employees or between employees and leadership, effectiveness and efficiency may be compromised. It is also a dangerous strategy for organizations to be isolated. Nurturing key relationships and building strong partnerships is a key factor in promoting organizational wellbeing and success.

Community: The communities in which we live and work have the capacity to both "nurture and sustain us" and directly impact our wellbeing. We rely on the infrastructure and resources of a community whether they are political, economic, social, or technological. Within some communities, people are disengaged and in others they are engaged and at times, even empowered to take action. Some work sites feel and behave as a community, whereas others feel and appear as silos where there is little connectivity and people work in isolation.

Environment: The environment we live in is crucial to our health and wellbeing. It is critical to ensure that our home and work environments are healthy and we are not exposed to hazards, such as polluted air, water, or toxins. We also need to consider our global environment and take steps to protect all our natural resources from contamination and depletion. One approach is the Natural Step Framework from Sweden, which has been used by numerous businesses, government agencies, non-profits, and individuals around the world to become environmentally responsible (and save money). Based on a set of sustainability principles, the framework focuses on connecting symptoms of un-sustainability with their root causes and taking action that is science based and in support of deep and long-term transformation (Natural Step). Within healthcare, the Healthcare Without Harm coalition sets similar goals, working to transform the healthcare sector so it is no longer a source of harm to people and the environment.

Another important factor in environmental wellbeing is access to nature. There is a preponderance of evidence that "Nature heals." Being in nature, or even viewing scenes of nature, reduces anger, fear, and stress and increases pleasant feelings. Exposure to nature not only makes you feel better emotionally, it contributes to your physical wellbeing - reducing blood pressure, heart rate, muscle tension, and the production of stress hormones. Roger Ulrich's pioneering research in this area has been supported by researchers around the world [27, 28]. Even a simple plant in a room can have a significant impact on stress and anxiety, according to research done in hospitals, offices, and schools [29, 30].

One of the most intriguing areas of current research is the impact of nature on general wellbeing. In one study, 95% of those interviewed said their mood improved after spending time outside, changing from depressed or anxious to calmer and more balanced [31]. Other studies show that spending time in nature or viewing scenes of nature is associated with a positive mood [32] and psychological wellbeing, meaningfulness, and vitality [33]. Furthermore, spending time in nature or viewing nature scenes increases our ability to take on new mental tasks and pay attention [34, 35]. Thus, organizations are likely to see employee wellbeing and productivity increase if they provide access to green space or add plants and scenes of nature.

Safety and Security: In both our personal and work lives, "fear incapacitates." People can have excellent physical health and a strong purpose in life, but if they live in fear, their sense of safety and security and overall wellbeing is eroded. Fear also diminishes joy and creativity and makes human flourishing impossible.

A deep understanding of the factors that promote and erode wellbeing and the urgency of addressing stress and burnout of the healthcare workforce provided the impetus to launch our wellbeing leadership program at the Earl E. Bakken Center for Spirituality and Healing at the University of Minnesota.

9.4 The Wellbeing Leadership Program: An Innovative Staff Development Initiative

The Wellbeing Leadership Program offered through the Bakken Center is a creative blend that includes 3 day-long retreats, independent study, and online learning. The program emphasizes personal and leadership practices that are simple, concrete, powerful, and inspiring. The series is based on the premise that leaders are needed at every level of the organization who have the knowledge, skills, and capacity to advance wellbeing. Competencies of wellbeing leaders are defined as follows:

- Understand the value of their own wellbeing, the wellbeing of others, and the impact this has on the organization.
- Develop and maintain wellbeing practices and leadership skills in the face of complexity and challenge.
- Recognize and work with patterns at a level of the whole person and whole system.
- Evoke innovative thinking and allow answers to emerge from diverse perspectives.
- Take adaptive action that transforms individuals, teams, the organization, and the larger community and leads to sustainable practices and results.
- Energize positive change by making wellbeing contagious!

Day 1 of the retreat series focuses on developing a personal plan for health and wellbeing. Participants do a self-assessment prior to the retreat using the assessment tool from the website Taking Charge of Your Health and Wellbeing (see: www.takingcharge.csh.umn.edu). Topics discussed at the retreat include the determinants of wellbeing, mindfulness and self-awareness, and behavior change.

Day 2 of the retreat series focuses on organizational wellbeing. Participants complete an organizational assessment in advance of the retreat and begin to identify strengths, gaps, challenges, and opportunities. A major focus is on developing strategies that leverage organizational strengths and overcome barriers.

Day 3, the final day of the series focuses on deepening leadership practices. Participants are introduced to the concept of whole systems leadership, social networks, social change, and gentle action.

The series draws heavily from three content areas: (1) Self-Awareness, (2) Whole Systems Healing, and (3) Whole Systems Leadership.

Self-Awareness

As a leader, a very critical skill is to be aware of one's own feelings, emotions, and intentions and to have the capacity to self-regulate. Scharmer [36] notes that successful leadership depends on the quality of attention and intention that the leader brings to any situation. He notes that two leaders in the same circumstances doing the same thing can bring about completely different outcomes, depending on the inner place from which each operates. Self-awareness enables a leader to regulate their emotions and responses and to develop acceptance and openness. When leaders have self-awareness, they have a deeper understanding of values which in turn helps them to accept others who may have differing values and views.

Mindfulness, often defined as present moment awareness, is an excellent way to begin to tap into one's feelings, thoughts, emotions, and bodily sensations. A way to begin to cultivate mindfulness is to simply notice what is going on in your body. Are you feeling open and relaxed or heavy and tight? How is your breathing? Often physical clues can help bring you into the current moment and help you recognize the emotions and thoughts you are experiencing. When you become more aware of your own emotional state, you are more capable of deeply listening to another person and perceiving what is going on around you. From a leadership perspective, this is critical. When you become mindful, you are also able to be less reactive in a situation and more able to choose how you want to respond [37].

Whole Systems Healing

Whole systems healing [38] is an expansive way to view the world. It is a way of addressing problems and cultivating the health and wellbeing of individuals, organizations, communities, and the environment by living and acting with awareness of the wholeness and the interconnectedness of all living systems. It requires an understanding of several critical key concepts:

- Complexity Science/Chaos Theory: All living systems, from individual humans and communities, to the ecosystem of the planet, are complex systems that are constantly adapting and evolving in response to changing conditions from within and outside.
- Social Networks: social structures made up of individuals or organizations that are connected or inter-related. The ties can be social, economic, or organizational.
- Social Change: a process, whereby values, attitudes, or institutions of society become modified.
- Gentle Action: as articulated by David Peat [39], gentle action is the use of grassroots efforts and collective intelligence to focus many small, coordinated efforts on the best point of leverage within a given system. It is the strategic implementation of highly coordinated, low intensity actions.

Whole systems healing is not only a way to address problems or resolve issues, it is an approach of shifting the culture within an organization.

Whole Systems Leadership

In describing the type of leadership that is now required in organizations, Kahane [40] notes that leadership must be systemic, participative, and emergent.

- Systemic: embedded pervasively throughout the organization.
- Participative: involves many people's ideas, energy, talent, and expertise.
- Emergent: able to move and adapt nimbly in a minefield of uncertainty.

Whole systems leadership embraces this approach and is a departure from conventional leadership as illustrated in Table 9.1. In the whole systems framework, leadership is viewed as a behavior that can show up any place in the organization. It is not tied to having a role or a position with authority. While a conventional leadership approach focuses on control and stability, a whole systems approach recognizes that disrupting habitual patterns may be just what is needed to move the organization forward. A conventional leadership approach may direct time and

Table 9.1 Conventional and whole systems leadership

	Conventional view of leadership	Whole systems leadership
Leadership is…	a position or role of authority	an activity or behavior that can arise anywhere in a human system
Leadership flows…	in one direction: from the top-down	in all directions
Leadership is exercised…	by individuals with special leadership traits	collectively by groups and/or by individuals informed by the collective
Effective leadership comes from…	accurately anticipating a predictable path to a predetermined outcome	recognizing and influencing patterns that are present in human systems at all levels
Leadership requires…	certainty, clear vision, and the power of persuasion and control	willingness to embrace uncertainty, listen to all voices and take adaptive action, often in collaboration with others
Leadership creates…	harmony and stability	conditions that are conducive to groups moving forward - which sometimes means disrupting the habitual patterns of engagement so that groups, communities, or organizations can set the conditions for a preferred future
The purpose of leadership is to…	fix problems and leverage opportunities to achieve goals	enable adaptability, learning, and innovation so that groups make progress on the issues they care about - even in unpredictable and changing conditions
Leadership can make a difference through…	one large strategic intervention designed to fix a problem or achieve a goal	recognizing emerging patterns in human systems and making meaning out of many small changes

Source: Earl E. Bakken Center for Spirituality & Healing https://www.csh.umn.edu/education/whole-systems-healing/whole-systems-leadership

attention to fixing problems and leveraging opportunities to achieve goals. While goal oriented as well, a whole systems approach would also be focused on assuring that the organization is building capacity for adaptability, learning, and innovation.

9.5 Whole Systems Leadership Competencies

Leaders who embody whole systems leadership have knowledge, skills, and attitudes that enable them to generate appropriate and effective responses to complex situations. The six core competencies include:

1. **Deep listening:** Conversations have the power to transform our understanding and generate innovative options for action. A key component of successful conversations is deep listening, which means listening to learn and temporarily suspending judgment.
2. **Awareness of systems:** Whole systems leadership understands communities, organizations, and groups as adaptive, changing systems. With an awareness of systems, you get a fuller perspective of the situation, which expands and refines your options for action.
3. **Awareness of self:** Developing self-awareness is the necessary beginning to developing skillful ways to respond to situations. If you are not aware of your motivations, feelings, and beliefs, you cannot make effective decisions about how to behave.
4. **Seeking diverse perspectives:** A whole systems approach thrives on the respectful inclusion of all voices. From this viewpoint, conflicting opinions do not present a problem; rather, they present a potential resource that can sharpen thinking and lead to innovative options for action.
5. **Suspending certainty, embracing uncertainty:** Suspending certainty enables you to see beyond your habitual lenses to get a broader and potentially more accurate view of what is going on. It also creates room for diverse views so that new or different knowledge can come forth.
6. **Taking adaptive action:** Adaptive action means learning from everything you do. It means taking time to recognize patterns and reflect on their meaning before jumping to a solution. It balances an inclusive, deep listening approach with a bias towards action.

Organizational Change and Transformation

In considering how to advance small or large system change, there is increasing interest in applying the principles of design thinking. "Design Thinking" as a practice has been well articulated by Tim Brown and the work of the international company IDEO. In the book *Change by Design* (2009), Brown discusses the importance of considering three factors highlighted in Fig. 9.2 in promoting a system change.

Fig. 9.2 Three factors promoting change [41]. (Source: Anna Martius)

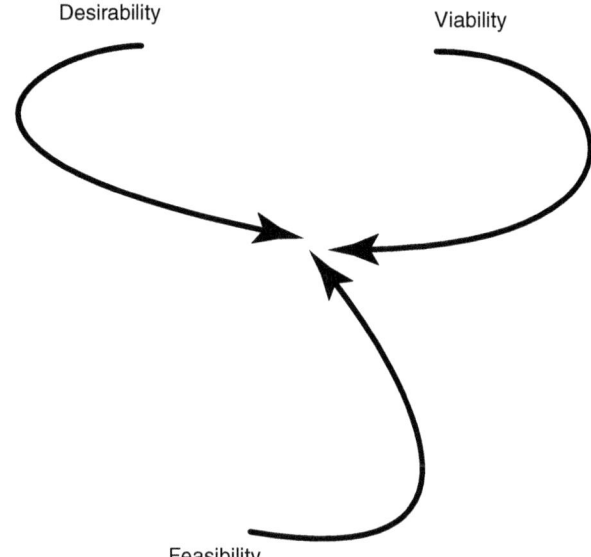

In launching organizational change, a beginning place is to understand what is desirable or needed. Understanding organizational needs requires deep listening and all of the skills and tools noted throughout this chapter. It requires suspending certainty and judgment so that you can see possibilities. It requires working with people with diverse views and perspectives and engaging people in a process of co-creation.

For strategies to be adopted and sustainable, it is also important to look at two additional factors: feasibility and viability. Feasibility relates to examining whether there are resources and infrastructures in place to support the proposed change. This may relate to human capital as well as tangible support including policies and leadership endorsement. Viability relates to sustainability and the question of whether sufficient financial resources are in place to support the change.

9.6 Summary and Checklist

Advancing wellbeing and human flourishing is a global need that transcends cultures and borders. It is a social change that requires an understanding of whole systems change and leadership. Within healthcare, there is an urgency to address personal and organizational wellbeing given the growing rates of stress, burnout, and early exit from health professions. Staff development interventions such as the wellbeing leadership program are needed that prepare leaders who have the knowledge and skills to create culture change that addresses the root causes of stress and burnout. The following checklist outlines the next steps:

- Convene a design team or guiding coalition for the organizational wellbeing transformation process and planning.
- Conduct an organizational wellbeing assessment and identify strengths, challenges, and opportunities.
- Create a thoughtful, organization-appropriate wellbeing plan with measurable outcomes.
- Implement the plan and enable action by highlighting early wins and leveraging strengths and opportunities.
- Celebrate organizational wellbeing learning and transformation!

References

1. Institute of Medicine. The future of nursing: leading change, advancing health. Washington, DC: National Academies Pres; 2011.
2. Maslach C, Jackson S. The measurement of experienced burnout. J Organ Behav. 1981;2:99–113.
3. Friedberg MW, Chen PG, Van Busum KR, et al. Factors affecting physician professional satisfaction and their implications for patient care, health systems and health policy. Santa Monica: Rand Corporation; 2013.
4. Shanafelt TD, Boone S, Tan L, Dyrbye LN, Sotile W, Satele D, West CP, Sloan J, Oreskovich MR. Burnout and satisfaction with work-life balance among US physicians relative to the general US population. Arch Intern Med. 2012;172:1377–85.
5. Kane L, Peckman C. Medscape physician compensation report 2014. 2014. https://www.medscape.com/features/slideshow/compensation/2014/public/overview#24. Accessed 7 Jul 2015.
6. McHugh MD, Kutney-Lee A, Cimiotti JP, Sloane DN, Aiken LH. Nurses' widespread job dissatisfaction, burnout and frustration with health benefits signals problems for patient care. Health Aff. 2011;30:202–10.
7. Salyers MP, Flanagan ME, Firmin R, Rollins AL. Clinicians' perceptions of how burnout affects their work. Psychiatr Serv. 2015;66:204–7.
8. Shanafelt T, Gorringe G, Menaker R, Storz K, Reeves D, Buskirk S, Sloan J, Swensen S. Impact of organizational leadership on physician burnout and satisfaction. Mayo Clin Proc. 2015;90:432.
9. Udod S, Care W. Walking a tight rope: an investigation of nurse managers' work stressors and coping experiences. J Res Nurs. 2013;18:67–79.
10. Berwick DM, Nolan TW, Whittington J. The triple aim: care, health and cost. Health Aff. 2008;27:759–69.
11. Bodenheimer T, Sinsky C. From triple aim to quadruple aim: care of the patient requires care of the provider. Ann Fam Med. 2014;12:573–6.
12. World Health Organization Preamble to the constitution of the World Health Organization as adopted by the International Health Conference, New York, 19–22 June, 1946, signed on 22 July, 1946, by the representatives of 61 States (Official Records of the World Health Organization, no. 2, p. 100) and entered into force on 7 April, 1948; 1946.
13. Antonovsky A. Unraveling the mystery of health—how people manage stress and stay well. San Francisco, CA: Jossey-Bass; 1987.
14. Kreitzer MJ. Spirituality and wellbeing: focusing on what matters. West J Nurs Res. 2012;34(6):707–11.
15. Clymer JM, Fielding JE, Rimer BK, Pronk NP. The guidebook for healthy communities and healthy states. America's Health Rankings: United Health Foundation. 2012. http://www.americashealthrankings.org/Reports. Accessed 6 Mar 2013.
16. Smith EE. The power of meaning. New York: Crown Publishing; 2017.

17. Nakamura J, Csikszentmihalyi M. Flow theory and research. In: Snyder CR, Lopez SJ, editors. Handbook of positive psychology. Oxford: Oxford University Press; 2009. p. 195–206.
18. Bronk K, Hill P, Lapsley D, Talib T, Finch H. Purpose, hope, and life satisfaction in three age groups. J Posit Psychol. 2009;4(6):500–10.
19. Diener E, Fujita F, Tay L, Biswas-Diener R. Purpose, mood, and pleasure in predicting satisfaction judgments. Soc Indic Res. 2012;105(3):333–41.
20. Kim ES, Sun JK, Park N, Kubzansky LD, Peterson C. Purpose in life and reduced risk of myocardial infarction among older U.S. adults with coronary heart disease: a two-year follow-up. J Behav Med. 2012;36(2):124–33.
21. Tanno K, Sakata K, Ohsawa M, Onoda T, Itai K, Yaegashi Y, Tamakoshi A, JACC Study Group. Associations of *ikigai* as a positive psychological factor with all-cause mortality and cause-specific mortality among middle-aged and elderly Japanese PEOPLE: findings from the Japan Collaborative Cohort Study. J Psychosom Res. 2009;67(1):67–75.
22. Hill PL, Turiano NA. Purpose in life as a predictor of mortality across adulthood. Psychol Sci. 2014;25(7):1482–6.
23. Holt-Lunstad J, Smith TB, Layton JB. Social relationships and mortality risk: a meta-analytic review. PLoS Med. 2010;7(7):e1000316.
24. Jaremka LM, Fagundes CP, Glaser R, Bennett JM, Malarkey WB, Kiecolt-Glaser JK. Loneliness predicts pain, depression, and fatigue: understanding the role of immune dysregulation. Psychoneuroendocrinology. 2012;8(8):1310–7. https://doi.org/10.1016/j.psyneuen.2012.11.016. pii: S0306-4530(12)00403-9.
25. Hawkley LC, Thisted RA, Masi CM, Cacioppo JT. Loneliness predicts increased blood pressure: five-year cross-lagged analyses in middle-aged and older adults. Psychol Aging. 2010;25:132–41.
26. Buettner D. Blue zones: lessons for living longer from the people who've lived the longest. Washington, DC: National Geographic Society; 2009.
27. Largo-Wight E, Chen WW, Dodd V, Weiler R. Healthy workplaces: the effects of nature contact at work on employee stress and health. Public Health Rep. 2011;126(Suppl 1):124–30.
28. Ulrich RS. View through a window may influence recovery from surgery. Science. 1984;224(4647):420–1.
29. Bringslimark T, Patil G, Hartig T. The association between indoor plants, stress, productivity and sick leave in office workers. Acta Hortic. 2008;775:117.
30. Park S, Mattson R. Ornamental indoor plants in hospital rooms enhanced health outcomes of patients recovering from surgery. J Altern Complement Med. 2009;15(9):975–80.
31. Mind Organization. Ecotherapy: the green agenda for mental health. London: Mind Publications; 2007.
32. Kim T. Human brain activation in response to visual stimulation with rural and urban scenery pictures: a functional magnetic resonance imaging study. Sci Total Environ. 2010;408(12):2600.
33. Cervinka R, Röderer K, Hefler E. Are nature lovers happy? On various indicators of well-being and connectedness with nature. J Health Psychol. 2012;17(3):379–88.
34. Berman MG, Jonides J, Kaplan S. The cognitive benefits of interacting with nature. Psychol Sci. 2008;19(12):1207–12.
35. Bowler DE, Buyung-Ali LM, Knight TM, Pullin AS. A systematic review of evidence for the added benefits to health of exposure to natural environments. BMC Public Health. 2010;10:456.
36. Scharmer O. The essentials of theory U. Oakland: Berrett-Koehler Publishers, Inc.; 2018.
37. Johns C. Achtsames Führen in der Pflege. Bern: Hogrefe-Verlag; 2018.
38. Center for Spirituality and Healing. 2012. http://www.csh.umn.edu/wsh/. Accessed 9 Dec 2012.
39. Peat D. Gentle action: bringing creative change to a turbulent world. Pari: Pari Publishing; 2008.
40. Kahane A. Solving tough problems: an open way of talking. San Francisco, CA: Berrett-Koehler Publishers, Inc.; 2004.
41. Brown T. Change by design: how design thinking transforms organizations and inspires innovation. New York: HarperCollins Publishers; 2009.

10

Stress Was Yesterday! Revitalising Care Is Today, by the Adoption of HeartMath® Interventions in Nursing within the National Health Service (NHS) UK: Facing the challenges

Sue Ann Smith and Gavin John Andrews

The National Health Service (NHS) is the state health service in the United Kingdom (England, Ireland, Scotland and Wales). Access to the service is via General Practitioner, hospital and emergency departments. The NHS in the UK is funded mostly through general taxation and National Insurance contributions. A smaller proportion is collected through patient charges, for things like prescriptions and dentistry. The NHS is staffed with a wide range of support, infrastructure staff and health professionals from many different settings including Medicine, Nursing, Community and Primary Care, Midwifery, Dietetics, Occupational Therapy, Physiotherapy, Podiatry, Chiropody, Radiography, Speech Therapy and more. The Royal College of Nursing analyse the shape and size and state of the nursing labour market each year and publish findings in the 'United Kingdom Labour Market Review' [1]. The report notes in 2021 that the Nursing and Midwifery Council (NMC) register shows there were almost 732,000 nurses and midwives on the register. In March 2021 74.9% registered as adult nurses, 12.5% mental health nurses, 7.3% registered as children's nurses and 2.3% registered as learning disability nurses. Nursing entry routes include the traditional university route or through a new degree-apprenticeship route. Registered nurses are a statutorily regulated profession and the standards for proficiency are set by the Nursing and Midwifery Council NM [2] (www.nmc.org.uk).

Nurse training requires nurses to be trained to degree level, Bachelor of Science in Nursing (BSc in Nursing) and 40–50% of time in the classroom at a university and 50–60% in hospital and community settings. The choice of route is BSc in adult, child, or mental health nursing. Midwifery training involves studying at

S. A. Smith (✉)
Choice Dynamic International Private Limited Company, Pontefract, UK
e-mail: drsue@choice-dynamic-int.com

G. J. Andrews
HeartMath UK & Ireland, London, UK

degree level, through an approved pre-registration degree or an approved degree apprenticeship in midwifery. Other options post-registration includes BSc's in Learning Disability, Public Health, School Nursing, Community Nursing and Health Visiting. A further point of entry is conversion from an undergraduate degree to a Post-Graduate Diploma in Nursing. This report concludes that the number of new entrants to the NMC register is now exceeded by the numbers leaving. The challenges faced by Nursing are outlined in the United Kingdom Labour Market Review (UKLMR) [1] and include decreasing number nurses in the workforce due to high numbers leaving rather than joining, high student attrition, age profile changes and increasing numbers of part-time staff. The number of people leaving the Nursing and Midwifery Council Register (NMCR) has dropped over the last year to 4.6%. In 2021, 18,880 registrants left the register and at the same time 19,745 new registrars joined (UKLMR 1). The student attrition from pre-registration clinical education programmes continues to be a long standing challenge. In March 2015 the Department of Health published a refreshed mandate to Health Education England [3] the national leadership organisation for education, training and workforce development. They set out actions to improve the quality of education and supporting healthcare students and trainees. A project called Reducing Pre-Registration Attrition and Improving Retention (RePAIR) was established as a result to reduce unnecessary attrition and reported in 2017 [4]. The main reasons identified for leaving the profession once qualified are: financial difficulties, academic pressures, personal problems, mental health issues feeling overwhelmed and stress. Buddying and transition into practice along with good preceptorship is reported as crucial to retaining students.

10.1 Staff Development: Revitalising Care of Staff and Patients

Less staff and high student attrition will be an increasing leadership challenge. Griffiths et al. [5] expressed concern that decreasing staffing levels in the NHS is associated with worse outcomes for both patients and staff, leading to stress negativity and low morale. Leaders will need to ensure there are mechanisms in place to build resilient teams who can cope with the challenges. The project described in this chapter relates to the training of trainers to deliver a one day workshop called Revitalising Care™ with the intention to deliver the workshop to Nursing and Healthcare professionals accross nine HealthBoards in Scotland starting 2012. The goal of the workshop and the related support of one to one coaching is to reduce stress, build resilience, help staff feel valued and revitalised, enhance teamwork and empowerment to create a more uplifting and harmonising environment and increase staff retention. The need for this type of development is supported by a review carried out by the House of Commons Select Committee UK ([6], p. 17) which made specific recommendations for a greater focus on retention driven strategies and an explicit commitment to making the Nursing workforce feel valued. In 2012 the

Scottish Government's Directorate for the Chief Nursing Officer, Patients, Public and Health Professions (CNOPPP), were visionary and commissioned and funded a project to train trainers in nine Health Boards to deliver a workshop for front line staff for 3 years called 'Revitalising Care™' [7]. It was part of a wider project to introduce accountability for achieving care and compassion in the workplace for both patients and staff. It was provided by Choice Dynamic International Private Limited Company [8] on licence from HeartMath LLC, USA [9]. The workshops were delivered by licenced staff development educators The goal was to address the retention of nurses and health professionals by promoting tools and techniques to build resilience to handle every day stressors.

Workshop Design: The workshop provides education about care and compassion, positive psychology, physiology of the heart, resilience, coherence and the opportunity to learn new tools and techniques to be able to calm stress reactions and take out the drama of situations more quickly. The result is better authentic care and compassion. The design of the workshop was carried out by the Institute of HeartMath (IHM) [10] which is a not for profit research and education centre based in California. Rollin McCraty is the Director of research and has conducted many studies for over 25 years exploring the heart–brain connection. Studies have focused on physiological mechanisms by which the heart and brain communicate and how the activity of the heart influences perceptions, emotions, intuition and health. During the early 1990s the research conducted at the IHM focussed on how stressful emotions affect the activity in the autonomic nervous system (ANS) and the hormonal and immune systems. Studies were conducted to assess the effects of emotions such as appreciation, compassion and care. These studies adopted many different measures such as electroencephalogram (EEG—which measures brain waves), skin conductance level (SCL—records autonomic system arousal), electrocardiogram (ECG which records heart rhythm and electrical activity), blood pressure (BP—which records blood pressure) and hormone levels, etc. Consistently, it was found that the heart rate variability or heart rhythms stood out as the most dynamic and reflective indicator of emotional states and, therefore, current stress and cognitive processes [11]. Studies indicate that there are health benefits of reducing stress: lowering of the blood pressure [12], impact on diabetes [13], impact on patients with congestive heart failure [14]. Building and sustaining resilience is dependent on the ability to more intelligently manage energy expenditures and recharge more quickly. Over 1400 biochemical changes are set in motion by changing the emotional state. Among these biochemical changes are two hormones 'cortisol', the stress hormone and dehydroepiandrosterone (DHEA), the 'vitality hormone'. Depleting emotions increase cortisol and renewing emotions increase DHEA [11] (Fig. 10.1). The goal is to work with participants to change their heart rhythm patterns from incoherence to coherence. See Fig. 10.1 which illustrates these two different patterns and Fig. 10.2 which is the monitoring technology emwave2 used by participants that they were given for personal use at home and work.

The goal in the workshop is to learn how to generate coherent 'smooth' heart rhythms through focusing on renewing emotions like appreciation, courage and

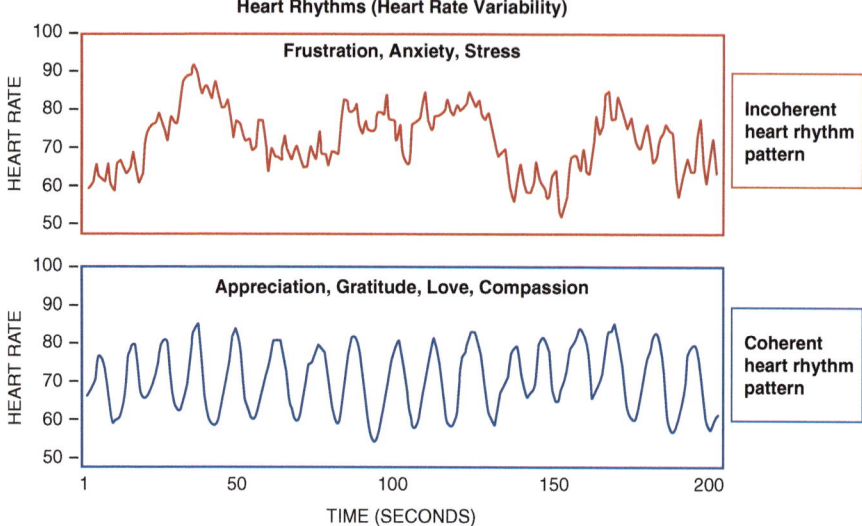

Fig. 10.1 Heart rate variability during frustration and appreciation. www.heartmath.org. (Copyright 1997 Institute of HeartMath). The top box in red shows irregular, jerky heart rhythm pattern typical of a stressful feeling like anger, frustration and worry, resulting in an incoherent heart rhythm pattern. The bottom box shows heart rate variability or heart rhythm pattern typical of appreciation and other positive feelings. This is called a coherent pattern

Fig. 10.2 Photograph of emwave2 technique

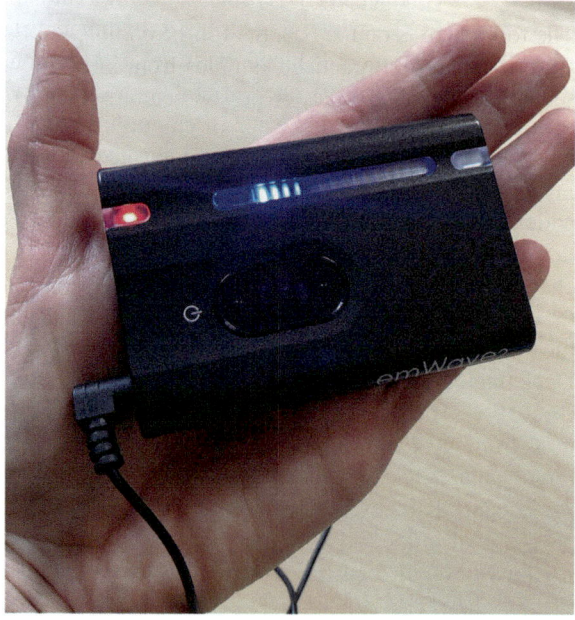

patience. Monitoring of heart rate variability (HRV) is achieved using emWave2™ [15] (Photo 1, Fig. 10.2).

The emWave2 collects pulse data through a pulse sensor placed on the ear lobe and translates the information from the heart rhythms into graphics on the computer or into easy to follow lights on the portable emWave2. Cryer [16] asserts that learning to manage emotional response to stressors is easier than people think. In order to break the cycle, the IHM has created several tools and techniques to help and examples are presented here.

- **EXAMPLE** Participants receive education in the working of the heart and coherence. They are advised to spend up to 5 min each day practising the tools and techniques learned on the workshop to increase the coherence baseline and ability to take charge of emotional reactions. Two main techniques provide the foundation. The first is 'Heart-Focused Breathing ™'.
- *Focus your attention in the area of your heart. Imagine your breath is flowing in and out of your heart or chest area, breathing a little slower and deeper than usual (inhale 5 s, exhale 5 s).*
- The second technique builds on the first and is called 'Quick Coherence Technique™'.
- *Focus the attention on the area of the heart. Imagine the breath is flowing in and out of the heart or chest area, breathing a little slower and deeper than usual (inhale 5 s, exhale 5 s). Then make a sincere attempt to experience a regenerative feeling such as appreciation or care for someone or something in your life, e.g. a pet, a special place.*

In the workshop, participants are encouraged to use these techniques when facing typical energy draining situations. For example, meetings, emails, financial issues, sleep disruption, making decisions, standing in traffic, workplace drama, overload and deadlines, challenging co-workers. They develop action plans, create buddy systems and have a coaching session over a 6 week period post the workshop.

Revitalising Care Project

Project design: Twenty staff development professionals attended a 4 day training workshop to gain accreditation to deliver 'Revitalising Care™'. The workshop included training in HeartMath™ tools and technique. Working in pairs they delivered one workshop in each of the 9 Scottish Health Boards to 127 people (approximately 15 participants per workshop). The demographic profile of participants included: 11 males and 115 female, 80% professional technical and 10% skilled clericals and 10% management. Over 50% held a bachelor's degree and 20% held a master's degree, 15% had been in post 6 months, 35% 2–5 years and 28% 10 years or more. A follow-up day 6 weeks later and one coaching session every 6 weeks, daily practice in the tools and techniques formed the basis of the interventions. The coaching session was to ensure the participants were able to use the technology and support them to apply the practice of the tools and techniques learnt on the workshop.

Evaluation: Completion of an online assessment instrument measured change over time which is a pre- and post-testing measurement—POQA (personal and organisational quality assessment). The measures include four key areas: emotional vitality, organisational stress, emotional stress and physical stress. Subscales of these four include emotional buoyancy, contentment, pressure of life, relational tension, intention to quit, anxiety and depression, anger and resentment, fatigue and health symptoms such as headaches, body aches, etc. Organisational quality scales are comprised of questions relating to areas of strategic understanding, goal clarity and work attitude.

Results

Emotional vitality scale: An overall measure of the degree to which employees feel a positive emotional energy that enables an optimistic and fulfilling life experience. Low scores on this scale suggest it is likely that the employees have low levels of emotional vitality, and, hence, may have limited emotional energy available to invest. The results suggest there was a 13% increase in emotional buoyancy (pre 30% post 43%) and a 23% increase in emotional contentment (pre 15% post 38%) (Table 10.1).

Table 10.1 Table with results from Organization's POQA-R4 profile N = 127

Organizational stress	% Pre	% Post	% Change
Pressures of Life	21	7	14
Relational Tension	26	17	9
How stressed have you been in the past month (100-point sliding scale)	51	19	32
Intention to Quit	12	5	7
Emotional Vitality			
Emotional Buoyancy	30	43	13
Emotional Contentment	15	38	23
Emotional Stress			
Anxiety and Depression	8	3	5
Anger and Resentment	4	0	4
Physical Stress			
Fatigue	37	11	26
Inadequate sleep	50	24	26
Body aches (joint pain, backaches, etc.)	35	22	13
Indigestion, heartburn, or stomach upset	17	6	11
Rapid heartbeats	14	4	10
Muscle tension	32	15	17
Headaches	19	8	11
Health Risk Factors			
Poor health perception	18	6	12
Low life satisfaction	7	1	6
Low Job satisfaction	15	6	9

Emotional stress scale: An overall measure of the degree to which employees report negative emotions, which they have difficulty controlling and which they feel impair the quality and effectiveness of their life experience. High scores on this scale indicate it is likely that the employees are feeling emotionally stressed, overwhelmed and/or frustrated by the present circumstances of their lives. The results suggest that neither of these scales were high in the pre-test score and there was a reduction of 5% in anxiety (pre 8% post 3%) and reduction in depression of 4% in the anger and resentment scale (pre 4% post 0%).

The organisational stress scale: An overall measure of the degree to which employees feel negatively pressured by stressors and conflicts at work and in their personal lives that not only detract them from work performance but may also lead them to want to quit their job. The results indicate there was a shift in each of the scales with a 14% decrease in pressures of life (pre21% post 7%), 9% decrease in relational tension, like co-worker conflict (pre 26% post 17%), 32% decrease in how stressed they have felt in the last month (pre 51% post 19%), 7% decrease in the intention to quit (pre 12% post 5%).

Physical stress scale: An overall measure of the level of physical symptoms of stress among employees. High scores on this scale indicate the employees may have low levels of physical and emotional energy and may also be experiencing precursors of significant health issues and problems. On each scale there is a reduction, fatigue 26% reduction (pre 37% post 11%), inadequate sleep 26% reduction (pre 50% post 24%), body aches and pains 13% reduction (pre 35% post 22%), indigestion and heartburn 11% reduction (pre 17% post 6%), rapid heartbeats 10% reduction (pre 14% post 4%), muscle tension 17% reduction (pre 32% post 15%) and headaches 11% reduction (pre 19% post 8%).

Conclusion

Analysis of qualitative interview data suggests that out of 127 participants there were only 10 who had not used the technology or undertaken their practice, 117 reported high value of the tools and techniques and practised them daily.

Twenty staff development facilitators continued over the following 2 years to deliver the one day workshops across the nine Health Boards in Scotland. Over 2000 staff attended up to 2015 and evaluation of impact data demonstrates high impact and change. In summary deliberately advancing organisational learning and developing capabilities in the use of tools and techniques was achieved.

10.2 What Others Can Learn from the Project

The Scottish Government's Directorate for the Chief Nursing Officer in 2015 handed over responsibility to all NHS Trusts for the continuation of the project. In 2019 half the trainers have retired and moved to new jobs. Sustainability rests with these NHS Trusts and some have continued, and others have not despite positive outcomes.

There are three key areas for improvement that would have helped to sustain the project beyond the 3-year contract.

- Commissioning of independent research that is published and marketed to motivate leaders to keep repeating the intervention.
- Support to staff development practitioners is essential to sustain the work and influence board level decisions.
- Commissioners of projects need to build sustainability plans beyond the project life cycle.

Guidelines for external providers working with government/cross regional projects

- Establish in a written contract of named accountable leaders who are responsible for communicating with external providers of the intervention. Identify the accountable officers for finance, project management, marketing and research.
- Ensure there is a clearly identified research and evaluation strategy in place before commencement of the project.
- Establish a self-managed learning system for staff development trainers, so that on completion of the project there is a system in place for ongoing continuing education.
- External providers should have in place a certification system and ways of attending updates and accreditation for practice. This can be achieved through a licence to practice fee paid yearly. This supports accountability to maintain good quality training and was created as part of this project.

10.3 Future Opportunities

Recent advances in technology are making the system more accessible to individuals through the new Inner Balance™ app which acts like the emWave2 but is accessed on a mobile phone using an ear sensor. Until now, The Inner Balance™ app using HRV biofeedback technology has been used to enable individuals to develop and measure personal coherence skills. More recently IHM has been researching Group and Global Coherence and have also launched an app called Global Coherence for measuring group and team coherence [17]. Coherence is an optimal state for learning, developing and utilising many of the skills and roles required of groups and teams; for example, collaboration, co-creation, conflict resolution and decision-making. These skills, and therefore group and team performance, are compromised by stress. The Global Coherence app can be used to create a private group of any size. This group can then practice coherence techniques together or remotely (anywhere in the world) and everyone can track both their individual coherence and the combined coherence of the group, in real time. One

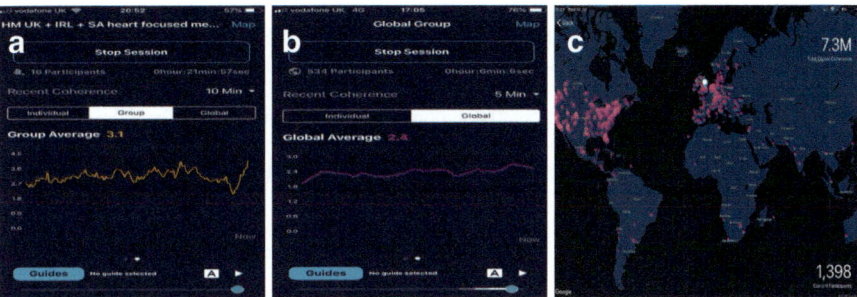

Fig. 10.3 (a) Data from a private group of 16 HeartMath coaches over a 10-minute period. Note how the coherence level fluctuates but clearly climbs over the first 7 minutes. There is then a decline in coherence from about 3.9 to 1.8 which occurred when the group leader interrupted the practice with instructions for the coherence technique to change. However, when the group had refocussed their practice the coherence level rose very rapidly back up to c3.9. (**b**) The Global Coherence app can be used for both smaller, private groups and large scale group events such as mass meditations. Figure 10.3b shows data from an open public coherence meditation session involving a very large group of 534 participants. The data shows the level of coherence over a 5-minute period. Note again how the coherence level fluctuates but that the average is clearly trending upwards, reflecting the increasing coherence level of the group. (**c**) Shows the global distribution of a very large group of almost 1,400 participants. Each person logged into the app appears as a highlighted dot on the map. Participant feedback reveals that many people enjoy this function and knowing that they are part of a larger whole

very powerful and important application of the app could be decision-making under pressure of time, or in ethical 'grey areas', or when there are multiple competing/paradoxical demands or outcomes. A decision made when most group members are highly coherent is more likely to result in a positive and ethical outcome, even when there may be significant costs to the decision. Stress makes smart people do stupid things. The Global Coherence app provides an opportunity for smart people to stay coherent even under stress (Fig. 10.3).

References

1. Royal College of Nursing, editor. United Kingdom Nursing Labour Market Review, UKLMR. Publication Code 007397; 2018.
2. Nursing and Midwifery Council (NMC). https://www.nmc.org.uk.
3. Department of Health. Delivering high quality, effective compassionate care: developing the right people with the right skills and the right values. A mandate from the Government to Health Education England: April 2015-March 2016. 2015. https://assets.publishing.service.gov.uk/government/uploads/system/uploads/attachment_data/file/203332/29257_2900971_Delivering_Accessible.pdf. Accessed Jun 2019.
4. RePAIR. Reducing pre-registration attrition and improving retention report, Health Education England. 2017. https://www.hee.nhs.uk/our-work/reducing-pre-registration-attrition-improving-retention.
5. Griffiths P, Ora D, Ball J. How many nurses: what does the evidence say? Evidence brief. Southampton: University of Southampton; 2017.

6. House of Commons Health Committee. Second report o*rdered by the House of Commons to be printed 16 January 2018* published on 26 January 2018 by authority of the House of Commons. 2019. https://publications.parliament.uk/pa/cm201719/cmselect/cmhealth/353/353.pdf sourced June 2019.
7. Revitalisng Care™. Workbook: creating an optimal healing environment from the inside out: HeartMath. 2011. www.heartmath.com.
8. Smith S. Choice Dynamic International Private Limited Company. www.choice-dynamic-int.com.
9. HearMath LLC is the for profit training company who licence 'Revitalising Care™ workshop published by the Institute of HeartMath 14700 West ParK avenue Boulder Creek California 95006; n.d.
10. Institute of HeartMath (IHM). https://www.heartmath.org.
11. McCraty R, Chidre D. Coherence: bridging the personal, social and global health. Altern Ther Health Med. 2010;16(4):10–24.
12. Alabdulgader A. Global advances in health and medicine. Glob Adv Health Med. 2012;1(2):54–62; www.gahmj.com.
13. McCraty R, Atkinson M, Lipsenthal P. HeartMath Research Centre, Institute of HeartMath, Publication no. 00-006, Boulder Creek, CA; 2000.
14. Luskin F, Reitz M, Newall K, Quinn TG, Haskell W. A controlled pilot study of stress management training of elderly patients with congestive heart failure. Prev Cardiol. 2002;5(4):168–76.
15. HeartMath emWave™ is a registered trademark of Quantum Intech, Inc. Quick Coherence is a registered trademark of Doc Childre. Revitalising Care and Inner-Ease are trademarks of Quantum Intech, Inc.; n.d.
16. Cryer B, McCraty R, Childre D. Pull the plug on stress. Harv Bus Rev. 2003;2003:102–7.
17. McCraty R, Atkinson M, Stolc V, Alabdulgader A, Vainoras A, Rafulskis M. Synchronization of human autonomic nervous system rhythms with geomagnetic activity in human subjects. Int J Environ Res Public Health. 2017;13(4):770.

Part III

We Are a Dream Team: Interprofessional Collaboration

Agile Working and Leading: New Approaches for Cross-functional Expert Teams in the Context of Precision Oncology

Sylvia Bochum, Christian Fegeler, and Uwe M. Martens

11.1 Background

Precision Oncology

In oncology, there has been a rapid increase in knowledge over the past 10 years. In particular, the development of next generation sequencing (NGS) technologies has heralded a paradigm shift in the treatment of cancer. Due to the increasing availability of molecular diagnostics, many tumor entities can now be subdivided into genetically defined subgroups, which means that systemic drug therapy can increasingly be adapted to the individual mutation profile of a tumor. This has been made possible by the parallel development of numerous new substances that can specifically inhibit cellular target structures or contribute to tumor eradication by activating the immune system.

These advances in the field of diagnostics and therapy of tumor diseases have created the basis for individualized therapy concepts. The pioneers of molecularly stratified precision oncology include chronic myeloid leukemia (CML), melanoma, and non-small cell lung cancer. For these tumor entities, targeted drugs for defined mutations are now available and their detection has already found its way into routine diagnostics.

However, the enormous increase in knowledge and available therapies inevitably leads to an increasing complexity of oncological therapy decisions and presents oncologists with a number of new challenges in terms of capabilities and available

S. Bochum (✉) · U. M. Martens
Cancer Center Heilbronn-Franken, SLK Clinics, Heilbronn, Germany

MOLIT Institute for Personalized Medicine, Heilbronn, Germany
e-mail: sylvia.bochum@molit.eu; uwe.martens@molit.eu

C. Fegeler
MOLIT Institute for Personalized Medicine, Heilbronn, Germany
e-mail: christian.fegeler@molit.eu

© The Author(s), under exclusive license to Springer Nature Switzerland AG 2022
R. Tewes (ed.), *Innovative Staff Development in Healthcare*,
https://doi.org/10.1007/978-3-030-81986-6_11

time in their workday [1]. This is because treatment options have not only become more complex and individualized as a result, but the management of therapy has also become much more dynamic. In order to derive the greatest possible benefit from existing knowledge and collected data and to improve the long-term chances of recovery for patients with tumor diseases, innovative IT solutions are urgently needed. On the one hand, these solutions must make knowledge available quickly and in a case-specific manner, and on the other hand, they must offer valid clinical decision support on the basis of existing data.

In the academic context, the German Federal Ministry of Education and Research (BMBF) is currently promoting the establishment of oncological data integration centers as part of its medical informatics initiative—but so far only at a few university hospitals [2]. At the same time, however, there are also considerable commercial interests in the collection and analysis of data in the context of oncological patient care. In order to promote the efficient, non-profit-oriented use of precision oncology data in routine care, and to make it available ubiquitously, the non-profit MOLIT Institute for Personalized Medicine has been developing innovative IT solutions on an open source basis for several years.

MOLIT Institute for Personalized Medicine

The MOLIT Institute was founded in Heilbronn, Germany, in 2017. The foundation was preceded by several years of scientific cooperation between the Cancer Center Heilbronn-Franken at the SLK Clinics Heilbronn and the GECKO Institute for Medicine, Economics and Informatics at Heilbronn University. The MOLIT Institute, which is run as a non-profit limited company, is funded by the Heilbronn-based Dieter Schwarz Foundation.

MOLIT is an independent research institution that aims to develop digital tools for precision oncology on an open source basis. The central development project in the MOLIT framework is the process-oriented information and communication platform VITU (Virtual Tumor Board), which supports oncological institutions across sites in the preparation, execution, and evaluation of molecular tumor boards [3]. This platform is used, among others, by the Zweckverband Personalisierte Medizin (ZvPM), in which seven cancer clinics at the Heilbronn, Ludwigsburg, Bruchsal, Stuttgart, and Esslingen sites are networked and conduct a joint Molecular Tumor Board. MOLIT also sees itself as an academic think tank that develops strategies for translational "bench to bedside to health care system" approaches (Fig. 11.1).

MOLIT employs ten permanent staff, including medical informatics specialists, molecular biologists, and physicians, as well as a larger number of working students from the fields of informatics and medicine on a regular basis. However, the development of the labor market in the health care sector is not only a challenge for hospitals, but also for research institutions such as the MOLIT Institute. It is not only nursing professionals who now have more career options, but also physicians and medical informatics specialists: these professional groups can currently choose the employer offering the best work conditions and the most interesting or meaningful projects. Indeed, more and more representatives of these professions are now looking for a work

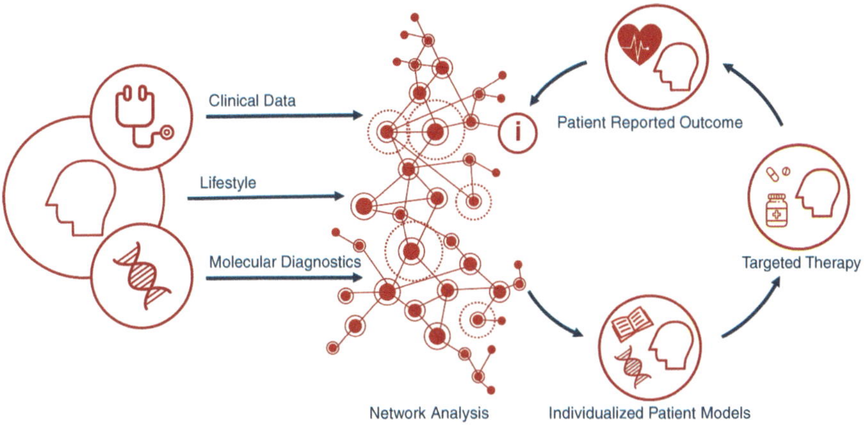

Fig. 11.1 From bench to bedside to health care system in precision oncology. (Source: author's own figure)

environment that offers them an alternative to the classic hierarchical and bureaucratic organizational constructs that still dominate the healthcare sector.

An additional challenge is that projects in the healthcare sector now require interdisciplinary teams to a large extent, as the areas of knowledge involved require qualifications that are too specialized for a single professional group to cover all necessary aspects. The intensive dovetailing of the disciplines of computer science, medicine, and molecular biology within individual project teams and the consistent establishment of an agile working method and leadership are therefore central pillars of the work environment and personnel development at MOLIT.

11.2 Personnel Development in an Agile Work Environment

Anyone who implements complex projects or develops innovative products needs organizational support and resources that allow flexibility and rapid learning in short iterations. Agile working methods, which are characterized by the constant alternation of short analysis phases with subsequent implementation phases, are a proven means for dealing with topics in which the various influencing factors are mutually dependent and the framework conditions can change quickly.

Agile methods accompanied by an agile work environment—triggered by technological change and digital transformation—are nowadays demanded by the majority of early career computer scientists. Even in the more traditional healthcare sector, including the clinical setting, digitalization, automation and the use of intelligent machines are recently on the rise, requiring, at least in certain disciplines, a work environment that deviates from fixed processes with rigid hierarchies and responsibilities. Ultimately, an agile work environment is not just about a change in mindset, but a fundamental cultural change that may have to be accompanied by far-reaching adjustments to the organizational structure in terms of working hours, work location, qualifications, collaboration, and completely new leadership models.

Agile Manifesto and Principles of Agility

Agility emerged in project management at the end of the 1990s as a countermovement to classic, hierarchically organized planning methods such as the waterfall model, with several sequential linear development phases not often leading to the desired success, especially in the IT environment. The lack of success could be attributed to rigid, long-term process planning and task structuring with intensive monitoring and control. Rigid control systems without flexibility are a hindrance to creative product development, and overly long development cycles prevent a rapid learning process triggered by user feedback.

Agility in the software environment was therefore a response initiated by software developers to numerous failed IT projects. In February 2001, a group of 17 well-known protagonists, including Jeff Sutherland and Ken Schwaber, the founders of the Scrumframework, published the so-called Agile Manifesto [4]. This programmatic declaration is considered one of the key milestones of the modern agile movement in that it takes up older management approaches to agility and generalizes and expands them with a view to project organization.

The **Agile Manifesto** comprises four core values:

- **Individuals and interactions** over processes and tools.
- **Working software** over comprehensive documentation.
- **Customer collaboration** over contract negotiation.
- **Responding to change** over following a plan.

The Agile Manifesto is supplemented by **12 principles of agility**:

1	Our highest priority is to satisfy the customer through early and continuous delivery of valuable software.
2	Welcome changing requirements, even late in development. Agile processes harness change for the customer's competitive advantage.
3	Deliver working software frequently, from a couple of weeks to a couple of months, with a preference to the shorter timescale.
4	Business people and developers must work together daily throughout the project.
5	Build projects around motivated individuals. Give them the environment and support they need, and trust them to get the job done.
6	The most efficient and effective method to conveying information to and within a development team is face-to-face conversation.
7	Working software is the primary measure of progress.
8	Agile processes promote sustainable development. The sponsors, developers, and users should be able to maintain a constant pace indefinitely.
9	Continuous attention to technical excellence and good design enhances agility.
10	Simplicity—the art of maximizing the amount of work not done—is essential.
11	The best architectures, requirements, and designs emerge from self-organizing teams.
12	At regular intervals, the team reflects on how to become more effective, then tunes and adjusts its behavior accordingly.

Agile Mindset

Although the principles from the agile manifesto originated in software development, they can be transferred to many aspects of collaboration in various industries. A study conducted by the Koblenz University of Applied Sciences under the direction of Ayelt Komus between 2012 and 2014 came to the conclusion that users of agile methods—both in software development and in projects without a particular IT connection—are significantly more successful and more satisfied within their roles than those who rely on classic project management [5].

The founders of MOLIT have consistently established the values and principles of the agile work methodology from the very beginning, thus promoting the development of an agile mindset among all team members. According to Hofert, this is "characterized by the ability to self-lead and self-update, basically the competence to 'update' at any time." An agile mindset thus represents a "logic of thought and action that focuses on the market and customers (...) and understands change as a permanent state" [6].

According to Jordan, this presupposes at the same time trusting that each individual wants to make a positive contribution within the scope of his or her abilities, that intellectually stimulating work is fun for employees, and that they thus give their best of their own free will. It is also assumed that people are happy to take on responsibility if they are provided with the appropriate framework and flexibility to make their own decisions. Pressure and control are replaced by freedom of decision, autonomous work, and extensive self-direction. The employees are thus responsible for finding the appropriate solutions within the set framework with the necessary freedom [7].

Agile Work Environment

In an agile work environment, work thus becomes more autonomous and less process-driven. Although neither the Agile Manifesto nor the 12 principles of agility contain an order or weighting, several aspects are of equal importance for team and personnel development as well as work organization in an agile work environment and are examined in more detail below:

Self-Management and Empowerment
All IT projects at MOLIT are carried out by self-organized teams. This also means that each team member is responsible to decide independently which tasks they will complete when and in what timeframe. Accordingly, the expectation for the team is that everyone is capable of self-management and takes responsibility for his part of the leadership.

Self-management is often seen as the opposite of hierarchy. Therefore, in agile teams a classic manager who is permanently present, defines and assigns tasks, grants budgets, and monitors and controls implementation, is unnecessary. However, this also requires that all team members are motivated to use their given flexibility in the interest of the customer and project progress and to take responsibility for their results.

The transfer of professional responsibility and decision-making authority (empowerment) also ensures that team members can act confidently despite ambivalent, complex, and rapidly changing information and situations [8]. The empowerment of MOLIT employees clearly goes beyond the mere delegation of a task. The respective area of responsibility is defined by the role each individual assumes in an agile team, which includes a defined set of rules and procedures. The role concepts in the agile setting also presuppose that no one is placed above the other, but that everyone in the organization is equal [6]. Empowerment is therefore associated with a high level of job satisfaction and has positive effects on employee performance and commitment, as well as employee retention [9]. Accordingly, the fluctuation of permanent employees has been minimal since MOLIT was founded—despite a highly competitive environment.

Interaction and Communication
Another focus of agile project management is also on exchange and interaction—both between team members and with customers or users. At MOLIT frequent but short meetings are therefore held within a development team for an efficient and effective transfer of information, usually face-to-face. Even with the close cooperation typical in an agile work environment, errors and conflicts cannot be completely avoided. Face-to-face communication is the most effective tool for an agile team to synchronize, share knowledge, critically analyze mistakes and their own performance, and make decisions. Direct face-to-face exchange in this regard can also take place in the virtual space without any problems, as the impact of the corona pandemic on the workplace showed. The communication in MOLIT's agile teams follows a clear structure and also includes the visualization of the work processes of all team members, e.g. with the help of a Scrum or Kanban board, which creates a high degree of transparency.

Reacting to Change and Interdisciplinary Cooperation
In classic project management, the first step is the comprehensive and complete clarification and definition of the requirements for the product. However, in the case of highly complex topics such as medicine, this is usually only possible with extreme effort. The agile approach, on the other hand, follows an iterative procedure in which the broad product vision is outlined at the beginning of the project, but the details of implementation only develop in the course of the project life cycle. This requires a high degree of adaptability from the team and a permanent willingness to work together with the customer or users and to take up their change requests and further developments even at short notice.

A decisive factor for the success of complex IT projects—especially in the healthcare sector—is the interdisciplinary collaboration of subject matter experts from a wide variety of areas with different expertise. Together they form a cross-functional team of experts, which means that all team members are not only specialists in their field, but also hold different functions within the project (e.g. IT architect, software developer, data analyst, product manager). The different perspectives promote the finding of constructive solutions to problems and new ideas. The users of the IT platform VITU developed by MOLIT, usually physicians and scientists working in oncology, therefore play a central role in the work of the agile teams and are actively involved in product development from the very beginning. This has already led to the formulation of several concrete requirements for VITU, such as the implementation of a search portal for clinical studies linked to the case registration for the molecular tumor board.

The regimented workflows in hospitals usually only allow for the direct integration of users into the project teams on a selective basis. However, it has proven essential for the successful implementation of a project that a project team has all the necessary specialist skills and disciplines available within its own ranks. Therefore, MOLIT's staff also includes physicians and molecular biologists who provide the important communication interface to the clinically active oncologists and who work closely together with the customers and the software developers as subject matter experts, process owners and testers throughout the entire duration of the project. In this way, possible conceptual errors can be averted and corrected at an early stage.

Strength Orientation and Reflection

Agile concepts are also about aligning with individual talents and strengths. MOLIT therefore enables its employees and working students to explicitly focus on topics and tasks that interest and inspire them. Further education and the possibility to acquire additional skills as well as the participation in scientific conferences are actively supported.

Not least because of this, MOLIT employees play a leading role in various national and international working committees such as the HL7 consortium, the HIGHMED consortium or the Consortium of Cancer Centres, and Oncological Work Groups in Baden-Wuerttemberg (ATO).

In order to increase creativity and innovation, MOLIT also propagates the composition of diverse teams within its IT projects, whose members have different qualities and expertise. Nevertheless, the focus in the development projects is not on the ability of the individual, but on the creativity and results of the entire team. This is another reason why the agile teams at MOLIT, which usually consist of 2–5 people depending on the project, go into retrospectives continuously and at fixed intervals. In doing so, they openly share feedback on what went well, what went poorly, and contribute ideas on how they can further optimize their collaboration in the future.

Employees from the fields of medicine and life sciences in particular are initially entering uncharted territory in an agile work environment. In hospitals, a hierarchical leadership and management style with top-down decisions and control is often still present. However, an agile approach cannot be learned in a workshop or from books alone. Instead, continuous trial and error, adaptation, and open dialogue between all team members are required, as well as a high degree of mutual trust and willingness to engage in conflict.

Agile Leadership

Leading at Eye Level

The role of managers is also important in the agile process. Particularly in cross-functional expert teams, a leadership style based on disciplinary power and control is no longer popular. Instead, managers must be prepared to relinquish responsibility since, in the agile context, they are no longer primarily supervisors and technical decision-makers, but rather those who provide the necessary infrastructure and drive personnel development. Accordingly, the founders of MOLIT do not interpret their understanding of leadership as a hierarchical model, but rather function primarily as coaches, moderators, designers, and role models, and provide orientation through the formulation of visions and goals.

At the same time, common challenges and values are defined in order to achieve the overall goal. "It is thought of as leadership from the side and no longer the ordering, managing, deciding and concretely prescribing the path, but the coaching, developing, moderating and supporting leadership that proclaims the goal at the end of the path or the vision beyond the horizon. (...) It gives impulses and challenges, as a partner and at eye level" [6].

Agile leadership also sees itself as a service provider for employees. The founders of MOLIT therefore relieve their expert teams of tasks that are not part of their core responsibilities. This also includes creating the appropriate framework in terms of budget, resources, infrastructure, marketing, and personnel development (servant leadership). Expert leadership roles in agile teams, however, are assumed by, for example, the product owner (mouthpiece of the customers/users, defines and prioritizes the requirements) and the scrum master (responsible for team building, conflict resolution and empowerment).

Further Development and Career Opportunities

With the definition of leadership as a role with clear tasks but without a disciplinary mandate, however, vertically oriented career paths typical in large companies or in hospital operations are eliminated in the agile work environment. On the one hand, this creates flat and permeable hierarchies, but on the other hand, classic career perspectives—and thus often the opportunities for a higher income—are lost.

"What do you attract young people with if it is not the next higher position? The tasks, the higher meaning of the activity and the goal—in other words, what drives people from within—are becoming more and more important" [6]. Intrinsic motivation is thereby primarily linked to three factors, which are explicitly addressed especially in the agile work environment [10]. In addition to the meaningfulness of a job, employees are motivated above all by autonomy, i.e. a certain degree of freedom to make decisions about their time, their scope of action, and the collaboration with others. Accordingly, working conditions with a high degree of flexibility have been created at MOLIT, which also means that employees largely decide for themselves where and when they work. Intrinsic motivation also arises from the opportunity to develop one's own competencies and to be able to contribute them in a goal-oriented manner. Therefore, MOLIT attaches great importance to the professional and

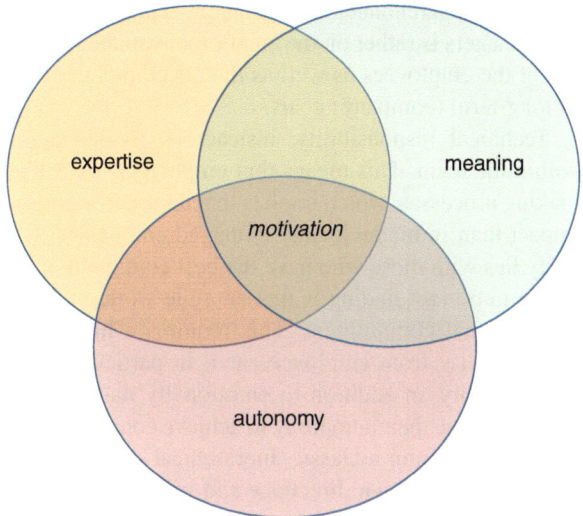

Fig. 11.2 Core factors of intrinsic motivation (modified by [10]). (Source: author's own figure)

personal development of the individual employees. The acquisition of new competencies can be achieved by trying out new roles or by deepening a role (e.g. subject matter expert in the development team, *Scrum Master, Product Owner*), but also by accompanying measures such as training or job shadowing. However, this further development deliberately does not follow a rigid, predefined *career path,* but is primarily oriented towards the interest and potential of the individual (Fig. 11.2).

11.3 Findings and Outlook

The digital transformation is currently leading to profound changes in many areas of work by breaking down existing thought patterns and structures—this also applies to large parts of the healthcare sector. New disciplines such as precision oncology are emerging and are accompanied by new tasks and requirements that make interdisciplinary working groups with physicians, molecular biologists, and medical informatics specialists a must in order to be able to determine the best possible therapy for the patient with the help of newly developed digital support systems.

However, these cross-functional interdisciplinary teams of experts with excellently trained and highly specialized employees require new working methods and work environments that differ from their classic hierarchical counterparts. An agile work environment like the one offered by the MOLIT Institute thus not only requires a change in the way individual employees think and work, but also requires a fundamental change in the organizational structure, the value proposition, and the understanding of leadership.

In contrast to the authoritarian leadership style, MOLIT provides leadership at eye level. This so-called lateral leadership means leadership without a superior function and a renunciation of content-related technical responsibility. The focus of the managers is rather on the creation of suitable working conditions and the coaching of the employees as well as the development of a strong vision and the setting of long-term (company) goals.

Technical responsibility, instead, is divided among various functional roles within the team. This means that employees are actively involved in the decision-making processes, which implies that their knowledge and experience have a greater impact than in hierarchically managed companies. Ultimately, technical responsibility lies with those who have the best command of the subject.

An important finding is that an agile work environment strengthens motivation and personal commitment. This requires a high degree of self-management and responsibility from employees and, in particular, their willingness to accept this responsibility, in addition to emotionally mature employees who can lead themselves and use their autonomy to achieve common goals. For supervisors, especially if they come from a classic, hierarchical organization, the essential task is to dispense with top-down directives and micromanagement and to focus their role on leadership and coaching.

The introduction and establishment of an agile work environment thus requires the willingness of all participants to consistently embrace the agile way of thinking and working. This is an indispensable, long-term learning process. In human resources development, it is critical to anchor the agile work mentality within the company. It should be built into all levels of organizational development and across all employee levels, from entry-level to leadership. In addition to a needs-based orientation of employee qualification, this also includes supporting managers in breaking away from a hierarchical understanding of their roles and instead acquiring competencies that enable teams to work autonomously. Another challenge for personnel development is to offer employees in an agile work environment a substitute for the classic career path. How do you reward technical and methodological expertise when you work in flat hierarchies without upward mobility? In order to attract and retain the technical specialists required in today's agile environment, it will be critical to develop alternative compensation and career models.

References

1. Wagner S, Serve H. Digitale Medizin in der Onkologie: clinical decision support, real world data und patient involvement. Dtsch Med Wochenschr. 2019;144:430–4.
2. Medizininformatik Initiative. 2020. https://www.medizininformatik-initiative.de/de/konsortien/highmed. Accessed 15 Sep 2020.
3. Fegeler C, Zsebedits D, Bochum S, Finkeisen D, Martens UM. Implementierung eines IT-gestützten molekularen Tumorboards in der Regelversorgung. Forum. 2018;33:322–8.
4. Manifesto for Agile Software Development. 2001. https://agilemanifesto.org/iso/de/manifesto.html. Accessed 15 Sep 2020.
5. Komus A, Kamlowski W. Gemeinsamkeiten und Unterschiede von Lean Management und agilen Methoden. Working Paper des BPM-Labors Hochschule Koblenz; 2014.

6. Hofert S. Agiler führen. Wiesbaden: Springer Fachmedien Wiesbaden; 2016.
7. Jordan D. Agiles Arbeiten: Das Wesentliche kurz erklärt. Kindle Ausgabe; 2020.
8. Nägele U, Vogler P. Personalentwicklung goes Agile. Hamburg: Tredition; 2020.
9. Seibert SE, Wang G, Courtright SH. Antecedents and consequences of psychological and team empowerment in organizations: a meta-analytic review. J Appl Psychol. 2011;96:981–1003.
10. Pink DH. Drive: the surprising truth about what motivates us. New York: Riverhead Books; 2009.

TeamProcessPerformance (TPP) in the OR with Gung Ho

Thomas Roehrssen and Klaus Wohlmeiner

12.1 Hard and Soft Success Factors of the OR Organization

The operating theater minute is becoming increasingly performance-dense, cost-intensive, and scarce. And OR process management is increasingly becoming a key success factor for the hospital. But the situation in hospital ORs is often problematic. Ohneiser ([1], p. 2) describes quite vividly the day-to-day problems that are evident in many hospitals and that are compounded by their interaction:

▶ "In many hospitals, the operating room business is disorganized and has gaps, (...). Physicians, nurses and OR technical assistants often complain about the waiting times they spend in a prepared operating room because either the surgeon, the anesthesiologist, the patient are not yet there or the patient's examination results are missing. This can collapse an OR schedule for the entire day. Operating rooms remain unused, overtime can occur at the end of the day, employee dissatisfaction grows, and idle time and personnel costs are incurred. The unwritten rule in (...) ORs indicates that each surgeon occupies 'his' room and determines at what time this occurs. The rest of the staff in the OR stand by. In addition to starting on time, efficient changeover times during the course of the day are essential for the economic provision of services. The prerequisites are exact scheduling and the interlocking of a multitude of processes. This complexity makes the changeover process susceptible to disruptions. Here, an intelligent and transparent process structure is needed within and between the professions involved." ([1], p. 2).

T. Roehrssen (✉)
Roehrssen Consult GmbH, Osnabrück, Germany
e-mail: tr@roehrssen-consult.de

K. Wohlmeiner
Deutsches Rotes Kreuz, Seniorenzentrum Henry Dunant gGmbH, Warstein, Germany
e-mail: Klaus.wohlmeiner@seniorenzentrum-warstein.drk.de

© The Author(s), under exclusive license to Springer Nature Switzerland AG 2022
R. Tewes (ed.), *Innovative Staff Development in Healthcare*,
https://doi.org/10.1007/978-3-030-81986-6_12

In the meantime, some of the key **success factors of an effective OR organization have** already been clearly identified:

- The establishment of a **professional OR management** (OR manager and OR coordinator with clear leadership profile and comprehensive authority to issue directives).
- A strategic and demand-oriented **service and capacity planning in the rooms**—without blanket territorial claims of individual clinics.
- The development of a **meaningful operation controlling and reporting**, in which figures are not only reported, but target-oriented measures are derived from them.
- The mastery of the **pre-stationary and pre-operative planning processes** in the outpatient departments with optimally used IT planning tools.
- Ensuring a **punctual start of surgery on the day of surgery** with synchronization of the processes in the area of clinics, wards, and the operating theater.
- The systematic analysis and treatment of **organizational and behavioral causes of changeover time delays as well as the introduction of a precise call-off management with the setting of a minute-precise start of the subsequent operation** (t_0).
- The implementation of a **binding system of rules** (statutes, service regulations, rules of procedure, etc.) including the consistent handling of critical deviations.

It is striking that in almost all OR projects in the hospital sector, the soft skills in the OR were rarely recognized as success factors and analyzed in their depth structure, although a lack of employee satisfaction and high sickness rates in OR areas have always been an issue and although everyday practice in the OR proves how perfectly the workflow functions with an OR team with team spirit. In our new opinion, an optimal OR organization is only present when the "spark has jumped over to the operating room." This "spark" lies in a special team dynamic that is supported by suitable framework conditions but cannot be evoked by organizational structures and processes alone.

In the microcosm of the operating theater, the organizational philosophy of a hospital can be seen "pars pro toto." But which organizational philosophies shape the hospital yesterday, today, and in the future?

12.2 Paradigm Shift: Organizational Philosophies in Historical Change

We believe that in the current upheavals in the OR organization, we must once again pay much more attention to cultural factors. In this context, the values and basic attitudes as well as the self-image, role expectations, and organizational philosophies in the minds of managers are of decisive importance. The change in the organizational philosophy of hospitals over the last 30 years can be described ideally in 4 stages:

- **The person-centered hospital 1.0 "Chief culture" (traditional organization)**
  In stage 1.0, a person-centered expert organization with authoritarian-directive leadership in medicine, nursing, and administration prevails. Chief physicians, nursing directors, and hospital managers dispense with defined strategies, structures, and processes. They lead by authority or personal charisma. As "assisting masters of their profession," they initiate, steer, and control the daily routine in their area. There is a "rule of man"— the values and rules depend on the person and change with the bosses who represent them. There is no delegation of tasks and responsibilities that cannot be personally withdrawn at any time. In the operating room, the surgeon is the "hero of the room." Some hospital organizations today still show relics from this time.
- **The responsibility-structured hospital 2.0 "Management by Objectives and Delegation" (modern structural organization).**
  In this stage, the principles of target agreement ("Management by Objectives") and delegation ("Management by Delegation") prevail from the top of the pyramid via the individual management levels downwards. The individual functions and areas of responsibility in clinical operations are defined and aligned with target agreements, regulations on tasks and competencies, as well as rules of procedure and business distribution plans. The "rule of man" phase now transitions to the new era of the "rule of law"; the rules are now above the managers. At this stage, responsibility is increasingly shifting from the top levels of management to the second and third levels of management. Middle management is finally being discovered as a previously "invisible high performer." Area, department, ward, function, team, and group leaders in nursing and administration, as well as section leaders and senior physicians in the medical service, are given their own profiled areas of delegation and competence that must be respected. Leadership is no longer simply accepted, but must prove itself. Leadership performance programs permeate the hospital. In the OR area, this phase sees the emergence of independent leadership responsibility of OR managers and OR coordinators with clearly defined organizational authority to issue directives on behalf of the management. The OR duty roster becomes the law in the OR.
- **The process-oriented hospital 3.0 "Quality management and process responsibility" (modern process organization)**
  With the focus on the external legal, economic, and professional requirements as well as the demands of patients, referring physicians, legislators, and cost units, a quality management system is developed in this phase that is aligned with external regulations and standards. Compliance as adherence to the numerous legal and operational requirements is defined as a new basic attitude that emphasizes social responsibility over and above loyalty to one's own company. In recent years, the focus has shifted from

normative quality management regulations (Hospital 3.1) to dynamic clinical process management (Hospital 3.2). Process maps and process documentation are created; clinical processes are analyzed, optimized, audited, and evaluated. New job descriptions and functions such as "process coordinators" and "case managers" complement the previous structural organization. In this phase, new control functions are also created in the pre-operative and pre-stationary outpatient departments with regard to the administrative and organizational planning and control of surgery, diagnostics, and admission management. In the outpatient departments, planning offices and centers are created for the planning of surgery and outpatient appointments. These planning functions can be considered "pre-operative schedulers," while the OR coordinator is the "dispatcher" responsible for the actual implementation of the OR program in the daily schedule, including the adjustment of sequences and room assignments.

In this phase, the OR coordinator continues to develop from supervisor and "trouble-shooter" to process manager with the goal of implementing efficient and reliable processes.

- **The postmodern hospital 4.0 "Agile teams and self-organization" (postmodern hybrid organization)**

Currently, the hospital landscape is once again undergoing radical change. The complexity of hospital organization with almost unmanageable process maps and interfaces continues to increase. The division of labor in the interaction of numerous professional groups, areas, and functions that must organize themselves around these processes is becoming increasingly differentiated. A process that has just been newly analyzed, optimized, and described must be called into question again within a short time due to new requirements. In many clinics, a confusing number of process documents develops, which have to be updated constantly. Quality management and clinical process management are facing a collapse of over-control and the end of digital process manuals is approaching. Added to this are the expectations of the new generations Y and Z, who no longer feel comfortable in the tight corset of classic management, structure, and process approaches.

In Hospital 4.0, only a few trigger processes are identified around which semi-autonomous teams organize themselves. The success of their work can be experienced—here and now—and is also transparent in simple key figures, which we call short-cut process goals. Freedom and organizational self-control are combined with a new team spirit. In upper and middle management, a value-oriented management style with a flat hierarchy and a high level of participation will prevail. At the grassroots level, the self-organization of semi-autonomous teams (hybrid organization) will develop. In the operation theater, OR managers and OR coordinators will focus more on designing and maintaining optimal framework conditions for the self-direction of clinic and OR teams as well as implementing new basic attitudes and lived values in the culture of the rooms.

For the new era of hospital organization, new views of culture, process design, teamwork, and leadership emerge, which we will concretize in the next chapter.

12.3 The Postmodern Hospital: Gung Ho, Self-Organization, Generations YZ, and Hybrid Organization

The story of the successful manager Peggy Sinclair, who achieved a turnaround in 1 year at the headquarters of an American corporation with the help of Gung Ho, a new team approach, serves as the basis of our postmodern organizational philosophy [2]. "Gung Ho" is the rallying cry of a particularly enthusiastic and high-performing U.S. Marine team that awakens team spirit.

The Gung Ho approach is based on three central core elements:

1. **Meaningful work ("Why"): Personal motives and missions, attitudes, and values that really make sense!**
   The first and most important question for the members of a team is the question "Why do I work here?" the question about the meaning and purpose of one's own activity in the company and in the department.
2. **Simple specifications ("what"): Tasks and rules, goals, and processes with plenty of room for maneuver!**
   The first, meaningful question is now followed by the second, structure-building question. As in a football team, it is now clarified who plays in which position, which rules apply to the team, and which results are to be achieved. Some standard situations still need to be practiced, but the "game" is then completely free, intuitive, and productive within this framework.
3. **Direct feedback ("how"):** Cheering with demand, promote, feedback.
   Enthusiastic teams thrive on timely feedback on success as well as daily recognition of the individual. In successful teams, team members challenge and affirm each other. They cheer each other on and celebrate their good results. The team establishes simple metrics by which team performance can be measured. And the team establishes feedback rituals in which individual performance, results, and skills are valued and potential areas for improvement are identified.

In view of the increasing shortage of skilled workers and current requirements in the recruitment and retention of new generations, the change in corporate culture in the direction of self-organization, agile teams, and Gung Ho is of great importance. We had just got used to Generation Y with their demand for "work-life-balance," and now the new, nimble Generation Z, born in 1995 or later, is arriving. They are being handed over to the hospital business by their helicopter parents, some of whom are overprotective. They want to work openly, honestly, transparently, freely, and uncontrollably—in self-organized teams and in Internet-based working-out-loud circles where they share their knowledge and experience with others. They live in at least three worlds: first in their private world, then still at their second home "on the job," and third as "digital natives" in the social network communities with which they spend a lot of time during the day. They are flexible and no longer feel such a high level of loyalty to their company compared to other generations. They live in a world of changing social groups and networks. For this generation in particular, we need new corporate worlds in which self-organization and digitalization are combined with a new style of leadership. Agile teams also need leadership, but a different kind than employees in peak-hierarchical companies.

After analyzing several successful business organizations of the postmodern era Frederic Laloux set out the new principles:

▶ "Postmodern organizations retain the managerial hierarchical structures of modern organizations, but pass the majority of decision-making to workers and employees, who can thus make far-reaching decisions without seeking management approval. The people who are directly involved with the demands of daily work know best the myriad of small problems in the workflow. Therefore, they should be trusted to find better solutions than experts who look at the situation from afar. (…). Implementing decentralization and empowerment in a large organization is difficult. Senior and middle management must share power with all employees and give up some of their control. (…). Employees are trusted to make the right decisions, guided by a set of shared values rather than thick rulebooks and agreements" ([3], p. 32f.).

In postmodern companies, hybrid organizations are gaining ground. These organizations are clearly structured at the top and middle management levels—but with rather flat hierarchies and opportunities for participation. At the grassroots, they are structured differently, namely within a defined set of rules, flexible, free, and self-organized. As with a hybrid engine, the primacy is initially on one engine (team under power = self-organization). If the primary engine is exposed to extreme demands and comes to a standstill or no longer has sufficient energy, then the secondary engine must step in (leadership provides fuel = systemic-transformational leadership). The secondary motor offers support and withdraws when the primary self-rotation is working again.

12.4 TeamProcessPerformance (TPP) in the Operating Theater

Based on our project experiences in recent years, we have now applied the approach of the postmodern hybrid organization to the hospital operating room.

▶ "TeamProcessPerformance is an answer to the meaningless, individualized and rigid service delivery found in many clinics, nursing areas and functional departments in modern hospital cultures. TPP supports a meaningful, team-oriented and agile work organization that emphasizes the basic motives of the individual, promotes his or her team integration and enables flexible action in the turbulent daily hospital routine" ([4], p. 47).

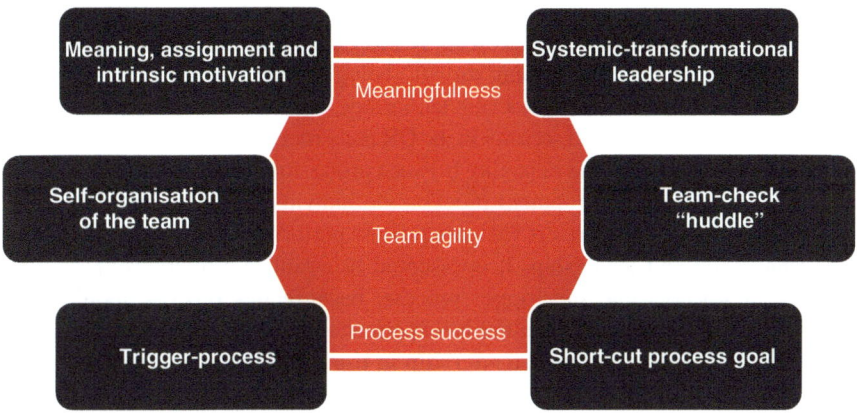

Fig. 12.1 TeamProcessPerformance Hexagon

In doing so, we also want to make it clear that team building in the OR should not simply happen in a group-dynamic manner disconnected from the organizational process. On the contrary: OR teams get their meaning and mission from the objectives of the OR in connection with their personal motives. Therefore, their soft skills are not to be developed free-floating in the group's own communication and relationship space, but are to be aligned with the operation process in terms of content. The OR process can be used to measure meaning for the individual as well as corporate success and quality in patient care.

We use our TeamProcessPeformance (TPP) to show how to model an appropriate development process using a hexagon (Fig. 12.1):

We divide the TeamProcessPerformance into three axes: **sense-making, team agility, and process success** ([4], p. 47).

On the first level lies the **creation of meaning**, the question of "Why?" of the activities in the OR. All activities are driven by the basic mission of the organization and the commitment of the individuals. Systemic-transformational leadership promotes the intrinsic motivation of individual employees as well as the spirit and self-organization of agile teams.

On the second level lies **team agility**, which on the one hand is characterized by a high level of team responsibility and self-organization and on the other hand is supported communicatively by team checks, which we call "huddles."

On the third level lies **process success** as the factual result of meaningful work, professional leadership, and agile teamwork. We focus on a very small number of processes, which we call "trigger processes," and we measure the success of trigger processes using immediately available process metrics, which we call "short-cut process goals."

1. **Meaning, mission, and intrinsic motivation**

    The basis for good team performance is first of all an intrinsic motivation of each individual team member, which results from reflection and identification with the task ("I recognize a meaning in my work and accept my task in the OR"). The motivational structures of individual team members on which TeamProcessPerformance can be built can be very diverse such as experiencing meaningful work, enjoying good quality in work, performing strongly, being independent and being allowed to take responsibility, enjoying social relationships in work, experiencing team cohesion, getting structure and security in the OR daily routine, experiencing good cooperation, commitment, and reliability between professional groups, etc.

Within a team development process, the individual motivations are worked out, reflected upon as drivers for team process performance and supported by the organization and leadership. It is essential to establish a relationship between these motivators and the trigger process, because this process should make deeper sense to everyone and not be experienced as alien.

2. **Systemic-transformational leadership in the operating theater**

With the new demands on self-organized teams, the role of the manager is also changing significantly.

> ▶ "The ability of teams to work is neither a matter of course, nor can it be achieved solely through a differentiated clarification of roles and a detailed set of rules for the individual process steps. What is needed is a sensitivity that goes beyond this for the implicit group dynamics that are always taking place. The almost always observable primacy of attention on the factual dimensions (...) often leaves the reality-determining, because emotionally particularly effective social dynamics in the blind spot of those responsible (meaning personal grievances, unequal distribution of influence, taboo subject areas, etc.)" ([5], p. 17).

In our view, the management literature of recent decades has suffered greatly from the fact that little account has been taken of the findings of the basic science of psychology, which is over 100 years old. In the future, we expect to see leadership approaches that are more evidence-based on the scientific foundations of psychology. Managers can be **supported** via training and coaching in the development of a psychologically based **systemic-transformational leadership approach.**

The systemic-transformational leadership style is based on four central principles:

(a) *Focusing on values, basic attitudes, and self-motivation*

The manager supports employees in finding their own meaning in their work. They promote the development of intrinsic motivation (self-motivation) and avoid, as far as possible, simply controlling desired behaviors by means of orders or external incentives and sanctions, because they are then not very sustainable.

Employees' work behavior is not simply confirmed or corrected superficially (praise and reprimand). Above all, the underlying basic attitude is worked out and—if necessary—questioned. Criticism talks are always connected with root cause analyses in the deep structure of the personality—its motives, competences, and views ("root treatment").

(b) *Emotionally intelligent leadership*
   The psychological concept of emotional intelligence developed in the 1990s (see [6]) should be understood and lived by leaders in postmodern organizations. Emotional intelligence includes five basic competencies:
   - **Internal self-awareness (introspection)**
     Emotionally intelligent leaders are always aware of their own bodily sensations (somatic markers), feelings (spontaneously felt overall evaluation), and thoughts (automated self-dialogues) in a parallel stream of consciousness complementary to external observation.
   - **Influencing one's own emotions (regulation)**
     Emotionally intelligent managers use their self-awareness as a basis for influencing themselves. They can control their own strong impulses, constructively change negative attitude patterns and ways of thinking (cognitive reinterpretation), and positively influence their own mood.
   - **Using emotions in dialogue in a targeted manner**
     Emotionally intelligent leaders can authentically bring in their (regulated) emotions and use them in a targeted manner to professionally manage the situation.
   - **Empathy**
     Emotionally intelligent leaders can grasp a person well internally via direct perception of their counterpart (unconscious mirroring of expression) or via perspective taking and cognitive reconstruction (Theory of Mind).
   - **Successful relationship building**
     Emotionally intelligent leaders use their empathic abilities to shape a dialogue in a recipient-oriented way. They hit and touch the inner world of the counterpart in the right places with their messages and thus achieve desired results.
(c) *Changing mental realities and cultures*
   A systemic-transformational leader knows that all people (including herself, of course) construct their own world in their heads. Views and convictions that have grown over many years provide security and are not simply thrown overboard. Rhetorical persuasion and behavioral instruction are of little help in changing cultures that are deeply embedded in the mind. That is why systemic-transformational leaders work with leadership and dialogue methods that challenge, question, and sustainably change stubborn views, beliefs, and attitudes.
(d) *Supporting the autonomous scope of action of the teams*
   Systemic-transformational leaders only intervene sparingly in the day-to-day business in an operational and regulatory way. They design the organizational framework for the autonomous scope of action of the teams and concentrate in their leadership work less on the factual and organizational control of the work and more on the motivation, basic attitude, and personality development of the individual as well as the relationship dynamics in the

team. They provide help for self-help and, as far as possible, do not allow speech delegation. The focus is primarily on emotional-motivational support as well as conflict management in the OR. Systemic-transformational leaders in the OR ensure that the operation theater teams see and tackle problems as common problems.

3. **Self-organization of the team**

   The self-organization of a team is a central key to success in hospital organization 4.0. Important characteristics of self-organization in the OR are:
   (a) Decentralization of planning and control processes in the OR—away from OR management and OR coordination to the OR room team.
   (b) Increased individual responsibility in the operating room team related to the performance of tasks and the achievement of goals.
   (c) Reduction of long information and coordination processes or time-consuming consultations with executives and functions outside the room.
   (d) Agile adaptation of the OR daily structure and OR procedures to the constantly changing requirements and turbulence in the OR daily program.
   (e) Increased job satisfaction through increased personal process control, team integration, and motivation to succeed.

   The following tasks are delegated to the operating room team:
   (a) Brief morning discussion of the OR program (team check 1/"huddle")—clarification of essential aspects in the work preparation for individual ORs/ if necessary also fine-tuning of the sequence and procedure in consultation with the physicians responsible for planning in the surgical clinic(s), anesthesia, and/or the surgeons to ensure optimal professional implementation and utilization in the OR; the proposed fine-tuning of sequences and procedures in the ORs are reported to the OR coordinator or coordinated with him;
   (b) Optimal integration of follow-up messages and emergencies in dialogue with the OR coordinator;
   (c) Implementation of the OR call management (call patient/operator) and the waiting time documentation in the operating room using the whiteboard (trigger process);
   (d) Controlled intervention in all secondary processes influencing the trigger process, such as patient preparation, patient transport, management in the holding area, airlock and recovery room, induction and discharge, room cleaning and preparation, storage, central sterilization, etc.;
   (e) Brief discussion shortly before the end of the service (team check 2/"huddle")—feedback on the surgery day with feedback on successes and potential for optimization; short outlook on the next surgery day.

   A team check is the equivalent of a huddle in American football. A huddle can take place at any time of the day. A huddle has already been tested in hospitals for the ward area and presented in the literature. However, the huddle can be implemented just as well in central emergency rooms and operating theaters.

   The concept of the huddle comes from American football. Before each play, the players briefly put their heads together (…) and discuss their tactics. The scoreboard provides clues: Is the team on track to win the game? How much time is left to influence the result? The key here is to look ahead together as a team, communicate purposefully and derive concrete actions. In a hospital setting, this means that a treatment team meets several times a day for a brief exchange. The term "huddle" is important to show how this differs from other meetings: A huddle is not a rapport or a meeting. And: you don't sit, you stand. This speeds things up.

The aim is to obtain an overview of what is happening based on key figures in a short time (maximum 7 min) together as an interprofessional team. The daily workload, deviations from the standard and special events are discussed. The huddleboard serves as a "scoreboard." If the performance in an area is not right or problems arise, concrete countermeasures are defined. "If a problem cannot be solved by the team within 24 h, it is escalated to the next management level" ([7], p. 98).

In a postmodern OR organization, team checks ("huddles") serve continuous team development and process improvement.

At the end of the OR day, the team gathers in front of the whiteboard in the room for a final maneuver feedback. The following tasks arise for this team check at the end of the OR day (final huddle):

(a) Evaluation of process efficiency based on delta deviations documented on the whiteboard between t_0 and t_1;
(b) Differentiated feedback to appreciate and recognize special individual contributions as well as overall team performance;
(c) Discussion of possible solutions and suggestions for improvement for the next OP days including agreement and delegation of appropriate measures;
(d) Identify problems that could not be resolved independently within the team within the last 24 h; report to OR management/coordination.

4. **Trigger process**

According to our definition, a trigger process is a process that is at the center of many other processes that are triggered and influenced by it.

The trick is to work out the appropriate trigger process on the basis of a joint analysis and to define it as simply as possible.

We have identified the trigger process of an operating room team as the process of precise planning, retrieval, and deviation documentation of a follow-up OR, which influences many processes in the OR and is a central aspect of change time optimization (Fig. 12.2). This process is described in the flow, responsibilities, and applicable rules. That's it!

The process is described as follows:

The operating room team determines when the next operation is to begin to the minute in an interprofessional room commitment (surgeon, anesthetist, operating room functional nursing, operating room anesthesia nursing) while an operation is still in progress, with an appropriate lead time for the next operation. The start is not the incision, but the first intervention of the surgical team on the patient after release by the anesthesiologist (e.g. positioning with the presence of the surgical team in the room). This is the planned start of the follow-up operation, which we call t_0 and which is documented on a whiteboard in the room,

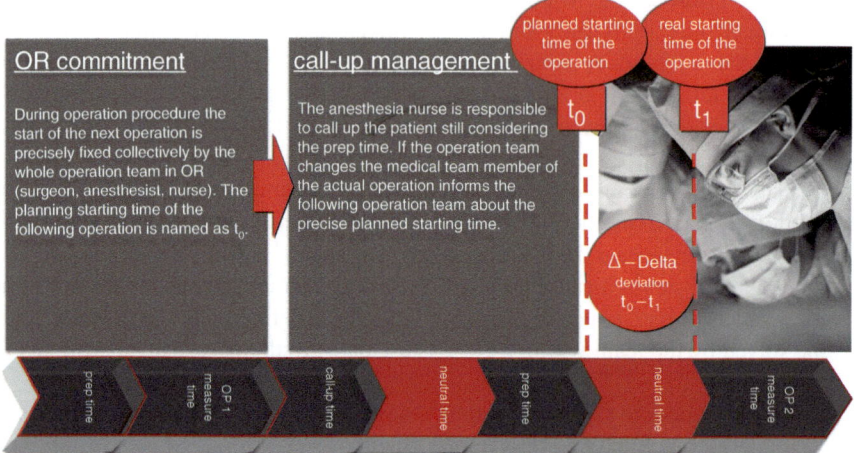

Fig. 12.2 Precise call-up management ([4], p. 50)

clearly visible to all. Call-off management then focuses on this point in time. Other preparatory processes are focused on this meticulously defined point in time. All other processes associated with room commitment and call-off management are not described (e.g. patient preparation, patient transport, holding area and lock management, induction and discharge, room cleaning and preparation, storage, etc.) in order to increase the free scope of action of agile OR teams. The determination of a time t_0 is not necessarily about the necessity of a precision landing, but rather about a precise planning parameter as an orientation, in which professional or "natural" fluctuations are accepted, but organization- and behavior-related absences are to be critically scrutinized.

5. **Short-Cut Process Objective**

   According to our definition, a short-cut process objective is a precise and measurable result of a process, which is measured directly after completion of the process using a simple key figure. The process objective is associated with a timely evaluation and motivation for success for the team. We have defined the punctual start of a follow-up operation as a short-cut process objective, and in doing so we work with only one key figure: the deviation (delta) between the planned start of a follow-up operation t_0 and the real start of the follow-up operation t_1.

   The operating room team documents the planning and realization of the short-cut process goal as well as the scope (in minutes) and the reasons for deviations (coded according to defined waiting time categories) on a whiteboard in the room. This gives the team a high and timely daily overview of the short-cut process goals and the related successes from OR to OR (Fig. 12.3).

   The systematic evaluation of the deviations is used for further process optimization in the OR. In the process, the deviation categories are filtered out that are more likely to be regarded as professional or "natural" fluctuations (e.g. incorrect estimation of OR duration, professionally necessary changes during the OR,

Fig. 12.3 Whiteboard system in OR ([4], p. 51)

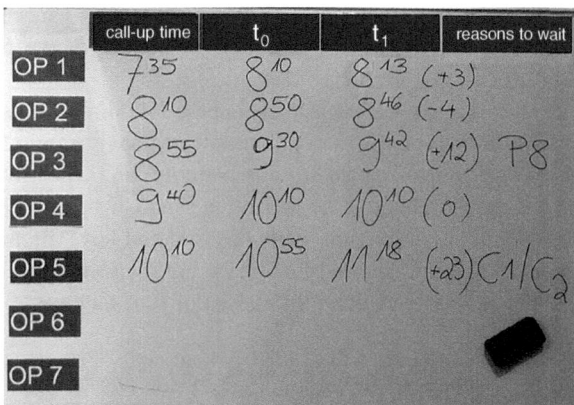

complications related to OR/anesthesia, etc.), so that ultimately only behavioral and organizational deviations are analyzed (e.g. delays in the area of inpatient patient preparation and transport, sluice congestion, inadequate patient preparation, missing or incomplete documents, waiting for anesthetist, waiting for OR nursing, waiting for surgeon, etc.).

In the agile OR team organization, problems are identified and analyzed promptly; joint approaches to solutions and measures are sought, planned, and agreed directly in the room (Plan). These are then implemented by individuals on their own responsibility (Do), then jointly reviewed (Check) and, if they work, incorporated into the routine (Act). Ideally, small Plan-Do-Check-Act cycles in the theater rooms, supported by huddles, occur repeatedly in the day-to-day business of the OR. The joint analysis and planning should not be too complicated and time-consuming; the implementation often corresponds more to a quick trial or a manageable spontaneous experiment ("Do it, try it, fix it"). A successful organization thus appears so to say emergently from the many small improvements in daily teamwork at the grassroots level.

12.5 The Subjective Success of TeamProcessPerformance

The short-cut process target as an objective parameter of changeover time optimization can be evaluated and measured well after the trigger process is well established. We have already been able to prove this in our projects on the basis of resulting productivity figures (in particular the reduction of changeover times).

But how do we measure subjective success from the perspective of the surgical teams? To this end, we have developed initial approaches based on the concept of "Core Self-Evaluations." This psychological concept was developed by Judge, Locke, and Durham at the end of the 1990s [8].

In our opinion, the success of OP optimization in terms of organizational psychology can be well measured by a characteristic that has been scientifically proven in relevant studies over the last 10 years to be a causal factor for psychological well-being, health, motivation, performance, and success in a professional context: the four-dimensional Central Self-Evaluations/Core Self-Evaluations—known as CSE for short ([9], p. 316 ff.).

The CSE approach assumes that the four dimensions are rather stable personality and attitude patterns in employees ("personality traits"). However, we assume that such basic attitudes and attitude patterns can be positively changed through the targeted development of organizational and team environments as well as through leadership, qualification, and coaching and have already measured these effects in relation to qualification measures using relevant questionnaires [10].

The core self-evaluations consist of four factors:

- **Locus of control**
  "I am at the center of my worklife and have control over it"
  A high level of dissatisfaction and demotivation arises in particular when the employee locates the locus of control outside of him/herself, i.e. he/she experiences him/herself as being determined by others rather than as a victim in relation to influential persons, critical events or problem situations in his/her work environment (external locus of control). A positive processing results when the affected person anchors the place of control in himself (self-control). He then sees that he can make decisions, take responsibility, and act in a self-determined manner (internal locus of control).
- **Perceived self-efficacy**
  "I can master requirements at the workplace with my competence or the social resources available to me."
  Dissatisfaction arises when the individual feels that he is no longer able to successfully cope with workplace problems on his own because of his ability and the resources in his work environment. Positive processing results when he is convinced that he has skills and opportunities in his work to cope successfully with problems. This can also happen through recourse to resources in the team or leadership.
- **Self-esteem**
  "I accept myself as I am and don't complain."
  When dealing with critical events at work, it is also important whether the person concerned is at peace with him/herself and has adequate self-acceptance. If the affected person's self-esteem is too hurt, his or her activities tend to focus on processing the hurt and compensatory self-esteem stabilization, rather than on successfully coping with the situation at work.
- **Emotional stability**
  "I am genuinely calm even in critical work situations."
  Emotional disturbance, lability, and neuroticism (fears, nervousness, worries, depressiveness, fear of the future, etc.) considerably limit successful stress and crisis management at work. Those who manage to recognize destructive emotional processes at the outset and to change them positively in crises by means of self-observation and self-control can concentrate more on coping with problems at work (see emotional intelligence).

We assume that it can be proven via surveys in the OR that an internal control conviction and a positive self-efficacy conviction among employees can be significantly improved with the introduction of TeamProcessPerformance. Furthermore, we believe that the self-esteem and emotional stability of employees are supported by a systemic-transformational leadership approach.

12.6 Implementation of the TeamProcessPerformance (TPP) in the OR

The implementation of TeamProcessPerformance within an OR initially starts with a kick-off workshop involving the medical, nursing, and support staff in the OR of a hospital. The workshop agenda focuses primarily on the values, rules, and self-organization of the operating room team:

- **Introduction to TeamProcessPerformance**
  How will self-organized teams change the hospital in the coming years?
- **Input: Presentation of the project goals**
  What goals are pursued by corporate management and OR management in increasing the self-organization of OR teams?
- **Moderation: My motivation and standards**
  What drives me personally? What values do I think the hall team should be guided by?
- **Input: Self-organized teams and processes**
  Team responsibility of the semi-autonomous operating room team, trigger process, short-cut process goal, whiteboard, and huddle.
- **Moderation: Development of a common set of rules**
  According to which rules do we want to work, inform ourselves and communicate in the room.
- **Commitment and implementation of team process performance**
  Goals, agreements, measures (action plan).

12.7 Project Results and Conclusion

In our OR projects over the past 30 years, we have primarily emphasized the aforementioned structural and process aspects of OR management. Ultimately, we have identified certain trigger processes that have a major influence on OR efficiency. However, we also found that although productivity can be significantly increased through appropriate process management, this did not lead to higher employee satisfaction in all ORs and ultimately the sustainability of the improvements in the long term was always questionable. This was, of course, an important learning experience for us.

For some time now, we have been working on the new TeamProcessPerformance approach, which integrates "hard" process factors and "soft" culture factors in the OR in a practical way. The operating room team becomes the "nucleus" of the OR workflow. Clinical process management is simplified to the maximum; it is the responsibility of agile teams. The team's success can be concretely measured from OR to OR by "hard" short-cut process goals. We have already been able to evaluate the optimization of the "hard" process factors via the trigger process and the short-cut process goal (reduction of the delta deviation between t_0 and t_1) through surveys.

The average waiting time per operation for each subsequent operation in an operating theater, for example, could be demonstrably reduced by an average of almost 10 min over a period of 2 months. In addition, in some ORs even higher values related to the first operation on the operation day result if synchronization problems in the clinical processes are also processed together. In total, this results in considerable optimization potential when extrapolated over the year (10 min × average number of operations per room/per day × number of rooms × 220 working days). Our evaluations show that the central factors for waiting times in the OR "Waiting for surgeon" and "Calling and transporting the patient" can be significantly reduced through team process performance. Just the introduction of a measurement of the short-cut process goals already leads to an effect from the first day, because through the recording and transparency, the OR participants automatically change their behavior in the direction of an improved self- and team organization. This so-called Hawthorne effect, known from experimental psychology, suggests that a considerable optimization potential already occurs with the start of the measurement, which cannot even be recorded. A corresponding measurement of this immediate onset effect is only possible if a reliable waiting time recording has already taken place in clinical IT in the past, which can also be evaluated according to comparable criteria. However, this is rather rare.

In the future, we also want to measure soft skills in the OR projects more precisely. We see the "Core Self-Evaluations" (CSE) developed from organizational psychology as measurable success factors for a satisfied, productive, and healthy employee culture in the OR as central factors of personality and culture that need to be measured. We are still in the very early stages of implementing a new team culture in the OR. The greatest challenges lie in building trust between the individual functions and professional groups in the OR, as well as in establishing room-related regular communication in the hectic daily routine of the OR. The daily structure in the OR offers little room for interprofessional short meetings ("huddles"), but these are essential and indispensable. We have learned that in the implementation of team process performance projects, hospital management must create a high level of acceptance among central managers in advance with regard to the goals and basic measures before a project can be started. Possible obstacles and resistance to change should be discussed in detail in advance and commitment should be ensured by means of a joint project contract between the managers.

References

1. Ohneiser A. Clinical structure and process optimization—change time optimization with precise call-off management and strategic OR capacity planning using the example of Ev. Krankenhauses Lippstadt gGmbH—Master thesis, Bielefeld; 2019.
2. Blanchard K, Bowles SM. Gung Ho! How to get any team in top form. Reinbek: Rowohlt Taschenbuch Verlag; 2003.
3. Laloux F. Reinventing organizations: a guide to designing meaningful collaboration. Munich: Verlag Franz Vahlen; 2014.
4. Röhrßen T, Stephan D. Leadership Performance Krankenhaus - Die Praxis der Führung für Ärztinnen und Ärzte. Berlin: Medizinisch Wissenschaftliche Verlagsgesellschaft; 2021.
5. Schumacher T, Wimmer R. The trend towards low hierarchy organizations. Organ Dev. 2019;2:12–8.
6. Goleman D. EQ—emotional intelligence. Munich: Deutscher Taschenbuch Verlag; 2011.
7. Walker D, Alkalay M, Kämpfer M, Roth R. Mehr Zeit für Patienten - Lean Hospital im Einsatz auf der Station und in der Abteilung. Berlin: Medizinisch Wissenschaftliche Verlagsgesellschaft; 2017.
8. Judge TA, Locke EA, Durham CC. The dispositional causes of job satisfaction: a core evaluations approach. Res Organ Behav. 1997;19:151–88.
9. Weiherl P, Emmermacher A, Kemter P. Gesundheitsmanagement, Präsentismus und Core Self-Evaluations. In: Richter PG, Rau R, Mühlpfordt S, editors. Arbeit und Gesundheit - zum aktuellen Stand in einem Forschungs- und Praxisfeld. Lengerich: Pope Science Publishers; 2007. p. 305–23.
10. Demir N. Evaluation of a leadership training at UNIVEG Deutschland GmbH—Bachelor thesis, Vechta; 2016.

Interprofessional Training Wards: Transcending Boundaries—Learning and Working Together

13

Christine Straub, Sebastian Bode, Lukas Nock, and Irina Cichon

13.1 Background

The ongoing discourse surrounding the future viability of the German health care system can be characterized by efforts to ensure that the requisite health care resources and services are in place to meet the needs of the country's increasingly aging population. In light of this development, particular challenges relate, inter alia, to increased patient numbers as well as a rise in the complexity of both cases and treatment options. As a result of this, the expertise of notably different health care professions is equally in demand. In this context, neither the needs of patients nor the increasingly complex requirements of modern care processes adhere to sectoral or occupational delimitations. In addition, many countries are already faced with a shortage of health care professionals, and Germany is not spared from this mass trend, with significant shortages across the health care and nursing professions in almost every German federal state [1]. According to a study commissioned by the

C. Straub (✉)
Department of General Pediatrics, Adolescent Medicine and Neonatology, Medical Center – University of Freiburg, Center for Pediatrics, Freiburg, Germany
e-mail: christine.straub@uniklinik-freiburg.de

S. Bode
Department of Pediatrics and Adolescent Medicine, Ulm University Medical Centre, Ulm, Germany
e-mail: sebastian.bode@uniklinik-ulm.de

L. Nock
Department of Social Work, Mannheim University of Applied Sciences, Mannheim, Germany
e-mail: nock@hs-mannheim.de

I. Cichon
Robert Bosch Stiftung, Stuttgart, Germany
e-mail: Irina.cichon@bosch-stiftung.de

German Council of Economic Experts, the current situation will only continue to worsen, resulting in a presumed additional need for just under 1.3 million full-time equivalent skilled workers for the year 2030 ([2], p. 4). At the same time, however, there is a steady growth in demands on all health care professionals, who must integrate major knowledge-based and technological progress into their work while simultaneously coping with a broader range of tasks.

In recent years, alongside primarily economic-driven approaches (cf. [3, 4]), technical innovations in patient treatment and care (cf. [5]), and ongoing professional development across the individual occupational groups that form the health care system, a new perspective has increasingly come to the fore in terms of overcoming the challenges outlined above: namely, interprofessional collaboration. The interprofessional focus reflects the problematic underdevelopment of interprofessional collaboration in health care. Instead, the dominant practice is toward segmented multi-professionalism. Critics of such an approach argue that this allows for coexistence, but not for any real cooperation between occupational groups (cf. [6]). Conversely, it is not simply care processes that are crucially dependent on the close interaction of actors involved. Successful collaboration and a positive social working environment are also key factors when it comes to recruitment and retention of staff. Numerous national and international studies have demonstrated the relevance of such "soft" factors, for example, in connection with nursing staff leaving the profession (for an overview, see [7]). Therefore, the concept of interprofessionalism relies on occupational groups involved in the provision of care "agreeing on a common goal and coordinating their work from this common perspective" ([8], p. 141).

In light of the institutional, structural, and legal nature of the health care system, however, the interprofessional integration of different health care professionals is dependent on multiple factors: On the one hand, there are historically developed and legally embedded asymmetries at play between the occupational groups (cf. [9]). As a result, medicine not only has wide-ranging rights of direction and delegation with regard to the health care professions, but it is also the case that the division of labor and the hierarchical structure—especially in the inpatient sector—are dominated by organizational principles that are largely medical in nature. This is reflected, not least, in the conceptualization of nursing, midwifery, speech therapy, occupational therapy, and physiotherapy as "auxiliary health care professions." The "predominance of medical tasks and culture" (loc. Cit., p. 289) formalized in this way makes interprofessional dialog more difficult. On the other hand, structurally induced time pressure and increased patient turnover intensify communication difficulties between the individual occupational groups in the health care system [10], promote tendencies toward task-related "subsystem optimization" (cf. [11]), and thus further promote occupational segmentation in the health care system. Finally, however, developments also arise from the professions themselves that further complicate participatory interrelations and how their collaboration with one another is shaped. The progressive professionalization and academization of the health care professions may inevitably contribute to improvements in qualification, as well as to greater specialized knowledge and proficiency for individual professions. Nevertheless, interdisciplinary goal- and solution-focused collaboration and communication are sometimes left by the wayside in the pursuit of specific professional interests, the setting out of claims to competence or control on the part of individual occupational groups, and the reclamation of responsibilities with regard to respective professionalization efforts (cf. [12], p. 201; [13], p. 55ff.).

In this context, an "interprofessional widening" of the health care system seems feasible only by involving the education system and promoting innovative professional development. Future physicians, nurses, physiotherapists, occupational therapists, speech therapists, and midwives need to be introduced to interprofessional teamwork at the point of their first professional socialization and to be equipped with the requisite skills for this. This can be done, for example, as part of interprofessional courses or on interprofessional training wards.

13.2   State of Development

Internationally, there are numerous successful approaches to interprofessional curricula and training courses across the different health care professions, although the degree to which they have been developed is largely heterogeneous [14, 15]. Countries such as Canada, Australia, Sweden, and Norway have a long tradition of interprofessional education and collaboration [16–18], which is why their health care and education systems are considered world-leading in terms of interprofessionalism. Of the German-speaking countries, Switzerland appears to be the most developed in this regard at present (see [19]). Walkenhorst et al. [20] and Herinek [21] provide an overview of the European state of development specifically relating to interprofessional project and networking activities in Germany, Austria, and Switzerland.

In Germany, there was and still is a historic separation between medicine and other health professions, both in practice and in education. It was only in the course of the Bologna Process around the turn of the millennium, and the resulting acceleration of the process of academizing non-medical health professions, that isolated approaches to interprofessional education began to emerge in Germany. Nevertheless, "interprofessional education and collaboration in Germany remained predominantly dependent on the initiatives of individuals or teams" ([16], p. 12). It is only in recent years that Germany has made significant progress toward catching up in this field, with a number of projects initiated and different interprofessional approaches tested and evaluated as part of the training and qualification of health care professions and in the study of medicine. In this context, a new training format—the Interprofessional Training Ward (IPW)—has been the focus for some time now of increased attention among both educators and students and trainees.

This training format originated in Linköping and was successfully implemented in Sweden as early as the 1990s. In 1996, the world's first "interprofessional training wards" were launched, which to this day are a mandatory part of interprofessional education for students of medicine, nursing, physiotherapy, occupational therapy, social work, and laboratory medicine in Linköping. On the training wards, responsibility lies with interprofessional teams of students in the final stage of their studies who, under the supervision of professionals, provide care and treatment to patients over the course of a 2-week assignment on an orthopedic or geriatric training ward. In the late 1990s, the Karolinska Institute adopted the Linköping model and other hospitals in Stockholm also introduced interprofessional training wards under the motto "learning together to be able to work together." Following the successful implementation of the model in Sweden, it has spread widely throughout Scandinavia via the "Nordic Interprofessional Network (Nipnet)" (cf. [22]).

Numerous challenges arose when it came to the design and implementation of the first interprofessional training wards in Germany (ITWs) after the Scandinavian model. These varied depending on the location as well as on the thematic focus and the participants involved [23]. The first ITWs were established in Heidelberg (HITW: Heidelberg Interprofessional Training Ward) and Freiburg (ITWP: Interprofessional Training Ward for Pediatrics) in 2017 with funding from the Robert Bosch Stiftung. Shortly thereafter, the MITW (Mannheim Interprofessional Training Ward) followed in Mannheim. The concept has proved itself and continues to spread. With support from the Robert Bosch Stiftung, the training format is currently being transferred to Munich, Bonn, and Nuremberg. Several other locations in Germany are also taking up the concept and have launched the necessary preparatory measures.

13.3 The ITWP Project: A Case Study

Institutional Framework and Conception

Integrated into a general pediatric ward, the Interprofessional Training Ward for Pediatrics: "Transcending boundaries: Learning and working together" (ITWP) has been in place since October 2017. The first stage was a preparation and conception phase that lasted around a year. Following this phase, the ITWP was launched as a collaborative project by the Center for Child and Adolescent Medicine at the University Medical Center, Freiburg (CCA) and the Clinic for Child and Adolescent Medicine at St. Josef's Hospital/the RKK Clinic Freiburg (SJH). With around 11,500 employees, the University of Freiburg's University Medical Center is one of the largest university hospitals in Germany. Approximately 2900 nursing staff and 1300 physicians provide care for around 69,900 patients per year. As a pediatric center, the CCA is responsible for the primary care of patients from 0 to 18 from Freiburg and the wider region and is also a central point of care for children and adolescents from all over Germany and abroad. The RKK Clinic is the largest non-university health care provider in the greater Freiburg area, treating over 26,000 inpatients per year. The Clinic for Child and Adolescent Medicine at St Josef's Hospital, along with the University of Freiburg's Center for Child and Adolescent Medicine, provides inpatient pediatric care close to home for those living in the city of Freiburg, the Breisgau-Hochschwarzwald area, as well as neighboring areas. Both pediatric hospitals share a joint chief medical director. St Josef's Hospital Freiburg is an academic teaching hospital as part of the Albert Ludwig University of Freiburg and has its own health care and nursing school, as well as a health care and pediatric nursing school.

The University Hospital Freiburg combines research, teaching, and patient care in its core mission. Those collaborating with the ITWP made sure to always take these principles into account, both when it came to the preparation and conception of the teaching project, as well as in its implementation. This was done to ensure good, patient-centered clinical care, as well as innovative interprofessional training in practice for health care and pediatric nursing trainees, as well as for medical students over the course of their year in practice.

A project steering group was set up in the summer of 2016 as part of the Research Group for Teaching and Teaching Research at the Center for Child and Adolescent Medicine at Freiburg University Hospital under the leadership of a pediatrics specialist and a social scientist with undergraduate training and professional experience in pediatric nursing. Alongside responsible parties from nursing and medicine at the SJH and CCA, health care and pediatric nursing trainees (HCPNTs), medical students on their placement year with elective pediatrics (PYMSs), nursing practice supervisors, and ward physicians were also involved in the process of planning the project from the very start. The participants engaged in coordinated interprofessional exchange. As a result of this, the following concept for the ITWP was developed, taking into account the experiences from the first funding phase of "Operation Team" supported by the Robert Bosch Stiftung [24].

The ITWP is integrated into a 16-bed general pediatric ward. On the ITWP, HCPNTs and PYMSs form interprofessional teams to care for 4–6 patients from 12 months of age. They are supervised by tutors from nursing and medicine. While the tutors bear professional responsibility, they help the HCPNTs and PYMSs to work as independently as possible (Fig. 13.1). Each team is made up of two PYMSs and two HCPNTs who are each assigned to the ITWP during their regular working

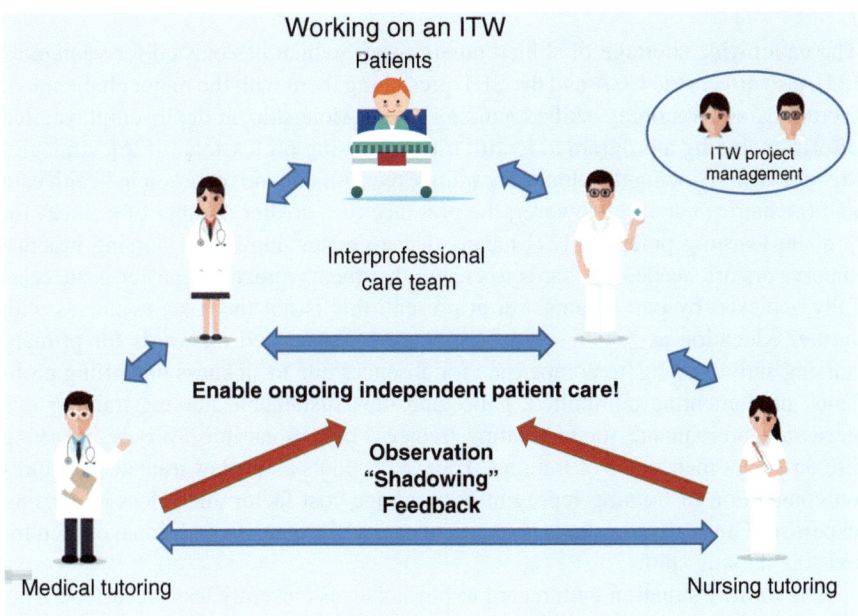

Fig. 13.1 Interprofessional learning, working, and tutoring on the ITWP. (Source: Bode & Straub, own representation, 2017. Design: media center/University Medical Center Freiburg)

hours and work together for a period of 2 weeks. These block placements are based on the HCPNTs' practice placement times and have proven to be effective. At night and on weekends, the patients are cared for by the regular ward team and the ITWP trainees are responsible for the handovers.

In order to focus on interprofessional collaboration, the ITWP team cares for patients with selected general pediatric pathologies. This is to ensure that the interprofessional teamwork and communication are the focus of their time on the ward and not discipline-specific work. The ward round is the most important part of the trainees' daily routine. First of all, the interprofessional ward round meeting takes place. Before a bedside visit can occur, everyone involved in the care process gathers outside the patient's room to discuss the patient's acute challenges and goals in advance. In-room discussions are led by the HCPNTs and PYMSs. Afterwards, the rounds are debriefed, and feedback is given, both by the trainees among themselves as well as by the tutors. Half an hour is reserved at noon for structured reflection or case-based peer teaching sessions.

Parents and patients are informed verbally about ITWP participation and also receive additional written information on the matter. No explicit consent to care needs to be obtained on the ITWP. Parents or patients do have the right to refuse, but this has not occurred to date.

Relevance for Professional Development in the Health Care Sector

The nationwide shortage of skilled nursing staff, which has existed for years now [25], also affects the CCA and the SJH, presenting them with the major challenge of recruiting and retaining skilled nursing staff. Alongside in-depth employee-led efforts, including a program to recruit trained nursing professionals [26], strategies are increasingly being developed for trainee recruitment and retention in health care and (pediatric) nursing. However, the presence of a greater number of trainees for "on-site learning practice" [27] means that a greater number of nursing practice supervisors are needed on wards to ensure that theory-practice transfer is successfully achieved by participants. Yet at present, this is not the case, as nurses with further education as practice supervisors are often needed on wards for primary nursing activities, e.g. to compensate for absences due to sickness or staffing problems. Implementing committed, good, and thus sustainable nursing training is a necessary prerequisite for facilitating trainees' transitions into everyday working life on-site at their place of training. Trainee dropouts as well as trainee departures on completion of training represent both a huge cost factor and a loss of nursing expertise. This leads to deficits in inpatient care and creates an additional burden for existing nursing staff.

The staffing situation with regard to physicians is currently less precarious. This is possibly as a result of the Working Hours Act entering into force on July 1, 1994, which prevented the widespread practice in the medical field of shifts of 24 h or even more and made it compulsory to adjust staffing ratios to guarantee medical patient care in hospitals [28]. However, a recent survey carried out by the Marburger Bund [Marburg Association] shows that placement year medical students feel like cheap labor, and that insufficient attention is paid to their training [29].

A critical challenge in the context of professional development at both the CCA and the SKH is to shape training and working conditions that allow the various occupational groups involved in inpatient care to synchronize and pool their expertise and competencies. This is the only way to simultaneously secure both effective, efficient, and patient-centered inpatient care alongside employee occupational satisfaction. The ITWP project aims to ensure that future nurses and physicians learn interprofessional collaboration in a structured manner during their respective time in training.

Potential for Innovation and Experiences of Implementation

Omachonu and Einspruch ([30], p. 5) describe innovation in health care as follows: "Healthcare innovation can be defined as the introduction of a new concept, idea, service, process, or product aimed at improving treatment, diagnosis, education, outreach, prevention and research, and with the long-term goals of improving quality, safety, outcomes, efficiency, and costs." The ITWP project is based on a new concept for the joint training of HCPNTs and PYMSs in practice. In particular, the process of developing a concept under the guidance of an interprofessional management tandem is innovative and bold. In light of the fact that interprofessional learning and teaching on the ITWP, as well as subject-specific instruction, take place directly amidst the everyday reality of life on the ward, it was absolutely essential that all actors involved from medicine and nursing were included in the project's conception right from the very beginning. A project environment and stakeholder analysis was carried out to identify the relevant people, as well as the structural and spatial conditions at play. This was necessary because effective and sustainable collaboration, especially where it transcends professional and institutional boundaries, does not happen organically, but must instead be initiated, negotiated, shaped [23], and repeatedly evaluated and adapted as part of the process. Thirty relevant persons were identified: The decision-makers from medicine (medical director/senior consultant/senior physician), nursing (nursing director/head of nursing/head of ward), and the head of the Health Care and (Children's) Nursing School of the SJH, HCPNTs, PYMSs, medical and nursing ward staff, nursing practice supervisors, a nursing instructor, and the senior physician instructor from the CCA. A joint workshop was held to discuss the goals, wishes, and fears within this group of people, working groups, work assignments, and work packages were set out, and the scheduling and communication structure was agreed. The workshop was moderated by an external professional moderator, which proved beneficial for dialog between members from different hierarchical levels and occupational groups. The "ITWP" topic was a new, previously unknown topic for the workshop participants. However, all participants were open to putting this new and promising project into practice.

From the start, all processes and project phases were designed both top-down and bottom-up. All stakeholders were involved in all stages of the project (initiation, conception, piloting, implementation, evaluation, adaptation). It was up to the project coordinator to establish and maintain transparent and structured communication between the members of the operational level ("steering group") and the decision-makers from nursing and medicine. The steering group is made up, interprofessionally speaking, of individuals from all the institutions involved and was responsible for all content-related and organizational tasks in the sense of a "learning organization" [31]. Minutes were taken at all meetings to ensure that communication between the members of the steering group was transparent and goal-focused. At regular intervals, the project management tandem sent a newsletter to decision-makers in nursing and medicine, as well as to the members of the steering group, detailing the current project status and the next stages of the project.

The ITWP project conveyed remarkably different occupational group-specific interests and goals, which, however, could only be achieved through interprofessional cooperation. For example, the persons responsible from both occupational groups were particularly interested in a successful theory-practice transfer for the participants on the ITWP. Through the coordinated cooperation of practice (ward management), as well as school (HCPN school), and academic educational institution (medical faculty), teaching and learning materials from medical studies and nursing training could be integrated for training on the ITWP, meaning they could be used as the basis for successful interprofessional theory-practice transfer in everyday inpatient work (e.g. giving and taking feedback, assessment tools, rounds scheme, handover scheme). Participants, patients, and patient parents benefited from this. The HCPNTs and PYMSs learn with and about one another directly in the form of practice. As a result, they gain active experience of their own role, responsibility, and expertise in relation to the role, responsibility, and expertise of other occupational groups. Ongoing dialog and work-related feedback under the guidance and supervision of trained tutors mean that information is not lost, and possible treatment errors are recognized, discussed, and acted upon in a timely manner. The IP team treating the patient involves the patients and their parents in the decision-making process, and nursing and medical aspects of care are always discussed jointly before being subsequently documented as per the requirements of each occupational group. This process saves time for both occupational groups while also serving patient safety in the context of inpatient care.

Another new and innovative feature is the support and supervision of the HCPNTs and the PYMSs by trained medical and nursing tutors (cf. [32]). Professional tutoring is provided at set points for specific occupational groups. Interprofessional exchange, the identification of interprofessional nursing and medical interfaces (e.g. interprofessional medical history and ward rounds), as well as ongoing support via "shadowing"[1] is carried out by the nursing tutors.

---

[1] Shadowing, or "hands-off" professional guidance, is understood to mean observing the actions and interactions of participants on an ITW, without any active intervention on the part of the tutors. This means HCPNTs and PYMSs should be given the opportunity to be the primary point of contact for patients and their parents, directly taking on medical and nursing care independently.

A major advantage lies in the integration of interprofessional competence acquisition into the practical training stage for HCPNTs and PYMSs. Up until now, the acquisition of interprofessional competencies is yet to take place intentionally during training, but rather is expected to occur implicitly after students have entered professional practice [33]. This is particularly applicable for interprofessional competencies that relate to how work is organized, teamwork, and team communication. With regard to the field of nursing, the Training and Examination Ordinance for the Nursing Professions (KrPflAPrV Annex 1. No.12 (to § 1 para. 1), [34]) requires that all competencies needed for later interprofessional collaboration should be taught during training. In terms of medical training, both the Master plan for Medical Studies 2020 [35] and the National Competence-Based Catalog of Learning Goals for Medicine [36] set out the necessity of acquiring interprofessional competencies during training as a key component of sustainable, patient-centered clinical care. In addition to new professional qualifications, the recommendations of the German Council of Science and Humanities [37] for all health care professions include relevant, cross-field qualifications, such as the ability to work together interprofessionally.

The ITWP offers an ideal basis and diverse learning scenarios for implementing the aforementioned requirements and recommendations, without requiring additional time in the respective curricula or syllabi. The participants learn and work directly in the daily clinical routine, are integrated into the regular processes of the ward, and assume responsibility for the inpatient care of up to six patients. Interprofessional learning does not take place in a theoretical context as a simulated scenario, but under real nursing and medical working conditions in practice. Such tangible practical learning experiences in an interprofessional team under the supervision and guidance of experienced tutors from nursing and medicine contribute to the strengthening of professional activities and understanding of professional roles and expertise. Through engaging in accompanying structured reflection on their own role within the interprofessional team in the sense of solution-focused advice (cf. [38]), the participants succeed in understanding and questioning their own and others' stereotypes and in transferring the results and experiences of this reflection to their everyday professional life. On the ITWP, HCPNTs and PYMSs are members of a team; they form a community of action with a common goal. This way, they learn to present their own perspective competently and to listen actively to other team members so as to jointly coordinate nursing and medical treatment plans and how work is organized.

Interprofessional care on the ITWP puts patients center stage. This means that all activities and feedback are geared toward working cooperatively with patients and their parents as long-term partners. This approach not only benefits the patients and their families, it also strengthens job satisfaction on the part of HCPNTs and PYMSs. Joint anamnesis discussions and ward rounds, as well as discharge management play a role here.

Between October 2017 and February 2019, five ITWP placements of 4 weeks each (two teams for 2 weeks each) were carried out. Further placements have taken place regularly. The concept was adapted according to the evaluation results and feedback following each placement. The project and the support provided by the ITWP were very highly rated by participants, ward staff, patients, and their parents. In particular, the participants' communication skills, the timely and comprehensible transfer of information, and the standard of professional nursing and medical care were positively emphasized.

The ITWP project was successfully integrated into the daily routine of the ward and succeeded in introducing the participants to their profession-specific responsibilities and roles in the interprofessional team. The training from nursing and medical tutors made it possible to focus on professional guidance, theory-practice transfer and, in particular, on interprofessional learning and teaching.

Transparent communication with all participants as well as clearly defined communication channels was crucial to the success of ITWP. Positive feedback from participants and, in particular, the excellent evaluations on the part of patients and their parents, helped to convince those initially rather skeptical of the feasibility of a pediatric interprofessional training ward.

The participants emphasized that the daily half-hour midday reflection session had played a major role in optimally shaping the learning process within the 2-week placement. The midday reflection was solution-oriented (cf. [39]). In a safe environment, the HCPTNs and PYMSs were given the opportunity to discuss successful interprofessional collaboration, as well as conflicts and uncertainties, and to work out joint solution strategies. Feedback, both from peers and tutors, was also very gladly received.

The interprofessional project management tandem played a key role in the successful transfer of the ITWP into regular operation. Above all, clear communication channels and role distribution were particularly advantageous. Support for the ITWP from nursing and medical management at the SKH and CCA, as well as from the HCPN school has been essential. By regularly internally training tutors on the basis of training concepts[2] developed for this purpose, the first people to disseminate the interprofessional training were found. Here, graduates from the ITWP, who now work as nurses and doctors at the SJH and CCA, also play an important role in interprofessional training and collaboration.

13.4 Findings and Transfer

First, the coordination of the steering group and stakeholders required significantly more resources in terms of both staff and time than planned. However, the importance of this work, and of regular, open communication, cannot be overestimated. It is important for an appropriate coordinator to take on the project coordination at an early stage.

---

[2] Sottas, B., et al.: Handbook for Tutors on Interprofessional Training Wards. Stuttgart 2020: Robert Bosch Stiftung. The handbook summarizes practical experience gained from the implementation of interprofessional training wards and corresponding training concepts across various locations in Germany and is a sound methodological tool for tutors on interprofessional training wards.

Training the tutors was essential, specifically as this kind of "hands-off" professional guidance is unfamiliar and requires a shift in mindset and a transfer of responsibility from all involved. It was advantageous to train nurses and physicians who were already well established in their professional roles as tutors and to offer in-depth support to tutors during their first placements on the ITWP.

The most significant finding from the ITWP project is that interprofessional training is possible in Germany on an interprofessional training ward as part of the regular operation of a general pediatric ward. It was not only participating HCPNTs and PYMSs who felt very positively toward their placements on the ITWP, but also patients and their parents, who rated care on the ITWP as excellent. It is essential to prepare and involve all stakeholders in depth, also to ensure long-term support for such an innovative project. Equally important is having a motivated and professionally experienced interprofessional project management team willing to cooperate "at eye level."

Projects such as the ITWP must always be adapted to meet local conditions, which is why it is strictly necessary to carry out an appropriate analysis at the start of the planning phase. The support of the ward team as well as the decision-makers at all management levels should absolutely be given. Resistance, even from individuals, can complicate or delay implementation. It is helpful to include all those involved as early as the project planning phase so as to address any fears directly and work out solutions together. Legal aspects, such as a vote by the ethics committee and the staff council, possibly patient information and consent forms, and access to patient data, in line with the General Data Protection Regulation and duty of confidentiality may require advance planning.

It is helpful to visit established interprofessional teaching projects and to observe such projects where necessary. The ITWP project management team was able to bring back a great deal of experience following a visit to an interprofessional training ward at Karolinska Institute in Stockholm, before adapting what they had learnt to local conditions. Once the project has been adapted to the location in question, engaging in further dialog with colleagues pursuing the same or similar projects is beneficial to reflect on ideas and experiences, to exchange ideas, and thus to further develop the project at hand. The interprofessional exchange that occurred as part of the "Operation Team" projects served as an outstanding framework in this area and contributed to the further development of all projects. A formative evaluation of the project should be a matter of course in order to identify and implement necessary changes.

With regard to professional development in the health care sector, practical experience from the previous implementation of the ITWP indicates that interprofessional training wards meet the individual wishes of prospective specialists for improved training and interprofessional teamwork and can thus contribute to increasing employer attractiveness. In fact, tutors and participants alike report positive effects on motivation and satisfaction, as well as on the professional, methodical, social, and personal qualifications of the future professionals. Therefore, interprofessional training wards can be conceptualized as innovative places of learning in the sense of interest- and aptitude-based, and thus sustainable, professional development.

References

1. Bundesagentur für Arbeit [Federal Employment Agency]. Statistik/Arbeitsmarktberichterstattung, Berichte [Statistics/labor market reporting]: Blickpunkt Arbeitsmarkt – Fachkräfteanalyse [Focus on the labor market—skilled worker analysis], Nuremberg, June 2018.
2. Augurzky B, Kolodziej I. Fachkräftebedarf im Gesundheits- und Sozialwesen 2030 [The demand for skilled labor in the health and social care sector by 2030]. Working paper 06/2018 of the RWI – Leibniz Institute for Economic Research. 2018. https://www.sachverstaendigenrat-wirtschaft.de/fileadmin/dateiablage/gutachten/jg201819/arbeitspapiere/Arbeitspapier_06-2018.pdf. Accessed 24 May 2019.
3. Buhr P, Klinke S. Qualitative Folgen der DRG-Einführung für Arbeitsbedingungen und Versorgung im Krankenhaus unter Bedingungen fortgesetzter Budgetierung. Eine vergleichende Auswertung von vier Fallstudien. [Qualitative consequences of the introduction of DRGs for working conditions and care in hospitals under conditions of continued budgeting. A comparative analysis of four cases studies]. Publication series of the Public Health Research Group. Research focus: work, social structure and the welfare state. Berlin: Social Science Research Center Berlin (WZB); 2006.
4. Simon M. Sechzehn Jahre Deckelung der Krankenhausbudgets. Eine kritische Bestandsaufnahme von Prof. Dr. Michael Simon, Fachhochschule Hannover [Sixteen years of capping hospital budgets. A critical review by Prof. Dr. Michael Simon, University of Applied Sciences Hannover]. Study commissioned by ver.di; 2008.
5. Hielscher V, Nock L, Kirchen-Peters S. Technikeinsatz in der Altenpflege [The use of technology in geriatric care]. Berlin: edition sigma, Nomos Verlagsgesellschaft; 2015.
6. Sachverständigenrat zur Begutachtung der Entwicklung im Gesundheitswesen [German Council of Economic Experts on the Assessment of Developments in the Health Care System] (SVR-Gesundheit [German Council of Health Experts]). Koordination und Integration – Gesundheitsversorgung in einer Gesellschaft des längeren Lebens [Coordination and integration—healthcare in a longer life society]. Special report 2009. Abridged version. 2009. http://www.svr-gesundheit.de/index.php?id=14. Last accessed 24 May 2019.
7. Hasselhorn H-M, Müller B-H, Tackenberg P, Kümmerling A, Simon M. Berufsausstieg bei Pflegepersonal. Arbeitsbedingungen und beabsichtigter Berufsausstieg bei Pflegepersonal in Deutschland und Europa [Nursing staff leaving the profession. Working conditions and intended career exits of nursing staff in Germany and Europe]. In: Schriftenreihe der Bundesanstalt für Arbeitsschutz und Arbeitsmedizin [Series of publications of the German Federal Institute for Occupational Health and Safety]. Dortmund: BauA; 2005.
8. Voelker C. Physiotherapie Berufliches Selbstverständnis [Physiotherapy professional self-image]. Berlin: Cornelsen; 2011.
9. Rohde JJ. Soziologie des Krankenhauses [Sociology of the hospital]. Stuttgart: Ferdinand Enke; 1962.
10. Nock L, Hielscher V, Kirchen-Peters S. Dienstleistungsarbeit unter Druck: Der Fall Krankenhauspflege [Care work under pressure: the case of hospital nursing]. Working paper 296. Düsseldorf: Hans Böckler Stiftung; 2013.
11. Zwack J, Nöst S, Schweitzer J. Zeitdruck im Krankenhaus. Individuelle Lösungsstrategien provozieren oft neue Probleme [Time pressure in the hospital. Individual solution strategies often cause new problems]. In: Arzt und Krankenhaus [Doctor and Hospital], vol. 2009(3); 2009. p. 68–75.
12. Sieger M, Ertl-Schmuck R, Bögemann-Großheim E. Interprofessionelles Lernen als Voraussetzung für interprofessionelles Handeln – am Beispiel eines interprofessionell angelegten Bildungs- und Entwicklungsprojektes für Gesundheitsberufe [Interprofessional learning as a prerequisite for interprofessional work-based on the example of an interprofessionally designed training and development project for health care professions]. Pflege & Gesellschaft [Care & society]. 15th ed, Vol. 3; 2010. p. 197–216.

13. Pfadenhauer M. Professionalität. Eine wissenssoziologische Rekonstruktion institutionalisierter Kompetenzdarstellungskompetenz [Professionalism. A sociological reconstruction of institutionalized competence representation]. Wiesbaden: Springer; 2003.
14. Cichon I, Klapper B. Interprofessionelle Ausbildungsansätze in der Medizin [Interprofessional training approaches in medicine]. Bundesgesundheitsblatt – Gesundheitsforschung – Gesundheitsschutz [National health care journal—health care research—health care protection], 2/2018; 2017. p. 195–200.
15. Reeves S. Why we need interprofessional education to improve the delivery of safe and effective care. Interface - Comunicação, Saúde, Educação. 2016;20(56):185–96.
16. Barr H. Interprofessional education. The genesis of a global movement. 2015. https://static.websitecreator.eu/var/m_f/fd/fd4/3631/153622-Genesis_of_global_IPE_movement_2015.pdf?download. Accessed 14 May 2019.
17. Dunston R, Lee A, Matthews L, Nisbet G, Pockett R, Thistlethwaite J, White J. Interprofessional health education in Australia: the way forward. Sydney: University of Technology, Sydney and The University of Sydney; 2009.
18. You P, Malik N, Scott G, Fung K. Current state of interprofessional education in Canadian medical schools: findings from a national survey. J Interprof Care. 2017;31(5):670–2. https://doi.org/10.1080/13561820.2017.1315060. Epub 2017 May 8.
19. Kaap-Fröhlich S. Interprofessional education for tomorrow's healthcare—a Swiss perspective. Public Health Forum. 2018;26(1):42–4. https://doi.org/10.1515/pubhef-2017-0074.
20. Walkenhorst U, Mahler C, Aistleithner R et al. Positionspapier GMA-Ausschuss – „Interprofessionelle Ausbildung in den Gesundheitsberufen" [GMA committee position paper—"Interprofessional education in the health care professions"]. GMS Z Med Ausbild [GMS Z Med Educ]. 2015;32(2):Doc22.
21. Herinek D. Projekt- und Vernetzungsaktivitäten in den DACH-Ländern [Project and networking activities in the DACH countries]. In: Ewers M, Paradis E, Herinek D, editors. Interprofessionelles Lernen, Lehren und Arbeiten. Gesundheits- und Sozialprofessionen auf dem Weg zu kooperativer Praxis [Interprofessional learning, teaching, and working. Health and social professions on the way to cooperative practice]. Weinheim: Beltz Juventa; 2019. p. 304–309.
22. Sottas B, Mentrup C, Meyer PC. Interprofessional education and practice in Sweden. Int J Health Prof. 2016;3(1):3–13.
23. Nock L. Interprofessionelle Ausbildungsstationen – Ein Praxisleitfaden [Interprofessional training wards—a practice guide]. Stuttgart: Robert Bosch Stiftung; 2018.
24. Nock L. Handlungshilfe zur Entwicklung von interprofessionellen Lehrveranstaltungen in den Gesundheitsberufen [Help for developing interprofessional courses across the health care professions]. Stuttgart: Robert Bosch Stiftung; 2016.
25. Blum K, Löffert S, Offermanns M, Steffen P. Krankenhaus Barometer – Umfrage 2011 [Hospital barometer—survey 2011]. Düsseldorf. P. 6 ff; 2011.
26. University Hospital Freiburg. Mitarbeiter-werben-Mitarbeiter-Programm. Ihre Empfehlung ist uns viel wert! Strategische Personalentwicklung. Stabsstelle beim Klinikumsvorstand [Employee Referral Program. We value your referral! Strategic professional development. Staff position with the hospital board of directors]. 2019. https://www.uniklinik-freiburg.de/index.php?id=13347&ADMCMD_editIcons=1. Accessed 15 May 2019.
27. Mamerow R. Praxisanleitung in der Pflege [Practice guidance in nursing]. 5th ed. Berlin: Springer-Verlag; 2016.
28. Ethikrat, Deutscher [Ethics Council, German]. Patientenwohl als ethischer Maßstab für das Krankenhaus [Patient well-being as an ethical standard for the hospital]. Statement from April 5, 2016. Berlin: Deutscher Ethikrat [German Ethics Council]; 2016.
29. Deutsches Ärzteblatt [German Medical Journal]. Verdruss im Krankenhaus [Exasperation in the hospital]. 2018;115(25): A-1209/B-1017/C-1012.
30. Omachonu VK, Einspruch NG. Innovation in healthcare delivery systems: a conceptual framework. Innov J. 2010;15(1):1–20.
31. Senge P. The fifth discipline. Stuttgart: Klett-Cotta; 1995.

32. Straub C, Duerkop A, Bode SFN Lernbegleitung auf einer interprofessionellen Ausbildungsstation [Tutoring on an interprofessional training ward]. PADUA - Fachzeitschrift für Pflegepädagogik, Patientenedukation und -bildung [PADUA—Journal of Nursing, Education, Patient Education, and Pedagogy] (accepted for publication May 2019); 2019.
33. Bode SF, Giesler M, Heinzmann A, Krüger M, Straub C. Self-perceived attitudes toward interprofessional collaboration and interprofessional education among different health care professionals in pediatrics. GMS J Med Educ. 2016;33(2):Doc17.
34. KrPflAPrV. Training and examination ordinance for the nursing professions; 2003.
35. Masterplan Medizinstudium [Master Plan for Medical Studies] 2020. 2017. https://www.bmbf.de/files/2017-03-31_Masterplan%20Beschlusstext.pdf. Accessed 3 Apr 2019.
36. NKLM (Nationaler Kompetenzbasierter Lernzielkatalog Medizin [National competence-based catalog of learning goals for medicine]). In: GMA, MFT, editors. Vol. 1. Kiel: GMA & MFT; 2015.
37. Wissenschaftsrat. Empfehlungen zu hochschulischen Qualifikationen für das Gesundheitswesen [Recommendations for higher education qualifications for health care]. Cologne; 2012.
38. Walter JL, Peller JE. Lösungs-orientierte Kurztherapie [Solution-focused brief therapy]. 6th unchanged edition, 2004. Dortmund: verlag modernes lernen; 1994.
39. Spiess W. Beratung: Definitionen, Klassifikationen, Modelle, ... [Advice: definitions, classifications, models, etc.]. In: Spiess W, editor. Die Logik des Gelingens. Lösungs- und entwicklungsorientierte Beratung im Kontext von Pädagogik [The logic of success. Solution- and development-focused advice in the context of pedagogy]. 2nd ed. Dortmund: Borgmann; 1998.
40. Ewers M. Interprofessionalität als Schlüssel zum Erfolg [Interprofessionalism as the key to success]. Public Health Forum. 2012;20(4):10.e1–2.
41. Ewers M, Walkenhorst U. Interprofessionalität in den DACH-Ländern – eine Momentaufnahme [Interprofessionalism in the DACH countries—a snapshot]. In: Ewers M, Paradis E, Herinek D, editors. Interprofessionelles Lernen, Lehren und Arbeiten. Gesundheits- und Sozialprofessionen auf dem Weg zu kooperativer Praxis [Interprofessional learning, teaching, and working. Health and social professions on the way to cooperative practice]. Basel: Belz Juventa; 2019. p. 20–37.

Interprofessional Teaching and Learning in Germany: The "Operation Team" Support Program

14

Lukas Nock and Irina Cichon

14.1 Background: Why Interprofessional Learning?

It is not simply in the wake of social change and demographic developments that demands on stakeholders in the health care system have grown. The increasing rationalization and mechanization of care processes, as well as an ongoing professionalization of the health care professions, have also played a major role here. Such developments pose particular challenges, such as in the form of rising patient numbers, shorter hospital stays, and increasingly complex treatment options and needs. As a result of such factors, the respective expertise of the various health care professions is in equal demand. In this context, neither patient needs nor the increasingly complex requirements of modern care processes adhere to occupational boundaries.

With a view to managing the aforementioned communication demands, a new approach has increasingly come to the fore in Germany in recent years: interprofessionalism. The interprofessional focus is cognizant of the fact that interprofessional collaboration in health care is only marginally developed. Instead, predominant practice tends toward segmented multi-professionalism. Critics argue that the latter practice allows for coexistence, but not for any real cooperation between the various health care professions involved in the care process (cf. [1–3]). Functionally speaking, however, the health care system, in particular, is a highly differentiated system and its performance is almost wholly reliant on the close interaction of all stakeholders involved. The concept of interprofessionalism depends, therefore, on the

L. Nock (✉)
Department of Social Work, Mannheim University of Applied Sciences, Mannheim, Germany
e-mail: nock@hs-mannheim.de

I. Cichon
Robert Bosch Stiftung, Stuttgart, Germany
e-mail: Irina.cichon@bosch-stiftung.de

occupational groups involved in the provision of care "agreeing on a common goal and coordinating their work from this common perspective" ([4], p. 141).

In light, however, of the institutional, structural, and legal nature of the health care system, as well as the shortage of staff and time in the practice of health care provision, the interprofessional integration of different health care professions is dependent on multiple factors—not least given that the subject of interprofessionalism is yet to play a prominent role in the context of training or studies.

Since 2013, the Robert Bosch Stiftung has employed a range of projects, including the Operation Team program, to continuously promote the development of interprofessional collaboration in the health care professions. The strategic starting point for this support is the education system that is to say the professional socialization of future professionals in nursing, medicine, physiotherapy, speech therapy, midwifery, and occupational therapy. Operation Team initiates, systematically networks, and offers ideal-based support to collaborative projects with the long-term aim of an interprofessional widening of the education system, whereby interprofessional learning becomes a fixed component across the curricula of the different health care professions.

To date, this has resulted in a range of different educational options unique to the German setting in the areas of training, studies, and continuing professional development. The projects supported offer a wide variety of different learning environments in which future nurses, physicians, and members of different therapy professions can learn with, from, and about one another. This could be on an interprofessional training ward or in simulation training in the field of clinical emergency medicine, in the form of student tutorials, through practicing joint ward rounds and case reviews, or as part of continuing professional development courses on culturally sensitive health care.

14.2 The "Operation Team" Support Program: A Review

Support activities as part of Operation Team date back to 2013. These can primarily be grouped into seven measures, some of which stand independently and some of which build on other measures:

- *First support phase (2013–2015)*: Joint projects with medical faculties and nursing and therapy profession training/study programs were funded at a total of eight different locations in order to jointly develop and implement an interprofessional teaching program.
- *Second support phase (2016–2018)*: Funding continued for seven of the collaborative projects from the first phase with ten additional projects added. The focus here was on the structural anchoring and curricular integration of the new teaching options on offer at the respective locations.
- *Third support phase (2018–2021)*: In the last step, previously developed and tested interprofessional teaching concepts were transferred to new medical faculties and training institutions for health professions which had not been involved up to this point. The third support phase includes a further seven sites and should be completed by the end of 2021.

- *Interprofessional continuing professional development (2015–2020)*: Concurrently, the interprofessional focus was expanded to continuing professional development in order to raise awareness of interprofessional collaboration among established professionals and embed the topic in the training catalogs of the health care system.
- *Interprofessional training wards (since 2016)*: With support from the Robert Bosch Stiftung, the first interprofessional training wards based on the Scandinavian model were designed and implemented in clinical environments in Germany. This has once again broadened the focus by allowing practical training to take place interprofessionally, thus supplementing theoretical teaching and continuing professional development.
- *National model curriculum for interprofessional collaboration and communication (2016–2019)*: With support from the Robert Bosch Stiftung and the active participation of many Operation Team projects, the German Institute for Medical and Pharmaceutical Examination Questions (IMPP) developed a model curriculum with the aim of anchoring interprofessional teaching in the German national medical examinations, thus ensuring its long-term curricular implementation in compulsory teaching at all medical faculties in Germany. As a result, an action plan for implementing interprofessional teaching across medical faculties as well as interprofessional examination content for the national examination is available.
- *ILEGRA PhD-program "Interprofessional Teaching in Healthcare—Mediation, evaluation, examination" (2018–2022)*: Finally, a total of 12 doctoral fellowships were awarded to young scientists from the health care professions, meaning fundamental research on the further development of interprofessional teaching will be funded until 2022.

Each of these support measures was directed at a different focal point and was carried out with the participation of different groups of stakeholders across various fields of action. The unifying central strategic goal of the Operation Team support program was, however, to improve interprofessional collaboration in the health care system by widening the training system in terms of interprofessionalism. More specifically, this means the compulsory nationwide curricular anchoring of interprofessional learning content in the study and training programs of the regulated health professions, in particular medicine, nursing, physiotherapy, occupational therapy, speech therapy, and midwifery.

14.3 Project Cluster

Interprofessional training wards
Here, trainees and students of medicine, nursing, and other health care professions jointly take on the independent care and treatment of patients in a clinical setting. Each case is handled as a team, and treatment plans are jointly developed. On the wards, participants are supported by nursing and medical tutors and receive regular and instantaneous feedback.
Example projects:
- HIPSTA—Heidelberg Interprofessional Training Ward
- IPAPÄD—Interprofessional Training Ward for Pediatrics (Freiburg)
- Kinder IPSTA—Interprofessional Training Ward at the University Hospital Bonn
- NIPSTA—Nuremberg Interprofessional Training Ward
- IPANEO—Interprofessional Training Ward in Neonatology (Munich)
- MIA—Mannheim Interprofessional Training Ward

Interprofessional core competencies
A number of different teaching formats have emerged as part of Operation Team that have made interprofessionalism and related issues explicit objects of learning in and of themselves. For instance, in order to promote the core communicative competencies required for interprofessional collaboration, typical prejudices and points of conflict were worked on, boundaries and shared objectives were discussed, communication techniques were tested out, and informal exchange was also encouraged.
Example projects:
- Valuing one another—providing care as a team: interprofessional care and therapy planning (Marburg)
- INTER-M-E-P-P—interprofessional teaching and learning in medicine, occupational therapy, physiotherapy, and nursing (Berlin)
- HEALTH&HUMAN—students and trainees from the HEALTH care professions and HUMAN medicine in interprofessional competence training (Hamburg)
- IPHiGen—interprofessional action in health care (Bochum)
- InterTUT—interprofessional tutorials (Berlin)
- InHAnds—Interprofessional Health Alliance Lower Saxony (Göttingen)

Interprofessional simulation training
With regard to mission-critical decisions, close interaction between the different occupational groups involved in the treatment process is particularly important. To promote interprofessional collaboration in prototypical everyday hospital situations where there is a high likelihood of errors—for instance, in emergency medicine or handover situations—a number of teaching formats have been developed which utilize *skills labs* and simulation settings to practice and coordinate key action plans.
Example projects:
- FinKo—promoting interprofessional communication (Munich)
- Cutting down barriers (Magdeburg)
- Cutting down barriers (Frankfurt)
- Cutting down barriers (Würzburg)
- GeLIS—joint learning of interprofessional skills (Regensburg)
- Improving patient safety by integrating interprofessional human factor training into health care profession training (Greifswald)

Cross-professional topics
Cross-professional topics that are of particular relevance to all professions involved lend themselves well as media for interprofessional learning. As part of the support projects that followed this approach, topics such as dementia, palliative care, and nutrition management, as well as joint examination techniques, for instance, were used as an opportunity to learn with, from, and about one another in theoretical-reflective learning units and practical exercises.
Example projects:
- GReTL2.0—interprofessional health care training in reflective and transformative learning (Halle)
- Understanding together—physicians and physiotherapists learning together (Mannheim)
- Interprofessional nutrition management in inpatient and at-home care (Düsseldorf)
- COMPIDEM—better competencies for interprofessional and individualized care for people with dementia (Lübeck)
- MEDPhysio in hospital and research (Osnabrück)
- OpTEAMal—optimal teamwork in medical teaching (Aachen)
- Carus interprofessional (Dresden)

14.4 International Comparison

Countries such as Canada, Australia, Sweden, and Norway have a long tradition of cross-professional collaboration (cf. [5–7]), which is why their health care and education systems are considered world-leading in terms of interprofessionalism. Of the German-speaking countries, Switzerland appears to be the most developed in this regard at present (cf. [8]). Walkenhorst et al. [9] and Herinek [10] provide an overview of the European state of development specifically relating to interprofessional project and networking activities in Germany, Austria, and Switzerland.

In Germany, there was and still is a historic separation between medicine and other health professions, both in practice and in education. It was only in the course of the Bologna Process around the turn of the millennium, and the resulting acceleration of the process of academizing non-medical health professions, that isolated approaches to interprofessional education began to emerge in Germany. Nevertheless, "interprofessional education and collaboration in Germany remained predominantly dependent on the initiatives of individuals or teams" ([5], p. 12). Operation Team was the first systematic attempt to establish interprofessional learning as a mandatory standard in the health-related education system throughout Germany. An evaluation was carried out at the end of the support program to analyze how the developments launched are perceived in a global context and how they can be classified as part of international comparison with other countries (cf. [11]):

- International visibility: From an expert perspective, the Operation Team brand and associated projects achieved a strong international presence. This is primarily understood in connection with various session and conference contributions, publications, as well as memberships and positions of responsibility in international professional societies, bodies, and committees on the part of stakeholders involved.
- International networking: The support program has led to the formation of international networks, particularly in light of funded visits abroad. In particular, there is active professional dialog with Sweden and Switzerland.
- Spill-over: Regarding the establishment of interprofessional training wards, international visits to Sweden proved particularly fruitful for German project locations. In turn, network partners from Switzerland were able to benefit from visiting the training wards now in place in Germany.

A lack of basic statistical data precluded an international comparison of the interprofessional status quo in Germany with Sweden or Switzerland, for example. However, the impact analysis from the Operation Team support program did reveal a number of development prospects (cf. [11]):

- Academized health care professions: Here, Sweden and Switzerland have a fundamental advantage over Germany, which grosso modo simplifies the nationwide implementation of interprofessional teaching. Namely, the academization of the health care professions has long been mandatory in the two countries. As

a result, many of the numerous hurdles relating to implementation that repeatedly arose in the projects supported by Operation Team in Germany do not arise in the first place (for example, with regard to divergent teaching and learning cultures, timelines, standards, etc.).
- Structural and legal anchoring: Although as of yet there is no nationwide program in Switzerland and there are some local differences in Sweden, interprofessionalism is much more firmly embedded in the training system in these two countries than it is in Germany. In Switzerland, for instance, interprofessional learning objectives are codified in the Federal Law on Medical Professions (Art. 6) and in the Federal Law on Health Care Professions (Art.16), which means they are mandatory accreditation criteria for universities. The same is true in Sweden, where some universities have even been threatened with having their licenses withdrawn by the Accreditation Commission in recent years because interprofessional learning objectives were insufficiently reflected in their courses.
- State funding: In Sweden, interprofessional learning has long been standard in university teaching and training practice and is therefore given regular state funding. The Swiss development process is also funded by the public sector, primarily from care funding (i.e. from the Federal Office of Public Health), but also from research funding from the Swiss Academies of Arts and Sciences (SAMS), and, as part of the Special Program for Human Medicine, from the State Secretariat for Education, Research and Innovation (SERI).

In light of the differences outlined here, while Germany, meanwhile, is at an advanced stage of development with regard to interprofessional education and teaching, these are still in need of in-depth advancement.

14.5 Summary and Outlook

Operation Team supplied proof of concept of the fundamental possibility of implementing interprofessional teaching, even among the most diverse of health care professions and despite numerous systemic, structural, and operational hurdles. In addition, the network of stakeholders that emerged as a result of the supported network of projects and at the level of professional, professional-political, and intermediary organizations also lent the topic of interprofessionalism a wide-reaching visibility and lasting presence. Therefore, the support activities succeeded, not least for this reason, in creating momentum through measures of strategic communication and networking. With the Master Plan for Medical Studies 2020[1] and the pending legislative initiative to amend the licensing regulations for physicians, a vote is now being held at the highest political level on whether interprofessionalism should be a mandatory component of medical curricula going forward, and thus whether sooner or later it should play a mandatory role in the training of other health care professionals. Should this be the case, it remains to be seen, however, exactly how

---

[1] A catalog of measures commissioned by the German government to modernize medical studies.

interprofessional learning will be implemented. This not only relates to questions regarding appropriate teaching concepts, suitable hourly volumes, or ideal scheduling. Rather the impact analysis has emphatically shown that somewhat diametrically opposed ideas of interprofessionalism operate under the same umbrella. The primary issue at hand, therefore, will be which basic understanding, which interpretation, will prevail.

In this context, the interprofessional widening of the health care system in Germany, as well as its training system, cannot be dependent on medicine alone, although the latter undoubtedly has a key role to play. Instead, professional societies and professional-policy representatives from the nursing, physiotherapy, occupational therapy, speech therapy, and midwifery professions are now also called upon to prove their professional validity and seize the opportunity to participate proactively in the development of interprofessional training and teaching at an early stage. Something for which Operation Team has laid the foundation.

References

1. Gesellschaft für medizinische Ausbildung [German Association for Medical Education] (GMA). Ausschuss "Interprofessionelle Ausbildung". Bedeutung und Aktualität des Ausschuss-Themas ['Interprofessional Training' Committee. Importance and topicality of the committee topic]. 2012. https://gesellschaft-medizinische-ausbildung.org/aktivitaeten/ausschuesse/interprofes-sionelle-ausbildung.html. Accessed 23 Mar 2021.
2. Sachverständigenrat zur Begutachtung der Entwicklung im Gesundheitswesen [German Council of Economic Experts on the Assessment of Developments in the Health Care System] (SVR-Gesundheit [German Council of Health Experts]). Koordination und Integration – Gesundheitsversorgung in einer Gesellschaft des längeren Lebens [Coordination and integration—healthcare in a longer life society]. Special report 2009. Abridged version. 2009. http://www.svr-gesundheit.de/index.php?id=14. Accessed 23 Mar 2021.
3. Salomon T, Rothgang H. Interdisziplinäre Kooperation der Gesundheitsberufe am Beispiel der Schlaganfallversorgung. Ergebnisse einer Systematischen Übersichtsarbeit [Interdisciplinary collaboration between the health care professions based on the example of stroke treatments]. Stuttgart: Robert Bosch Stiftung; 2010.
4. Voelker C. Physiotherapie Berufliches Selbstverständnis [Physiotherapy professional self-image]. Berlin: Cornelsen; 2011.
5. Barr H. Interprofessional education. The genesis of a global movement. 2015. https://static.websitecreator.eu/var/m_f/fd/fd4/3631/153622-Genesis_of_global_IPE_movement_2015.pdf?download. Accessed 23 Mar 2021.
6. Dunston R, Lee A, Matthews L, Nisbet G, Pockett R, Thistlethwaite J, White J. Interprofessional health education in Australia: the way forward. Sydney: University of Technology, Sydney and The University of Sydney; 2009.
7. You P, Malik N, Scott G, Fung K. Current state of interprofessional education in Canadian medical schools: findings from a national survey. J Interprof Care. 2017;31(5):670–2. https://doi.org/10.1080/13561820.2017.1315060. Epub 2017 May 8.
8. Kaap-Fröhlich S. Interprofessional education for tomorrow's healthcare—a Swiss perspective. Public Health Forum. 2018;26(1):42–4. https://doi.org/10.1515/pubhef-2017-0074. Accessed 23 Mar 2021.
9. Walkenhorst U, Mahler C, Aistleithner R, Hahn EG, Kaap-Fröhlich S, Karstens S, Reiber K, Stock-Schröer B, Sottas B. Positionspapier GMA-Ausschuss – Interprofessionelle Ausbildung in den Gesundheitsberufen [GMA committee position paper—"Interprofessional education in

the health care professions"]. GMS Z Med Ausbild [GMS Z Med Educ]. 2015;32(2):Doc22. https://doi.org/10.3205/zma000964, URN: urn:nbn:de:0183-zma0009647.
10. Herinek D. Projekt- und Vernetzungsaktivitäten in den DACH-Ländern [Project and networking activities in the DACH countries]. In: Ewers M, Paradis E, Herinek D, editors. Inter-professionelles Lernen, Lehren und Arbeiten. Gesundheits- und Sozialprofessionen auf dem Weg zu kooperativer Praxis [Interprofessional learning, teaching, and working. Health and social professions on the way to cooperative practice]. Beltz Juventa: Weinheim; 2019. p. 304–9.
11. Nock L. Interprofessionelles Lehren und Lernen in Deutschland. Entwicklung und Perspektiven [Interprofessional teaching and learning in Germany. Development and perspectives]. Stuttgart: Robert Bosch Stiftung; 2020.
12. Wissenschaftsrat [German Council of Science and Humanities] (WR). Neustrukturierung des Medizinstudiums und Änderung der Approbationsordnung für Ärzte. Empfehlungen der Expertenkommission zum Masterplan Medizin-studium 2020 [Restructuring of medical studies and amendment to the licensing regulations for doctors. Recommendations of the Expert Commission on the Master Plan for Medical Studies 2020]. Cologne: Office of the German Council of Science and Humanities; 2018.

Part IV

We Are Future: Innovative Staff Development

Bold Future of Human Resources Development in Healthcare

15

Renate Tewes

15.1 Introduction

Courage Is Good

▶ When you dare, your courage grows. When you hesitate, your fear. (Mahatma Gandhi)

Courage is good and has many facets. Too much of a good thing is pride and arrogance. Too little of a good thing is humility and poverty. Courage lies practically exactly in the middle and is therefore neither too much nor too little. In pride, humility is lacking. Superciliousness can be reckless, negligently taking risks that affect others. Humility alone can cause passivity.

For Anja Förster, courage is "having the drive and perseverance to put extraordinary things into action, without a net or a false bottom" ([1]: 34). Courage can be understood as a daring trust in one's own strength [2].

A courageous act always involves overcoming fear, according to psychologist Patrick Herrmann [3]. Courage pays off! Courageous employees are more likely to tackle problems and make better decisions. In contrast, fearful employees are expensive. In a long-term study, Winfried Panse and Wolfgang Stegmann [4] researched what it costs companies when their employees come to work with fear. They distinguish between existential fears (fear of old age, illness, impoverishment), social fears (fear of superiors, colleagues, expression of opinions), and performance or failure fears. If employees regularly experience fear, this has a negative effect on the body and/or the psyche and becomes expensive for the company [4].

R. Tewes (✉)
Crown Coaching International, Dresden, Saxonia, Germany
e-mail: tewes@crown-coaching.de

Fear has a negative effect on decision-making. One study determined the accuracy of X-ray findings. Anxious employees were less accurate in their diagnoses [5]. Instead of confronting fear, employees develop fear defense strategies that narrow perceptions and make poor decisions more likely [4].

In order to acquire courage, the comfort zone must be left behind. Personal development means going where the fear is [6]. Getting out of the securities that our society brings with it and overcoming fears instead. The whole safety net of western industrialized nations has made us unlearn courage. Children are no longer allowed to try things out indefinitely, but must grow up "safe." Germans seem to have a special need for safety and spend more money on insurance than other countries in a European comparison [7].

It can be courageous to stand up for your own values or to have a separation discussion with an employee who needs to be fired. Enduring embarrassing moments can require courage just as much as admitting one's mistakes. It is especially courageous to forgive someone [8] (Fig. 15.1).

Changes in the health care system require courage. It is necessary to give up the comfort zone and to endure the neutral zone in which the old is already gone but the new is not yet there. Only in combination with self-reflection does courage unfold its special power. Otherwise it could have been over courage that happened to end happily. "Without self-reflection, courage is worth nothing" ([9]: 47).

Fig. 15.1 Image "Courage" of the artist Fiona Dowling

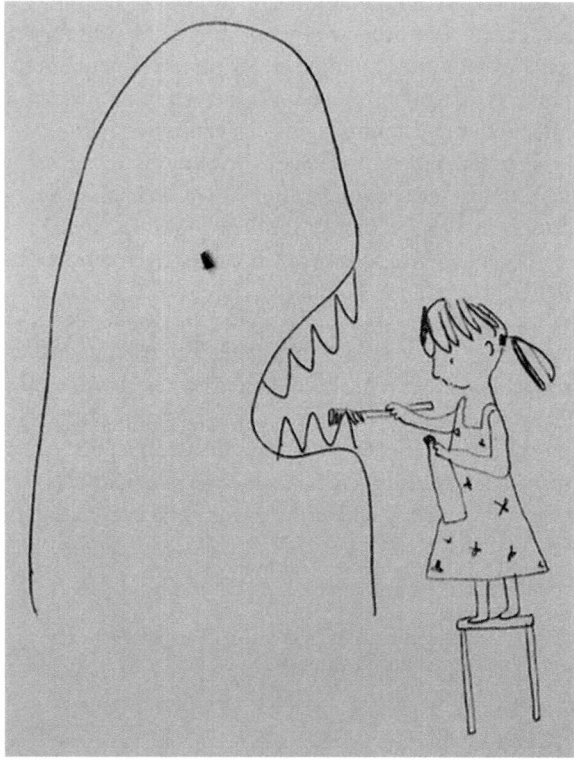

Manfred Kets de Vries, an economist with psychoanalytic training, says "If you want courageous employees, you must allow them to disagree and fail" and soberly states that there is a very fine line between courage and stupidity ([10]: 49).

The Health Industry as a Growth Engine

▶   The future belongs to those who believe in the beauty of their dreams.
    Eleanor Roosevelt (1884–1962).

The healthcare industry is one of the strongest growth drivers. In Germany around 5.6 million people are employed in the healthcare sector, i.e. every eighth employee [11]. If the definition of health care is defined a little more broadly and wellness and health tourism are added to it, it is even 7.6 million people and thus every sixth employee [12]. With a view to the 20 million baby boomers who will retire in the next two decades, the need for nursing and health care will increase significantly once again [13]. A real challenge for human resources management and development. Bold innovations are needed here.

What will the future be like? Pessimistic people tend to perceive problems first, and there are a number of them, such as the increasing shortage of personnel and the simultaneous increase in the need for care. Those with a cheerful nature may say: *"It's still all going well."* Futurologists take their cue from megatrends and develop scenarios. The question remains: can we trust science in this? In fact, scientists do a worse job of predicting the future than science fiction authors. Futurologist Bernd Flessner explains this fact by saying that scientists often have tunnel vision and are thus blind to their own work, whereas the authors of science fiction novels see the bigger picture since they always have to create a completely coherent world in their books [14] (http://www.welt.de). The future doesn't just happen, it is created. It is clear that change is coming, but how we deal with them is likely to vary. While winners take this new world into their own hands and shape it, losers are more likely to let themselves be shaped, according to futurologist [15].

In addition to the goals of knowledge transfer and skill development, today's personnel development focuses more than ever on attitude change. The change of perspective and attitude plays a central role in staff development. In the ideal case, this attitude is expressed in the company's goals and becomes the driving force in the development of personnel. Three areas need to be considered here: (1) further training and qualification of staff, (2) team development (interprofessional cooperation), and (3) organizational development (structures and processes). The current situation of personnel development is determined by three dimensions: (1) acceleration (temporal), (2) digitalization (factual), and (3) globalization and networking (social), according to Hans-Joachim Gergs, who accompanies change processes in the free economy ([16]: 18).

The development of personnel is particularly successful, when the positive result is not just a feeling, but measured by data. An example of this is an evidence-based personnel development project with the aim of increasing the hit rate of triaging in the emergency department. Whereas previously 26% of patients were not triaged or were triaged incorrectly, after the Emergency Severity Index training it was only 9.3% [17].

In the following section, I will explore the challenges of personnel development in the healthcare sector and explore possible solutions. The central focus here will be on the necessary competencies that need to be developed.

The most important challenges include technical progress, generational change (keyword: demographic change), traditional miscommunication, the tendency towards individualism, the increase in complexity and accelerated change processes, as well as the danger of international crises.

Possible solutions require a social change with a new understanding of communication as an economic factor and a focus on relationship-based work. The new technology, like care robots, must be researched and used sensibly (keyword: data protection), and genuine interprofessional cooperation must be learned. We need a new understanding of leadership, which enables both temporary leadership and autonomous teams, as well as real influence at all levels, including the level of health policy.

The most important competences that will be needed in the future include the ability to reflect, technical, emotional, and moral competence, the ability to cooperate interprofessionally, the ability to manage crises, changes and networks in a sustainable way, and to take responsibility (Table 15.1).

Table 15.1 Challenges, solutions and requirements of human resource development of the future

Challenges	Solutions	Requirements
Technical progress – Cyber attacks – Digitalization	Technology as a future driver – Research on technology – Data protection	Technical and ethical competence
Generation change – Baby boomer retire – Future of gen Y/Z	Focus on relations – Relationship-based care (RBC) – Person-centred care	Emotional and generational competence
Communication mistakes – Main reason for treatment mistakes	Communication as revenue-relevant – Consequent training – Value soft skills like hard skills	Communicative and reflexive competence
Individualism – Stimulates selfish and demanding behaviour	Success by interprofessional collaboration (IPC) – WHO framework – Promoting IPC and IPE	Collaborative and network competence
World gets more complex – Need of simple solutions – Waste of resources	Transition management – Project citizen involvement – Welfare economy	Transition and sustainability competence
Crises become bigger – Disadvantage of globalization	Criris as an opportunity – Taking influence – Culture of courage	Crises and responsibility competence

15.2 Technology as a Future Driver in Health Care

> **Looking into the crystal ball**
> *With a slight "ping," the personnel manager Samira Pfefferkorn becomes aware of the incoming call. On the wall in her office appears the name of the new team leader of the outpatient clinic: Paul Smith. A smile flits across Samira's face. She really likes Paul's British politeness and is proud to have poached him straight from a London clinic. He has committed himself to a 2-year project here in Berlin and will lead the change process in the outpatient clinic.*
>
> *No sooner has Samira uttered the magic words "Accept call" than Paul appears life-size holographically in her office. "Hi Paul, what can I do for you?" Paul clears his throat and makes an effort in German with an unmistakable accent, "Good morning Samira, I need your help. The triage assistant Rob TA 17 needs to be programmed with Swahili. We have a patient from Mozambique who is due in the OR in half an hour and needs to be informed about his illness in advance."*
>
> *"I'll take care of it" says Samira. "Thank you" says Paul.*
>
> *Samira instructs her computer, "Set Rob TA 17 to record mode." The computer replies, "Rob TA 17 ready." "Good" says Samira, "Load Swahili basic and advanced vocabulary focus on health." On the wall appears the image of Rob TA 17, a really good-looking robot with a sonorous voice that inspires confidence in patients. In front of him lies a young man with an arm injury on the mobile stretcher. Rob opens his eyes and greets the patient in Swahili: "shikamoni!" The patient smiles with relief and asks Rob TA 17 questions about his treatment, which the triage assistant can now easily answer in his language.*
>
> *Paul also follows the events on the office wall, which happen at the same time in his ambulance and says "thank you Samira." "You're welcome Paul."*

Technology in the Fast Lane

▶ If people acted according to their own rational interest, the world would be a paradise compared to its actual state.
  Bertrand Russel

Technological developments will completely change the entire healthcare market within a very short time. The new knowledge culture is described as a megatrend. Crucial for the success of these new technological advances is the trust patients and health care employees have in them. Building relationships with patients will become even more important than before.

With its digital strategy, the Federal Ministry of Education and Research of Germany has set out to steer the upcoming far-reaching processes of change. The digital strategy is intended to serve people, with a focus on their autonomy and security (data protection). The digital electronic patient file is identified as the core element for the healthcare system, which, as a personal data repository, will store all information from healthcare providers in the future. Later, this data can be supplemented with personal records (wearables, such as smartwatches) (BMBF, [18]). For nursing, a nursing innovation center has been named, as well as four practice centers focusing on: home care, inpatient care, intensive care, and nursing service center (http://www.pflegeinnovationszentrum.de).

Collecting and Evaluating Large Amounts of Data

Big data here means that incredibly large amounts of data are collected in decentralized structures, the analysis of which leads us to new insights. For more and more people, their own health stands for a good life, which needs to be protected. With pedometers and smartwatches, records are made of one's own movement status, apps can be used to control daily nutrition, and telemonitoring (RPM) has been developed for patients to monitor vital parameters. In the future, all of this information will be stored in centralized large databases to develop algorithms that can then be used to make new unimagined connections. This will result in new methods of diagnosis and therapy that no one has any idea of today.

In order to derive meaningful results from these large data sets, several innovative blockchain startups have been founded. We actually know the term blockchain from cryptocurrency, but in healthcare it goes far beyond Bitcoin and Co [19]. Here, data records are stored in blocks and then chained together to form meaningful chains. The advantage of the blockchain is that new blocks can only be appended if their content is compatible with the previous blocks, i.e. does not contradict them. In order to avoid misinformation, only certain people are authorized to append meaningful new blocks. It is important to ensure data autonomy for patients. The Israeli start-up *patient-first* with the founders Suter and Aharonovsky has developed a solution for this. If patients agree to feed their data into the system, they themselves can determine which companies are allowed to access it, thus regulating, for example, that a pharmaceutical company gets access in exchange for payment [19]. Other startups only allow doctors and hospital staff to access the data. This is the case, for example, with *SimplyVital Health*, founded by Kat Kuzmeskas, who only intends to make her blockchain available to patients at a later stage of development [20].

Individualized Patient Support

A dream come true! Immediate access to patient data through telemonitoring and forwarding to practices and clinics enables immediate intervention. Vulnerable patient groups, such as cardiac patients, can use intelligent technology not only to better monitor themselves, but also to transmit their data simultaneously to their healthcare partners (family doctor, outpatient nursing service, cardiac clinic). Doctors and nurses could compare this individual data with big data without wasting time and derive immediate interventions. This avoids inconvenient visits with long stays in waiting rooms or emergency rooms.

A whole range of different sensors were investigated as part of the *MoreCare* project, with the aim of improving activating care in outpatient care. The sensors are sewn into clothing, pictures on the wall, tablets, mobile phones, and smartwatches. These are light, sound, and environmental sensors. All devices are intelligently networked and feedback the patient's movement. In this outpatient rehabilitation project in a rural area, all participants (speech therapists, physiotherapists, nursing staff, physicians, etc.) were given access to the system for specific occupational groups so that relevant information could be retrieved in real time. The partially automatic documentation is experienced as particularly relieving. The technology used was continuously reviewed and improved during the project and adapted to the everyday conditions of a rehabilitation patient [21].

Electronic communication and information technology must target two areas in particular: (1) supporting people to live independently in their own homes for as long as possible and (2) contributing to counteracting the shortage of skilled workers [22].

Further examples of technical product development for healthcare can be found in Pfannstiel et al. [23], among others. For widespread use of such technology, the entire healthcare workforce needs to be retrained. Two areas are of particular importance here. (1) The focus needs to shift away from disease more towards prevention and (2) the attitude of healthcare workers needs to change from focusing on ordering to coaching the patient. So it's not enough to hand obese patients a flyer for a weight loss support group or tell smokers they just have to quit. Health workers must take on more of an educational role here and directly support patients in changing their behavior. Heart attacks can only be prevented if not only patient data is collected and communicated, but active work is done with the patients on their health behavior. Here the normal play instinct can be used. Through interactive games in the social network with like-minded people, members can encourage each other to change their behavior. Thus, on the one hand, they experience that they are not alone with their high blood pressure or obesity and, on the other hand, they can take action against it in a playful way. In comparison with others, the human ambition is often awakened to also create it or even to become better.

The method of motivational interviewing is recommended here. It was initially developed especially for addicts who found it difficult to change their behavior and the usual conversation techniques did not have any effect. Today, motivational interviewing is used when the goal is to stabilize behavior or change behavior [24]. All people in healthcare should be trained with it.

The Future Institute (Zukunftsinstitut), founded by Matthias Horx in 1998, predicts that by 2040 individualized medicine will have been implemented and drugs and therapies will only be used after prior genetic testing, thus avoiding individualized and expensive complications (http://www.zukunftsinstitut.de). In his books Sven Gabor Jánszky describes our possible future and combines science fiction with scientific data [15, 25].

Patient-Controlled Examinations

Many examinations are unpleasant for patients. For example, many women experience their mammogram as painful and often feel at the mercy of the situation. GE Healthcare has launched the *Senographe Pristina*, a mammography device that is controlled by the woman being examined. Using a remote control, the patient can control the compression of the breast during the image. This patient autonomy reduces stress and anxiety, which has a positive effect on image quality (http://www.3.hehealthcare.de).

The New Era of Care Robots

A whole range of different care robots are currently conquering the healthcare sector. They are called, for example, Pepper, Dinsow, Terapio, Paro, or Robear, and they support care in very different ways. There are two types of robots: (1) assistance robots, which are created to perform physical work, and (2) companion robots, which entertain patients or residents and reflect their emotions (Fig. 15.2) [26].

The robot Pepper was designed more for the clinical area and helps to make appointments, train patients, and evaluate vital signs and laboratory parameters in a medical context. Pepper speaks directly to people and guesses, for example, the age of the person in front of him. He is one of the humanoid robots and sees people through cameras in his eyes. Pepper answers questions and is used, for example, at the University Hospital in Halle for the MRI reconnaissance interview. Pepper takes over the informative first part of the conversation, so that doctors only have to answer final questions afterwards.

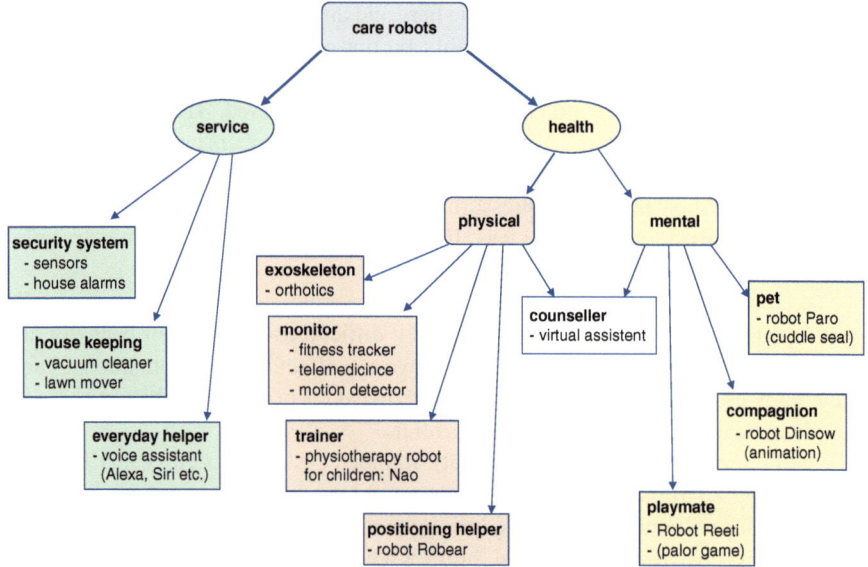

Fig. 15.2 Types of care robots (Tewes, own representation)

Terapio looks more like a green trash can and assists with rounds. He recognizes patients by their faces and provides the corresponding examination results. At chest level, there is a flap from which Terapio delivers tools such as tweezers and bandages, as well as a range of medications. The conversation between patient and staff is recorded by Terapio so that possible ambiguities can always be traced back [27].

The companion robots, such as Dinsow, are already quite advanced. It was developed for lonely people and is suitable for use in nursing homes. Dinsow encourages residents to do physical exercises, reminds them to take their medication, and encourages self-care.

The cuddly robot Paro was modeled on a baby seal and makes corresponding noises when it is touched. Paro is about 60 cm long, weighs 3 kilos, and has cuddly white fur. Paro can open and close his big googly eyes and is very popular with dementia patients. While care scientists appreciate the benefits of this offering, ethicists warn that it is a numbing world (http://www.welt.de). A team of Australian researchers has demonstrated that the use of Paro has a pain-reducing effect on dementia patients [28].

With its 140 kg, the Robear robot is one of the larger devices. It can carry people and still touch them gently. Robear has already been revised several times, so that the first "teething troubles" have already been technically eliminated. Robear supports the nursing staff in mobilizing patients when they need to be transferred or placed in a wheelchair. This is a useful way of counteracting a major cause of back pain among nursing staff (http://www.rinken.jp).

It is interesting to note how quickly society is becoming accustomed to robots. For example, as early as 2016, 83% of Germans in a representative Forsa survey stated that they would like to use service robots in their own households in old age so that they could live there longer [29].

What Scientists Predict for Us

Adrian Monti and Claire Coleman asked leading health researchers in 2016 for the Telegraph what the future holds [30] (http://tgr.ph/futureofhealth)

Professor John Moore-Gillon of the British Lung Foundation, for example, believes that an effective vaccine against asthma will be available very soon. He predicts a great future for immunotherapy, which will put radiation, chemotherapy, or surgery in their place.

Sonia Trigueros, group leader of Nano-Bio-Systems at Oxford University, is convinced that nanotechnology will make it possible to cure congenital blindness. To do this, nanoparticles 100,000 times smaller than a newspaper page are inserted into DNA, altering its genetic expression. The scientist predicts that already within the next 10 years nanostructures can be attached to the drugs of chemotherapy, in order to then effectively act only against the cancer and not harm healthy tissue any more.

Dr. Emily Burns, responsible for research communications at Diabetes UK explains that in the future, pancreas transplants will no longer be necessary, but diabetes can be cured by stem cell therapy. In diabetes, the beta cells of the pancreas attack the immune system. By means of stem cell therapy, protective layers will be placed around the beta cells in the future, so that diabetes patients can look forward to a healing future, says Burns.

Prof. Peter Johnson from Cancer Research UK wants to revolutionize cancer therapy. On the one hand, this is to be achieved through early diagnosis, as in future cancer will be identified through blood samples. On the other hand, it should be possible to visualize the cancer site more precisely, which means that higher doses of radiation can be applied to the malignant areas without damaging healthy tissue http://tgr.ph/futureofhealth.

Artificial Intelligence in Germany

In Germany, too, a lot of research is being done to develop technology for the healthcare sector and to make processes more efficient and successful. At Essen University Hospital, radiologist Felix Nensa heads a working group on artificial intelligence (AI) to develop the "Smart Hospital Information Platform." This joint project of radiology, nuclear medicine, and central information technology aims to consolidate and structure all patient data. Among other things, it must be determined who is allowed to access which patient data. Nensa already foresees the next stage of this technology, where patients can still be monitored by their doctors after discharge, for example, with a weight app that can indicate the development of dangerous edema in patients with kidney disease [31].

Internet of Things (IoT)

The Internet of Things (IoT) can already be predicted to be an industrial revolution. These are electronic systems that interact with people. These include the so-called wearables, i.e. portable mini-computers such as smartwatches. With IoT, relevant information from the real world is automatically linked and made available on the network. This is practical when changes in condition are determined, such as temperature, pulse, or the amount of medication.

A study by Aruba Networks [32] concludes that over 60% of healthcare organizations are already using IoT devices, and the demand is growing daily. For example, time and stress can be saved in emergency situations by using Bluetooth Low Energy location technology to find a device that someone had misplaced.

HeartMath Technology

The experience of positive relationships influences our perception. In an experimental study it was shown that the assessment of the height of a mountain to be climbed is significantly influenced by whether the test persons stood in front of the mountain with good friends, strangers, or even alone. The better the relationship quality (relationship duration, relationship closeness, cordiality), the lower the distance and mountain height were estimated. For test persons who estimated the summit height

Fig. 15.3 emwave®2 biofeedback device

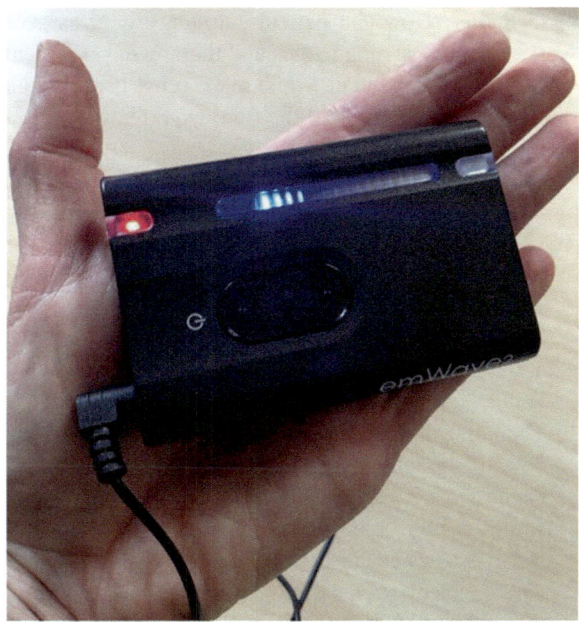

with strangers or alone, this was greater and the climb thus more difficult [33] (Fig. 15.3).

HeartMath has developed the practical biofeedback device *emWave®2, which* indicates the success of stress management methods by means of a coherence value. An ear sensor is used to measure heart rate variability, the ability of the heart to adapt to changes. By training techniques such as *Quick Coherence* or *Shift & Lift*, it is possible to return to the coherent range more and more quickly, even in stressful situations. With the free *Inner Balance App, the* current state can be determined via the ear sensor. The traffic light system shows red for stress and green for optimal adaptation of the heart. For more information, see the chapter "Stress was yesterday" by Sue Smith and Gavin Andrews in this book.

The *Global Coherence App* can connect a virtual group of people to meet at a specific time to practice the stress management techniques they have learned together. The participants can be in the same room or they can connect internationally. When practicing together, coherence scores increase faster than when the exercises are done alone. This app can also be used to determine a team's ability to engage in coherence with one another. For example, McCraty [34] demonstrated that synchronizing the heart rhythm of group members together increases group coherence, which in turn reduces stress. This is the first time that the relational work of teams can be determined and makes collaboration transparent.

In addition to technical competence, ethical competence is particularly in demand. Which data may be viewed by whom? Which networks are created by data links? Who bears the responsibility for autonomous decisions of the so-called blockchains? How can patient autonomy be preserved when data is fed into networks to improve diagnostics and therapy development?

A 70/30 arrangement would make sense here. For each technical training or continuing education, 30% of the time would have to be set aside for the development of ethical competence.

15.3 Generational Change and Relationship-Based Working

Samira Pfefferkorn arranged to meet some colleagues from the house for lunch at the enjoyment-center. When the glass doors to the center open silently and Samira looks around for familiar faces, the new head of research, Tino from Thailand, is already waving at her. He has chosen a nice seating area with colorful upholstered chairs and looks up from his tablet, where he had just been reading. "Hi Tino, how are you?" opens Samira the conversation. Tino smiles at her: "Great! Have you heard about our new game?" Samira raises her eyebrows curiously, "what new game, Tino?" Behind them Paul from the ambulance clears his throat, nodding amiably and joining them. Isabelle from data protection has also arrived and they all look at Tino promptly.

But before Tino could start, the attractive service person Rob SK 31 appears on the 3D monitor in the middle of the table. She greets everyone personally and takes the order. "Tino, can I get you some Thai rice with sweet and sour vegetables?" Tino nods in the direction of Rob SK 31. She also makes individual suggestions to everyone else, based as well on the daily scan values of the visitors (which are automatically determined at the entrance, with the consent of the staff) as on the tastes of the people (which are derived from the orders of the last weeks and varied anew). For each person she has a photo of the meal, which appears on the display of her upper body. It doesn't take 2 min and there are dishes on the table for everyone. The kitchen's new 3D printer makes it possible. The basic substances of the respective meal are inserted into the printer as a small cartridge and within seconds the printed meal appears.

"Delicious" raves Samira about her Indian fish dish with saffron. Paul enjoys his roast beef and Yorkshire pudding, while Isabelle opts for the colorful salad.

"Have you prepared a gig?" Paul asks in the direction of Tino. He grins broadly: "Yeah, sure." "Then let's get started," Samira encourages Tino. With a quiet click on Tino's tablet, a short video now appears in the middle of the table, playing in 3D. Some of Tino's colleagues can be seen developing clever research questions with each other. Each question asked appears on the wall of the research lab and can easily be moved back and forth with small hand movements. The best question of the day for the project is chosen and played to an international audience of researchers worldwide. Today it is, "What composition of proteins and minerals unleash the strongest healing function in 120-year-old heart patients?" The research community is a lively one around the world and welcomes challenging research questions. Fast forward the gig and 10 min later answers from Mexico, Senegal, Australia, Iran, and Russia reach the Berlin research lab. Now Tino's colleagues start to evaluate the different hypotheses. For each suggestion, a test tube is set up with the corresponding mixture of proteins and minerals, and the elemental substance of 120-year-old heart patients is poured in. The reactions will now be scientifically checked and the international colleague who has supplied the correct answer will be allowed to join the group of publishers. As soon as the result is available, the data will be forwarded to Rob Script 19, who will write the text and publish it on behalf of the participants. Paul nods appreciatively, "that's a cool game you've created!" Tino nods amiably and gets serious: "honestly? I'm really glad that the international research community is getting involved with these games and collaborations instead of competing with each other. An older colleague told me what it used to be like when research teams spied on each other. That must have been awful!"

Now Isabelle intervenes, who has been following the whole thing closely. "Yes, my father was also active in data protection for a time in his life, as I am today. He sometimes told me things that I couldn't believe. Even today, there are still thieves who hack into networks to sell the data to the highest bidder. But the prosecution of the perpetrators has become so successful that it's hardly worth it anymore. My father told me that back then they sometimes didn't even catch the hackers because data protection simply wasn't that far advanced yet." The others nod in agreement.

"Dessert?" asks Samira to the group. And immediatly the good-looking Rob SK 31 appears in the middle of the table. "Samira," she starts, "I have a delicious buttermilk muffin for you today." Now Samira remembers that when she entered the pleasure center, she was scanned and recommended several proteins to ingest. Hence, buttermilk, I guess. "Okay" Samira admits defeat, "but please Rob SK 31 make it look and taste like chocolate." "I'd love to," Rob SK 31 replies with a smile and disappears. Samira exhales audibly "I think she's over committed today!" Suddenly Rob SK 31 reappears in the middle of the table and announces towards Samira, "I heard that!" and disappears again. Perplexed, Samira asks around the table, "who programmed her to respond to that addition without addressing it by name?" Isabelle from data protection grins broadly and confesses: "sorry but I was in a programming mood today."

The Consequences of Generational Change

▶ The problem today is not nuclear energy, but the heart of the human being
Albert Einstein

Demographic change is leading to a generational shift in companies. Many of the baby boomers who are now retiring hold management positions that now need to be filled. Fewer births are reducing the number of younger people, and the large cohort of baby boomers (the generation before the pill crunch) is leading to a large increase in the number of older people.

While in 2013 27% of the population was older than 60 years, the population forecast for 2030 assume 35% (13th coordinated population forecast). This development has major implications for the healthcare system. The increase in very old people (80+) with the typical accompanying symptoms of physical complaints and dementia is becoming a real challenge. Conversely, the number of employees in the health care system, especially in nursing is decreasing, it is precisely these who are urgently needed.

Shifts are emerging in diseases, as the Global Burden of Disease study shows. While heart disease, apoplexy, and breast cancer are on the decline among women, we are seeing an increase in back pain, depression, and COPD. Men are less likely to develop cirrhosis of the liver. Heart disease, lung cancer, and apoplexy, however, remain the most common causes of disease, while diabetes and depression are increasing [35].

There will also be a major shift in the care provided by family caregivers. Currently, about two-thirds of those in need of care are cared for by relatives at home. Due to the aging of the baby boomers, there is an exponential increase in the number of people who are dependent on nursing care and can no longer be cared for by their own family members. There are various reasons for this, such as too big distance between parents and children or the increase in the number of women working. The undervalued status of social professions in our society may also contribute to the fact that it seems less attractive to take care of sick relatives.

The generational shift in healthcare is leading to a new discussion of values. For baby boomers, functions, titles, or hierarchy-conscious tasks are important, they take responsibility for the entire organization (step in if someone drops out) and live to work. Generation Y is highly tech-savvy and world-wide connected. They work accordingly effectively and question pointless activities. In addition to work, their personal lives are important to them and thus they work to live. It becomes clear that worlds collide here and thus tensions are pre-programmed [36].

Despite the looming leadership gap, however, the departure of the baby boomers can also bring an opportunity. For the younger generation, leadership is not necessarily a lifetime task, but can also be temporary, such as project management. The good networking potential and the focus on getting things done effectively can lead to new teamwork in which roles are not fixed but are constantly redistributed depending on the task at hand. Cooperation should also be fun, and one's own participation should be experienced as a success.

Paradigm Shift for Personnel Development

For personnel development, this means that in future qualifications will be based less on fixed roles and more on the respective knowledge required for the next area of responsibility.

Like the pilots who have to train again when they change aircraft types, for example, from a Boeing 747 to an Airbus A 350–900. For this purpose, they receive all technical data and information on the new aircraft with a program installed on their tablet, which must be processed and then passed with a test. This ensures safe flying when pilots fly other routes and/or other aircraft. This retraining measure including the test takes place online.

Leadership training should not only be offered to managers, but to all those who are interested in leadership tasks from time to time. This breaks through the rigid top-down thinking and enables those involved to be deployed more strongly than before according to their competencies. So we move away from the question "who can do this?" and towards "who can do that?"

Megatrend: Relationships

With the increasing dominance of technology in our lives, the need for typically human things such as contact and relationships is growing. So it is no wonder that in the health care sector there is a great demand for methods that focus on people and their relationships. In the USA "Relationship-based Care" in short RBC has become one of the most successful change management programs (see Wessels et al. in this book). In this program the following six aspects in the organization are analyzed for relationship-based working: Leadership, Teamwork, Interprofessional Collaboration, Care Structures, System Design, and Evidence. Through various programs, such as "See me as a Person" or "Re-Igniting the Spirit of Caring," the entire culture of an organization is reflected upon in interprofessional teams and strategically changed together [37, 38]. Every 4 years, leaders and staff from hospitals that have successfully implemented RBC come together and share their incredible results at a symposium. Time and time again, participants report how much new life has been breathed into the organization as a result of RBC and how staff dissatisfaction has been transformed into a new form of satisfying collaboration. For example, the 638-bed Mississippi Baptist hospital in Jackson reports that the introduction of relationship-based care reduced nurse turnover, saving about $1.64 million in 1 year alone. The cost of temporary workers dropped from $4.65 million to $0, meaning RBC's investment paid off many times over (chcm.com).

In Europe, the "person-centered care" approach is gaining ground, which started in Ireland and has since found resonance in many European countries (McCormack et al. in this book). Brendan McCormack is himself active in teaching and research and has not only described the practical implementation for his person-centered approach, but also developed a theoretical model for it [39]. This model has already been researched and developed further by academics in Holland, Norway, and Scotland [40]. The Norwegian Ministry of Health has even decided to introduce the person-centered approach nationwide with the aim of guaranteeing the dignity of all citizens [41].

And the policy in Lower Austria has decided to introduce person-centered care in all nursing homes. This project was and is being researched by the nursing scientist Hannah Meyer (http://www.noebetreuungszentren.at). The person with his or her needs is the focus of attention and satisfies both: the residents and the staff.

For this purpose, the Protestant University of Applied Science, Dresden offers a Bachelor's degree course called "Practice Development," which teaches the concepts of Person-centered Care (http://www.ehs). Here, nursing professionals study alongside their work and learn to change their professional practice systematically and with a view to the employees and patients. The focus on people and relationships is put into practice and does not remain as an empty bubble on mission statements.

Studies with Generation Z (born after 1995) show that they attach great importance to social support in the team and a good corporate climate. They rate these cultural and social aspects in organizations as significantly more conducive to health than, for example, stress management training or sports activities [42].

Integrative Methods Have a Future

Society as a whole is developing a greater interest in its own health and, in addition to conventional medicine, integrative methods are increasingly in demand. These are methods that complement conventional medicine, such as homeopathy, aromatherapy, pranic healing, and much more. Here, too, the focus is on the individual, which patients are happy to take advantage of, as health care workers are finding less and less time for them. Thus, both the International Integrative Nursing Symposium and the Integrative Medicine Congress are very popular. More and more renowned universities are opening their own research department for Integrative Care, such as Harvard or Stanford. More about this in the chapter "Pearls of Wisdom" by Emily Witrak Nowak and Val Lincoln in this book.

The necessary prerequisites for relationship-based and person-centered work are emotional and generational competences. Both can be learned and require a great deal of reflection. A good guiding question for this is: "what do I carry inside me that bothers me about you?"

15.4 The Secret of Success: Communication

Samira stares thoughtfully at the feedback results from the surgical team. The new hand surgeon, Dr. Abdul Darzi, is doing anything but well. He conducts his operations from Medina in Saudi Arabia and has never been to Germany. His knowledge of hand surgery is impressive and Samira was happy to have him for remotely assisted complicated procedures. But she had already guessed that it would not be easy with him. Abdul had not earned a reputation as a team player and was considered headstrong and arrogant by staff. All the team members in yesterday's surgery had given him poor marks for cooperation. Immediate action was needed here.

She got an overview: of the total of three operations carried out with Abdul as team leader, two were mediocre in the assessment of cooperation and yesterday's was questionable. In total, three people (Martin, Mia, and Svetlana) and three robots had worked with Abdul. She registered a group call with the three colleagues concerned and asked for appointment suggestions. Instead of a suggestion, Svetlana immediately came forward. A glowing dot with her picture, name, and work location appeared on the office wall. Samira exhaled once deeply and accepted the call. "Svetlana, how nice of you to get back to me right away!" Svetlana looked grimly at the display. "I'm still angry, Samira! Abdul took out his bad temper on Rob OP 33 yesterday. Even though the good girl is a robot, I caught the whole dialogue and asked Abdul several times to be more respectful. But nothing helped."

"Yes, Svetlana, that's annoying. Tell me, what's your assignment schedule today? Can I come by?" Svetlana reads the upcoming appointments off her glasses and replies, "The next surgery starts in 4 minutes, but I could set up time with you at noon today."

"Great, Svetlana, I'll pass the date on to Martin and Mia right away. It would be great if we could talk about it together!"

At noon Samira sneaks into the OR as arranged and is met by Martin and Swetlana in the meeting room. "Mia has another online training and will join us in 8 minutes" says Swetlana. Unprompted, Martin sets out a soy soft drink for all three of them and comments, "it's good for our nerves."

"Thank you very much Martin! Then you must have prepared the meeting room as well?" Samira asks. The room is wrapped in warm light tones and offers a view of a stylishly landscaped courtyard, where a fountain gurgles away. The holographically visible patio with trees and beautiful hedges in all shades of green lends tranquility and strength. It is obvious that someone wanted to initiate a calming mood here. Martin smiles caught: "something relaxing can't hurt."

Samira is prepared and brought some information with her. Dr. Abdul Darza had also worked with two of the clinical contract partners over the past few years, with whom they help each other with staff. Evaluations are available from both of them. Out of a total of 32 surgeries, Abdul has received feedbacks ranging from good (8×), quite okay (14×) to mediocre (8×) to questionable (2×) regarding his competence in team work. They look at the types of operations, team constellations, and times of day to analyze if there are any similarities. In all ratings of "good" and "quite okay," it is noticeable that the OR staffing was almost exclusively male.

To better understand the pattern, Samira calls out additional biographical data. His recent congressional contributions appear, as well as details from his family. Abdul had witnessed his brother injured in a car accident as a child, losing a hand. At the time, his older sister had been driving. He had then decided to become a hand surgeon. As one of the best in his field, he later succeeded in helping his brother to get a well-functioning replacement hand.

"Okay," Samira puts in, let's hypothesize. Martin speaks up, "apparently Abdul can't communicate well when women are present." Samira asks in the direction of Svetlana and Mia, who had joined them by now, "Are there exceptions?" Mia puts in thoughtfully, "come to think of it, his comments only became disrespectful when I made suggestions on how to proceed. That may have come across to him as me getting behind the wheel like his sister did back then." "True," Svetlana follows up, "I too saw him as friendly at first. That only changed when the good colleague Rob OP 33 suggested exposing the tendons first and then taking care of the epidermis."

Samira summarizes, "This sounds like unprocessed trauma. What do you suggest as solutions?"

"We can assign only male colleagues and male robots for his operations in the future" suggests Mia. "Can we do that?" asks Samira. Now Martin intervenes: "We can do that. But I have another idea. Abdul is giving a talk at a conference in London in six weeks. I would also like to attend. Maybe I can talk to him personally and carefully draw his attention to the topic of trauma therapy. I have done trauma therapy myself, after people died in front of my eyes during a flood disaster on a journey, whom I could not save. These images in my head kept me busy for a long time and limited me in my everyday life. Since the therapy I can face challenges again without fear. If the right moment presents itself, I might bring this up with Abdul."

Samira nods appreciatively, "That would be great, of course, if you could share that personal experience with Abdul."

Mia smiles at Martin: "Thank you very much for this suggestion. It is really commendable. Nevertheless, I ask not to be assigned together with Abdul in the future."

"But sure," Martin puts in, "we'll stick to using only male personnel in any further operations with Abdul.

Svetlana smiles, "Great then I can finally drink coffee again instead of soothing soy soft drinks."

Faulty Communication Produces Treatment Errors

▶ In the beginning was the word. Immediately after came the misunderstanding
Reinhard Sprenger

The most common reason for treatment failures is poor communication [43, 44]. "Every minute, five people die worldwide from preventable treatment errors" according to WHO Chief Tedros Adhanom Ghebreyesus [45] (http://www.who.intent) [46]. Forty percent of patients experience harm during outpatient procedures and 10% in hospital. In surgery, failure to follow safety procedures leads to complications in about 25% of patients, which are fatal for about one million people. Treatment errors are expensive. Medication errors alone, for example, are estimated to cost an additional $42 trillion annually in the USA. The key to greater safety lies in greater patient involvement, according to the WHO (http://www.who.intent).

The Swiss theologian Markus Ronner calls communication science the study of misunderstandings [47]. Successful communication is therefore needed. The present health care system is strongly oriented towards the linear thinking of a cause–effect logic, which is expressed, for example, in the word "order." The emphasis is on following and obeying. What is needed, however, is dialogue, which corresponds to a circular pattern of thought. This talking to each other, listening to each other, expressing interest in the other, showing understanding and empathy is the prerequisite for successful communication.

Communication is the means of transport for professional work and thus an essential part of so-called professional competence! This does not fall from the sky, but it can be learned.

In more technical areas, such as intensive care units or operating theaters, even less importance is often attached to communicative competence, which has fatal consequences. Conflicts increase here, which on the one hand endanger patient safety and on the other hand increase costs [44, 48]. In a study of 7498 ICU participants from 24 countries, 72% reported experiencing conflict in the last week. Of these, half of the participants (53%) described the conflict as serious and damaging to teamwork. 44% even state that during the experienced conflict the survival of patients was potentially threatened [49].

In a study of communication in the operating room, 30% of communication errors were found to compromise patient safety [50]. In the USA, patient death from medical error is the third leading cause of death, after heart disease and cancer [51].

Understanding and Changing Communicative Demotivation

The health care system would be greatly helped if the employees working there were not constantly demotivated. Unprofessional communication, especially by managers, is at the top of the list of motivation killers.

Often the supervisors themselves are not aware of the effect their words have. For example, if the manager comes out of a meeting with top management and tells the team, "You won't believe the stupid things they've come up with up there again..." This suggests to employees that top management doesn't know what they're doing, with the result that employees have a hard time identifying with their organization. After all, who wants to be part of a company of incompetents. At the same time, identification with the organization is the strongest intrinsic motivating factor, which is ruined by this above fatal sentence of the manager. As long as managers choose such careless phrases, any training for employee motivation makes no sense.

In this case, personnel development means training managers to position themselves in meetings with top management and to actively participate in the decision-making process. Workshops on targeted negotiation management or strategies for exerting influence can work wonders here. Ultimately, active engagement with management also expands the scope for action, which has a positive effect on professional autonomy and thus on job satisfaction.

However, there are also situations in which managers have to communicate decisions to their team that they themselves do not support. Here, it is necessary to maintain composure, think through the information, and "digest" it until it can be communicated in a reasonably value-free manner. This requires real emotional work and needs some training. The necessary emotional intelligence can be learned.

The widespread top-down thinking is fed by hierarchical structures that are no longer up to date.

Conflicts due to poor communication between the different professional groups are responsible for serious burnout symptoms, both among nurses and physicians [52].

What Communication Has to Do with Hormones

Another example of unprofessional communication is allowing bitching and whining. Professional communication in the team is a leadership task. This means not only that superiors set a good example, but also that they guide their team to communicate professionally. Overstrained managers often complain that "it's like kindergarten." In doing so, they distance themselves from the team and at the same time they show their lack of appropriate leadership tools to intervene in a meaningful way.

Complaining is not only exhausting for all involved, but also shrinks the brain. This is the conclusion of several studies that examined the effect of stress on the brain. Post-traumatic stress, for example, shrinks a specific site in the hippocampus that stands for memories and rational decision-making by up to 26% [53] and by 16% in the case of early childhood sexualized violence experiences [54].

Complaining is negative thinking and complaining can become a habit that damages the brain in the long run [55]. Natalie Marchant and her research team have

Fig. 15.4 Brain physiology of negative thoughts

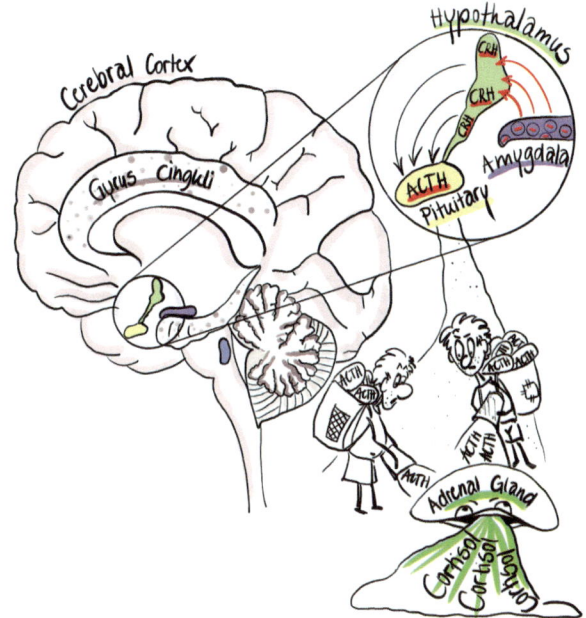

shown that repeated negative thinking positively influences the development of Alzheimer's disease in people aged 55 [56] (Fig. 15.4).

To understand the influence of positive and negative thoughts, let's take a little trip into physiology. Practically every thought triggers a whole cascade of physical reactions [57].

First, information from the environment arrives at the cerebral cortex via sensory perception. From there, it is transmitted to the limbic system, which is also known as the center for emotional intelligence [58]. Here, the information is compared to previous experiences and evaluated. If the incoming data is evaluated negatively, the amygdala becomes active, which stores all negative experiences throughout life. The firing amygdala causes the hypothalamus to produce hormones such as CRH (corticotropin releasing hormone), which causes the pituitary gland to release neurotransmitters such as ACTH. ACTH docks with the adrenal gland, which then releases cortisol. When we not only think, but actually express our thoughts, the body reacts with corresponding intensity. Normally, the cortisol stops the hypothalamus. But when negative thoughts occur too often, as with frequent whining, depression, burnout, or PTSD, this emergency brake can no longer be activated. Then the body releases high doses of cortisol, which harm the body [59, 60]. In this regard, it is also interesting to note a study conducted with family caregivers who are caring for a family member with cancer. It is not the interaction with their sick family member that leads to elevated cortisol levels in family caregivers, but their repeated negative thinking [61]. And high stress-related cortisol levels limit thinking skills that affect memory, organization, and visual perception, which was demonstrated in a study of 2000 participants [62] (Fig. 15.5).

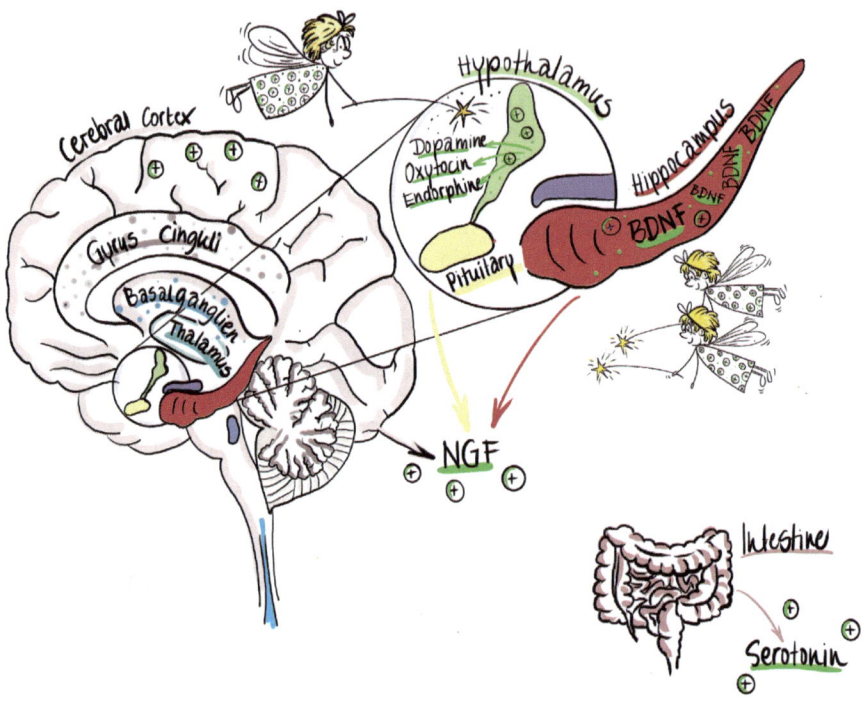

Fig. 15.5 Brain physiology of positive thoughts

Thoughts arrive at the cerebral cortex in the form of sensory perceptions and are then evaluated in the limbic system. When these are now evaluated positively, a whole series of reactions occur in the brain. The hypothalamus now produces dopamine, oxytocin, and endorphin. The intestine is activated to produce serotonin by messenger substances from the pituitary gland. We know these substances as the so-called happiness hormones. They give us a good feeling, make us satisfied or even happy. By exercising we can raise our serotonin levels and by setting and achieving realistic goals we can raise our dopamine levels. Dopamine is linked to the reward center and makes us feel satisfied when rewarded.

But even more exciting is what happens in the hippocampus (also a part of the limbic system). Here, two growth factors are now released that have an incredible effect on our body. They are called BDNF (brain-derived neurotropic factor) and NGF (nerve growth factor). The increased release of BDNF and NFG leads to an increase in the connections between nerve cells (synapses) and increases the functional performance of the nerve cells. The proliferation of nerve cells by these two messenger substances has also been proven. BDNF protects neurons and synapses and promotes the growth of nerve cells (called neuroneogenesis). Since NGF is very important for our body, it is also produced in other places, such as the basal ganglia, the pituitary gland, or the spinal cord.

NGF regulates the immune system, reduces neuronal degeneration, and is more abundant in lovers. It is also effective against Alzheimer's disease, but must be injected intracranially because NGF does not cross the blood barrier [63]. We can also control the production of NGF ourselves. A study by scientists at the Medical University of South Carolina was able to prove that NGF can be increased through yoga (Omchanting and Pranayama) [64].

In summary, information that is negatively valued by the limbic system (e.g. negative thoughts) slows brain coordination, impedes creative abilities, reduces brain activity, and negatively affects mood, memory, and impulse control. Whereas information considered positive strengthens synapses, causes neurons to grow, enhances attention and memory skills, improves information analysis and problem solving skills, and increases creativity. Stress hormones, such as cortisol, damage the body in the long run, while happiness hormones, such as oxytocin, endorphin, or dopamine, are good for the body and support healing processes.

Why Complaining Is Harmful

If you whine in front of an audience and someone else notices, their body will react accordingly. Every whining from colleagues must be understood as an invitation to whine along or to get out. When whining, the stressful processes in the body are triggered. This is also often noticeable: after an extensive bath in the whining pool the involved ones often feel powerless or energy-less and worry rather than having cheerful thoughts. As soon as whining occurs, energy get lost. The longer or more often whining is done, the more powerless the people involved become. Regular whining leads to a depletion of one's own energy. But even if you don't complain, the complaining of others can be annoying and increase the cortisol level.

This pathophysiological process by which we damage our bodies through complaining needs to be understood so that it can be changed. Employees can learn not to respond to whining offers and thus maintain their energy instead of wasting it. For managers, the attitude of a mentor or coach is needed here to practice professional communication with team members.

Whining can also be a sign of an unreflective victim role, which is supposed to offer protection from responsibility. We see this attitude in teams that have been led in an authoritarian manner for a long time. Here it takes some patience on the part of the new leadership to gradually get the team used to the benefits of self-responsibility.

Because professional communication is so important to patient safety, employee satisfaction, and the economics of healthcare, it is gaining prominence. The long occupied place of only being a soft skill and therefore a nice-to-have is being abandoned in favor of a serious position as a hard cost factor and thus becomes a must-have.

Why We Blaspheme

Experience shows that employees in the healthcare sector find it difficult to constantly change, which is expressed in the phrase "but we've always done it that way." How can this be explained?

Everyday professional life in the healthcare sector is like a cauldron of emotions. Patients are in pain or fearful of upcoming procedures. Serious accidents disrupt their lives and lead to unexpected worries and distress. Uncertainty mobilizes fears that healthcare workers are constantly confronted with. This also triggers feelings in staff, but these are rarely reflected upon and processed. This is because health care does not offer places to work on feelings. Exceptions to this are regular supervision in psychiatric wards or depth psychological discussions in hospices and oncology departments. As a rule, the unpleasant feelings triggered by patients are repressed and projected onto others. Instead of reflecting which emotions patients trigger in me (e.g. helplessness, powerlessness, anger) these are idealized (I am a good person and have no bad feelings) and projected onto others (preferably the evil management or the incompetent politicians). Thus, widespread blasphemy in organizations can be understood as a defense mechanism against the anxiety-producing insecurities employees face [65, 66]. Projection was confirmed as a preferred defense mechanism among both nurses and physicians in one study [67].

The lack of confrontation with one's own feelings has a long tradition in healthcare and leads to rigid behavior patterns in teams [68]. Thus, the permanent uncertainty in healthcare is compensated for by controlling and ritualizing everyday life. This suggests that the unpleasant feelings can be managed with control mechanisms. It is not for nothing that quality controls determine everyday professional life. The unconscious dynamics in organizations stress employees and promote unconscious defense processes [65, 66].

Dealing with Stressful Emotions

How can the common big blind spot be reduced? First of all, it needs the insight that the emotional shifts (wanting to protect patients and blaming management or politicians for this) are an inappropriate waste of energy. After all, every time we rant, whine, or bitch about others, cortisol is produced, which has a lasting effect on mood and saps energy. We must learn to live with uncertainty rather than repress it. The idea that rigid control helps against flooding emotions must be exposed as an illusion. And the favorite mechanism of projection must also be sacrificed. The soft skill of reflection must become a prerequisite for work in the health sector.

To achieve this, we need methods and places for reflection. Or to speak with Gary Hamel and Michel Zanini [69]: "Build a platform, not a change program." Some of the best known methods of reflection in health care are case review, supervision, reflecting team, coaching, Ballint group, flashlight, or mood barometer. Common to all these methods is their application in a group. This enables a change of perspective and expands one's own field of vision. Honest and appropriate feedback can be practiced and blind spots can be reduced. Through reflection, frustration, fears and insecurities can be worked through and their energy used in a targeted way to eliminate sources of anger and to change things instead of complaining about them.

In addition to group methods, there are also instruments for reflecting on one's own actions alone, such as mirror work ([70]: 144ff). However, these methods are only recommended for people who are extremely reflective, as most people tend to use rose-colored glasses in their self-assessment instead of holding up a mirror to themselves honestly and unsparingly.

"The more unstable the environmental conditions are, the more important a company's ability to reflect becomes," according to continuous self-control expert Hans-Joachim Gergs [16]. Reflection creates distance and thus enables an overview that is easily lost in the frenzy of heavy workloads. Distance must be understood as an important thinking tool in this context ([71]: 35).

So there is a need for places where pauses for thinking and feeling are not only permitted, but explicitly desired. Working through unpleasant feelings together enables honest and trusting cooperation and reduces talking about each other. Looking to the future, Gergs sees self-reflection as a meta-principle that lays the foundation for an effective error and feedback culture ([16]: 56).

The lack of self-reflection in the leadership of some companies fosters their narcissistic arrogance and cements top-down thinking in organizations. We know from studies of communication in the operating room that strong hierarchies in teams cause the error rate to skyrocket [50, 72]. This is because those lower in rank often see what is going wrong earlier, but do not dare to communicate it. The courage to talk back is internationally referred to by the concept of "challenging authority" and has been well studied for the OR [73]. In teams working in partnership, it is easier for everyone involved to share feedback, which has a positive impact on error rates. Business researcher Hans Hinterhuber warns that narcissistic top managers pose a risk to the organization [74]. Especially companies in crisis looking for a savior fall for self-promoters who are ultimately only concerned with their own well-being. But it is precisely in times of crisis that discussions at eye level and the participation of the workforce are important.

Communicative and reflective competence is the most important basis for cooperation and should not be taken for granted. The good news: both can be learned and should therefore be trained throughout life and thus be included in all further training and education.

15.5 Interprofessional Cooperation as a Decisive Factor for the Future

> Paul from the ER appears holographically in Samira's office and clears his throat. "Paul, how nice to see you" Samira greets him friendly. "Hello Samira, I'd like to do some leadership training. My British soft skills are passable but sometimes I don't understand my team. While Lina from the Philippines reacts anxiously when I express my expectations to her, Jens asks me almost daily to critically mirror his behavior. Patrick from Nigeria seems to be in competition with me, at least he constantly tells me what I can do better. I would need a program where I can learn about personalities and culture."

Samira nods, "Yes, I can well understand that. When I came here from India, I not only had to familiarize myself with German culture, but I was also part of constantly changing international teams. And every colleague has his or her own idiosyncrasies. By the way, we have a great leadership trainer who offers practical personality training. Her name is Tabea Groß and she gets the best evaluations from the participants." From her display she reads, "practical, instructive and humorous!" and continues, "We have three new employees who have come to us from other countries. Christopher is a surgeon and comes from New Zealand, Samantha is leading a project to link physiotherapy from the inpatient, rehabilitation, and outpatient sectors and comes from Uganda. And Tino has taken over the research department for 2 years and has Thai roots." "Yes" Paul hooks in "I already know Tino from the welcome party. His game-changing research methods are really impressive."

"Right" says Samira, "should I check with the three of them to see if they have a need for the subject as well or would you rather have one on one training, Paul?"

"A small group would be fantastic. Then I'll also get to know the new colleagues better."

"Great idea Paul, I'll get back to you as soon as I know more."

"Thank you so much, Samira."

The hologram with Paul disappears and Samira registers a videocall with Tabea Groß. The display shows the information: "I'll be there for you in 27 minutes." "Okay," Samira thinks, "I'll send the new colleagues an offer first. I'll also make a short video to address all three of them personally.

Samira pulls up some of Tabea's training papers on the display and switches them over to her office wall.

"Video recording now! Individualize speeches" says Samira and stands in front of her office wall.

"Speech 1: Hello Christopfer, Speech 2: Hello Samantha, Speech 3: Hello Tino."

"Paul is our new team leader in the outpatient clinic. With a wave of her hand, a photo of Paul appears next to her. He has just inquired if you would also like to do a training with a focus on understanding culture and personality. I'm trying to mobilize a small group for this, so you'll be no more than 4 participants." The names of each of the other three new colleagues appear in a scroll bar, along with their respective departments. Samira shows a video message from Tabea. Here Tabea introduces herself and reports in her typically humorous way that she loves talking to people about human stuff and likes to make her workshops interactive. With a movement of her arm Samira draws different personality models on the wall one after the other and reports that the selection of the respective models is adapted to the questions of the group of participants. Samira shows a short video of a participant who reports on how much she has benefited from the training with Tabea and which of the aspects she has learned she now takes into account in her everyday professional life.

Finally, Samira smiles at the camera and says, "If you feel like joining, just get in touch with me." Samira's contact details appear in the scroll bar.

"Stop video recording" says Samira and looks at the clock on the display. The entire recording with interludes now takes 3 min and 12 s. "Well" Samira thinks to herself, "a bit long, but okay. Next promotional video I'll try to get to exactly 2 minutes 55. Because that's how much time everyone has to watch the message." With a few key combinations, she sends the individualized videos and sends Paul a copy.

A "ping" sounds and a call from Tabea is announced on the wall. Samira answers immediately and Tabea appears holographically in the office. "Hello Samira, you are looking good! Are you training for the swimming championships again?" Hello Tabea, no swimming is not so important right now, I have other plans." Demonstratively she stands sideways and strokes her belly. Tabea looks incredulous at first and then beams all over her face. "How nice, you're pregnant! This is really a surprise!" "Yes"" smiles Samira, "we are also very excited about this addition." With a wink Tabea asks "and, did your Steffen get to be active or did you guys go for the freezer variety?" Typical Tabea, always cheekily direct. I wonder if that's what they teach you in psychology school. But with her incomparable charm, you just want to tell her everything. Still, Samira hesitates and changes the subject, "Where are you right now?" Tabea points to her brightly colored sandals and says, "I only ever wear those in Shanghai. Here you can walk around as colorful as you want and nobody raises an eyebrow. Tomorrow I have my last day of life coaching and then I'm coming back to Berlin." Samira sees her chance: "A very nice colleague has just started as a team leader in our outpatient clinic. Paul asks for a personality training with you."

That's when Tino's message "I'm in" appears on the wall. Samira comments further, "And also Tino, the new research director would like to be there." Tabea frowns and calls up her calendar entries. "I see," she says, "it's going to be tight." Samira lays it on again, because negotiation is something she's learned, "If you offer life coaching for my new people, I'll also tell you the secret of wonderful insemination." "Great, well then!" Tabea gets down to business, "Tell the two gentlemen to go ahead and prepare themselves first. I have created some video modules on the subject. I'll send you the first two. They are 30 minutes each with subsequent reflection, for which another 30 minutes should be planned. They can send me the excerpts of the joint reflection in a short message. They can do this together live or via video talk with each other. Then you should contact me and I will make an appointment with them. Maybe we can even do it live. I'll see what I can do." Then comes that mischievous look from Tabea again, "and, who will be the godmother?"

Interprofessional Cooperation as an Economic Adjusting Screw

▶   Those who work alone add, those who work together multiply.
Arabic proverb.

The successful collaboration of all professional groups is being researched internationally under the term *Interprofessional Collaboration*, or IPC for short. Scott Reeves has initiated and conducted many studies on this subject and in 1999 founded the *Journal of Interprofessional Care*.

Interprofessional collaboration (IPC) means that the various professional groups in the healthcare sector meet as equals and join forces to make decisions together. This sounds simple, but it is a real challenge in an age characterized by individualism and entitlement behavior. At IPC, solutions are developed through genuine dialogue, without one person or one professional group being dominated or given more decision-making rights. In a world of "orders," IPC amounts to a paradigm shift. The typical hierarchical structures of hospitals often work against true togetherness. Even in operating rooms, where we classically speak of an OR team, there is often still the idea that hierarchical working prevents errors. In fact, the opposite is true. Studies show that hierarchy in the OR is the most common reason for miscommunication, and miscommunication in the OR is in turn the most common reason for increased morbidity and mortality rates among surgical patients [44].

In addition to the different professional groups, it will also be necessary to cooperate with the new robot colleagues in the future. The importance of successful human–machine collaboration (HMC) will strongly influence the future of healthcare. Thus, interpersonal collaboration (IPC) always includes to human–machine collaboration.

There are many good reasons why *interprofessional collaboration* (IPC) should be embraced in healthcare. Here are the most important ones:

- Increases patient safety [75–77].
- Reduces treatment errors [44].
- Reduces the costs of medical errors [78].
- Increases quality of care [76, 79, 80].
- Reduces employee sickness and turnover [81].
- Significantly reduces patient mortality in intensive care units [78].
- Reduces conflicts [49].

The research results on IPC prove that it is no longer a nice-to-have option, but urgently needed. Once cooperation has been learned, it is fun. This is because genuine collaboration triggers resonance experiences that increase the joy of good work and performance [82].

Why Cooperation Has Not Worked So Far

If cooperation between the professional groups pays off so much, the question naturally arises: why is it so difficult to ensure? The greatest potential for tension lies in the health care system between the two professional groups of nurses and physicians. Hibbeler [83] speaks of a chronic conflict in the German Medical Journal. Both professions are missing something crucial that is necessary to work together. To understand this, we need to explore the concept analysis on interprofessional collaboration (IPC) by Laura Petri [75]. She identified the preconditions that are necessary for IPC to become possible.

In addition to organizational support (structural empowerment), role clarity and interpersonal relationship skills are needed [75]. While nurses lack role clarity, physicians lack interpersonal relationship skills.

First, regarding nurses: the lack of role clarity leads to a lack of self-protection mechanisms in situations that are experienced as attacks.

Care professionals experience time and again that their limits are exceeded. This includes, for example, disrespectful behavior, being put under pressure, rude behavior, or being very demanding. In the moments when this happens, care professionals often do not draw a line and thus do not protect themselves. Instead of saying, "excuse me, but I don't want you to talk to me in that tone," they often "keep quiet," only to gossip about it with colleagues afterwards. However, for the person who used the wrong tone, such no-reaction behavior means "okay like that, keep it up." The nursing staff often do not give any feedback after an inappropriate communication, to the "boundary crosser." With this missing feedback, however, the behavior of the boundary crosser is unfortunately confirmed. For the latter it is therefore: "that was okay, keep it up."

Role clarity is a crucial factor in interpersonal collaboration [84, 85]. The clearer one's own role is, the more strongly it can be represented externally [86]. Uncertainty about professional boundaries thus transfers to the management of personal protective behaviors. Interestingly, the shared interprofessional education of medical professionals, nurses, and therapists strengthens professional identity [87–89]. With George Herbert Mead, one could formulate here that only with a counterpart does one's own self become clear [90].

Now let's turn to physicians. They unlearn their ability of empathy through their studies at University and also later in their careers, which many studies have shown [89, 91, 92]. Empathy among physicians is a critical prerequisite for collaboration and patient-centered care [93]. The good news is that empathy is re-learnable for physicians. Fifteen of 18 studies have demonstrated that physicians show significant improvements after empathy training [94] (Fig. 15.6).

It can therefore be summarized: in order to close the communication gap between nurses and physicians, nurses must learn to give clear immediate feedback and physicians must (re)train their empathy. Only when these conditions are met it is possible for both professions to resonate with each other and establish true collaboration. This resonance can even be technically measured using the *Global Coherence App*

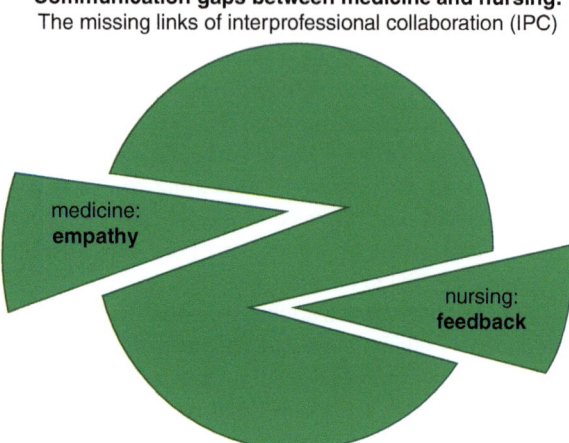

Fig. 15.6 Communication gap between nursing and medicine (Tewes, own illustration)

from the HeartMath Institute. More about this in the chapter "Stress was yesterday" by Smith and Andrews in this book.

What Does It Take for Interprofessional Cooperation to Succeed

When interprofessional collaboration (IPC) succeeds, it not only reduces treatment errors and saves costs, but has a host of other positive effects, such as: Good team climate and the ability to identify with both: one's own profession and the team [95], collaborative leadership, interprofessional conflict resolution, person-centered care [85], relationship-based working, constructive feedback culture, strengths-based practice [96], and communication characterized by seeking to understand each other, as well as helping the other to make sense [97].

The good news first: interprofessional collaboration can be learned [98]. However, IPC does not succeed if the organization is not willing to invest in training on interprofessional collaboration [99] and if physicians cling to hierarchical structures and entrenched communication styles or time is not allocated for real collaboration [100].

The company must also make its contribution so that IPC can be lived. This is because power struggles demonstrably occur at the expense of patients when constructive collaboration between healthcare professionals is not structurally supported and encouraged by the respective organizations [95, 101]. It is not enough for CEOs to say "I expect you to work together" if interprofessional collaboration is not structurally embedded.

Although leadership and management structures have a great influence on interprofessional cooperation, there are hardly any studies dealing with how nurses and physicians in leadership roles are prepared to lead with each other [102]. On the contrary, eyes have often been closed to status struggles and the consequences of poor collaboration have not been considered from an economic perspective. It is therefore not enough for management to simply expect or demand good cooperation. Structures must also be created to make this possible. Employers often act contradictorily here. If, for example, on the one hand it is expected that the various professional groups should pull together, but on the other hand competition is rewarded at the same time. This is the case, for example, when chief physicians receive special bonuses for a certain number of certain procedures or examinations and the rest of the team gets nothing, although they are significantly involved in these procedures or examinations. Motivation through bonuses for chief physicians often leads to overtime, which affects the entire team and unnecessarily increases the workload of all. What is needed here is structural empowerment, in which past practices of staff development are systematically analyzed. All the usual meetings, rules, and procedures must be put to the test to find out whether they promote cooperation or competition. Only the structural orientation of the organization for collaboration and against competition makes interprofessional teamwork possible. It is the only way to avoid saying one thing and doing another. This structural empowerment is largely responsible for the success of Magnet clinics.

When implementing IPC, it is advisable to first determine the initial situation. A variety of instruments are available for this purpose. For the German-speaking world, Fabio Vittadello, Maria Mischo-Kelling and their team [103] translated the Interprofessional Cooperation Scale. A nice comparative overview of other English-language instruments can be found in Sue Bookey-Bassett and her collaborators [104].

In order to better understand interprofessional teamwork, the following four focal points should be considered [76]:

1. relational (professional power, hierarchy, socialization, team composition, team roles, team processes),
2. processual (time and space, routines and rituals, information technology, unpredictability, urgency, complexity task shifting),
3. organizational (organizational support, professional representation, fear of litigation),
4. contextual (culture, diversity, gender, political will, economics).

In this figure, it is clear that Interprofessional collaboration needs to be centrally supported by management and requires a common direction among all professions to be formalized so that it can be internalized. In their study, Samuelson et al. [105] found that the factors of trust, respect, and collaboration competence have the greatest impact on interpersonal collaboration.

In the following section three practices are required to implement interprofessional collaboration (IPC) in healthcare [106, 107]:

1. Corporate decision-making to systematically implement IPC with established necessary structures (empowering and rewarding teams that practice IPC instead of individuals for their individual performance).
2. Training of managers with a focus on interprofessional collaboration.
3. Interprofessional education and training as a rule.

If organizations do not systematically support constructive cooperation between the various professional groups in the health care system, power struggles occur in which, in case of doubt, the well-being of patients is accepted [101].

Need for Interprofessional Education (IPE)

The joint continuing education and training of all professional groups in the health care system is, of course, a decisive prerequisite for error prevention and enables better cooperation. However, the foundation for learning technical language, professional culture, and professional pride is laid during initial training. The differences internalized here are difficult to reconcile later.

A meeting of the health care professions on an equal footing is only possible if the nursing profession is also fundamentally academicized and medical and nursing students already take joint modules during their studies. The increase in quality through academicized nursing increases professional satisfaction [108]. The increase in nurses with a bachelor's degree has been shown to reduce patient falls and infection rates [109]. Academized nursing directly affects quality of care [110] and pays off in reducing burnout rates [111], costs due to errors in care [112], costs of patient falls [113], and medical costs due to needlestick injuries [114]. Only people who have never approached nursing science like to regularly bring up that a nursing degree is distant from practice. The success of joint education of medical, nursing, pharmacy, and other health professions students has been extensively described elsewhere [115]. In addition to performance orientation, an interprofessional we-orientation must be systematically established and given weight [116].

The development of communication skills is crucial in joint training to improve interprofessional cooperation [46]. These include asking meaningful questions; reflecting on one's own part in debriefing; positively reinforcing team members; genuinely listening without prejudice; being able to explain contexts; showing oneself vulnerable; starting interactions and bringing them to a positive conclusion; asserting one's influence and negotiating persuasively [117]. None of this can simply be taken for granted, but requires regular practice.

The communication of the different professional groups with each other is determined by different influencing factors that need to be analyzed and interpreted. Thus, each *person* brings his or her individual "rucksack" into the interaction, which is "packed" with experiences, knowledge, motives, attitudes, personality, feelings, age, and gender. *Situational factors* include roles, rules, culture, language, spatial environment, hierarchy, common avoidance behaviors, and dominance structures. The *communication goal* also plays a role. Thus, it makes a difference whether the goal is of high importance, time limited, precision is significant, or instruments of goal achievement have been worked out in the past. The *mediating processes* include both cognitive skills, such as the ability to get to the point, to make and implement decisions or to grasp the context, and affective skills, such as striking an appropriate tone or balancing tensions in the team. Other influencing factors are the ability to give appropriate *feedback* and an understanding of personal and human perceptual capacity [117].

Celebrating the successes of interprofessional collaboration requires both collaborative and networking skills. A prerequisite for this is that nurses learn to give immediate, clear, and direct feedback when someone has crossed their boundary and that physicians learn to empathize with the other professional groups. This doesn't fall from the sky, but it can be learned. To do this, the management of the organization needs to change their reward system and in the future reward team performance, rather than individual performance. This is more fair, because often an entire team is behind a performance with which an individual team member stands out. Research shows the benefit of interprofessional training wards [118].

15.6 Success Factor Transition Management

> Samira leaves her apartment in Berlin—Treptow and is asked by the front door: "secure everything?" "Yes," Samira replies, "secure everything." This information is passed on from her front door to all the apartment technology, so that the devices such as screens, stove, heating, apartment butler go into an economy mode, while the cleaning devices such as the vacuum cleaner or bed ventilator become active and the data security is armed.
>
> The ordered car stops punctually in front of her. The door opens with an iris scan and Samira makes herself comfortable on the sofa. She now has 31 min to her office in the clinic and can check her e-mails in peace and call up the news that is relevant to her for the day, which her personal robot has compiled for her. These self-driving cars are really a pleasant way to get around. The driving customers can do whatever they want: eat, sleep, do gymnastics or arrange to travel together with colleagues who have a similar driving route.
>
> In the diary, "Net" is marked for today, the short form for Networking Day. "Okay," Samira talks to her robot, "then I'm going to make nice contacts with my networking partners." In Mumbai, people have been awake for 4.5 h, a good time to check in with her friend and colleague Sheila. They studied "International Human Relations" together in London and shared a flat during that time. An unforgettably wonderful time, during which Sheila fell in love with Jay from Mumbai. When Sheila got pregnant, the couple decided to go back to Mumbai together to give their parents the joy to live with their grandchildren.
>
> "Call Sheila from Mumbai," Samira instructs her display. Sheila appears on it lying in a hammock. "Hi Sheila" Samira smiles at her friend "I would love a hammock right now too." "Oh Samira, how nice to see you! Just taking

a lunch break. It's 39 degrees here, so it's nice to put my feet up. Where are you right now?" Samira visibly fades in for Sheila, "lounging on the couch in the car right now, heading to the hospital. How's your treasure of gold Leela?" Sheila smiles her proud mother smile, "you should see her, at 3 years old she is a very lively child. Learning comes easy to her, so much so that she is learning Thai, the language of her nanny, in addition to English and Hindi in kindergarten. After she was rather >mouthy< until half a year ago, Jay and I decided to go for the Cognition Implant. Just a small injection with a big effect. Since then, she's been learning with great joy and talking like a waterfall."

"I see," Samira says skeptically. "Samira, I didn't think we would decide to take this step either. Now we're glad we did, though. It's amazing what you have to deal with as a parent. I'm looking forward to hearing from you about the decisions you have to make with Steffen. Are you doing well in your pregnancy?"

After the two exchange personal matters, Sheila gets down to business, "Before you ask, I have something for you!"

"What?" blurts out Samira. "I met Malou from Senegal at the International Security Day. She's a data security officer and, at 32, has an impressive career. She's been to Los Angeles and Sidney and God knows where, but best of all, she's pregnant!"

"Uh-huh," comes hesitantly from Samira.

"And guess who from?" puts in Sheila. "I know Malou's partner?" asks Samira.

"That's right" trumpeted Sheila, "he works for you in the ER and his name is Patrick."

An adrenaline rush runs through Samira and she suddenly sits bolt upright on the sofa, which turns into a kind of office chair with a light touch of the sensor. The staff schedule appears in front of her and with one glance she can see that Patrick has signed on for another 1.5 years.

Curious, Samira asks: "Are there any chances of family reunification in Berlin?" Sheila laughs, "you should ask her yourself. Here's her contact details." A photo of Malou Abara appears on Samira's display with her CV and address details.

"You're a sweetheart" gloats Samira. "I know" smiles Sheila.

No sooner has Samira arrived at her office than she places a call with Malou. Once she is in headhunter mode, nothing can stop her. Samira puts all the photos of employees and their children on the office wall to make a good visual impression on Malou. And of course, pictures of Patrick are conjured up on the wall as well. It's a good thing that they have a first-class company kindergarten at their hospital, she'll be able to score points with that. If both parents work at the hospital, the chances of retaining employees for longer are increased. A pregnant applicant is a gift and will be treated as such. Now it's time to be quick before other hospitals beat her to it.

Transition Management

▶ Egypt wouldn't be that far. But until you get to the south station
Karl Kraus

Thanks to the technical revolution (digitalization) and social change (Generation Y,Z), changes in companies will be driven forward even faster than before. For this reason, transition management will be an important focus, especially in human resources development. While the term transformation describes the result of a change process, transition refers to the transfer from one state to another. The great art of accompanying change management processes lies on the one hand in controlling emotions and on the other hand in maneuvering through the so-called neutral zone [119]. In any change process, there is a need to let go of something old and invite the new. However, the "neutral zone" is right in between. The old has lost its validity and the new is not yet truly visible. Like sailing on a ship, I leave the shore behind and find myself on the open sea for some time before land comes into view again. And this time "on the open sea" is difficult for companies in the change process. Employees are expected to give up what they are familiar with, what they have grown accustomed to, and perhaps what they have grown to love, without knowing what is ultimately to come. Giving up certainties and accepting the loss of control demands a lot from everyone involved. The accompanying uncertainties can awaken fears and lead to excessive demands, which then show up in sick leave or fluctuation. While complexity increases, the need for simple solutions grows. This is where good transition management is needed.

The Three Reasons for Resistance to Change

Transition processes cause resistance among employees. There are three reasons for this: (1) changes cost energy (more than before), (2) they take longer, and (3) the new initially feels unfamiliar and therefore not right.

Changes are exhausting because our brains have to produce new synapse circuits. Old, well-worn sequences of action are neurally well networked and cost us little energy as routines. Experienced drivers already react unconsciously to traffic and do not have to think about it again. But it is exactly this rethinking and new wiring in the brain that is necessary when learning or developing something new, and that of course costs energy. While we still react with tiredness after our first driving lessons, it is no longer an effort for us as experienced drivers. The unlearning necessary for this is also an active process. Once we have learned something and "wired" this info appropriately, this knowledge immediately jumps to mind when we come to the subject. So we have to actively ignore outdated knowledge and use further energy to recall the new knowledge.

Until we have become accustomed to new courses of action, they initially take longer, because we lack the routine for this. This is often the "killer argument" in healthcare, because time is a sensitive factor here. While the old procedures were routine and therefore time-saving, the new ones have to be practiced first. It takes longer until the new procedure is integrated into the daily routine, because it is always necessary to think again before the new behavior is "in."

But the third aspect that leads to resistance is particularly "mean." Because our actions are accompanied by emotions and new things often don't feel right at first. Routinized action gives us the feeling that it is "okay" because we are used to it. Changed actions cannot yet "produce" this feeling. Since we as humans are emotional beings, we often allow ourselves to be "unconsciously" controlled here. Until a new behavior feels right, there is a dry spell (neutral zone) to walk through.

Change takes energy, takes longer, and doesn't feel right. Three good reasons not to do it. Transition management requires leadership and emotional labor. To take a team on this journey, cognitive explanations are not enough. In the neutral zone, employees should be actively involved. Here, it is important to find out together which new roles are necessary, which rules will make sense in the future, and which knowledge is required to navigate anew on the "high seas." Part of the transition is also to give room for feelings. It is permissible to mourn when cherished things have to be given up. Fears may be addressed when aspects of the future are still uncertain. Anger also has its place when a lot of commitment has been put into an activity that is now no longer needed. If managers don't take these emotions seriously or dismiss them as kid's stuff, it will fall back on them later. Emotions also want to travel with change. However, they move at a different pace than the mind. Leaders are challenged to endure this and to bear it. Distancing oneself from these unpleasant emotions or blocking them out leads employees to let this emotional cauldron explode elsewhere. For example, in slandering the top management. In this way, employees distance themselves from the manager, which is accompanied by a loss of trust. But trust is particularly important in change processes, because loss of trust blocks the process.

Emotion work is a great art to learn. Unfortunately, few management courses qualify people for this skill. The idea of some change managers that with the right plan they can manage a change without losing control must be exposed as an illusion. Addressing the neutral zone with open cards may "shock" at first, but is less frustrating in the long run for employees who expected an orderly plan only to be disappointed. Bridges and Bridges [119] recommend seeing the neutral zone as something normal and describing it accordingly. Strong leadership is required and is characterized by keeping promises, listening carefully to employees and understanding what is important to them, soliciting feedback on one's leadership, and building trust. Here, more than ever, the rule applies: if you want to lead, you have to listen.

Sustainability of Change Processes

Transition processes are easier to endure if the result is lasting. Sustainability is becoming a high value in our fast-moving times. For this reason, the Federal Ministry of Health Germany has presented a departmental report aimed at creating more sustainability in the health care system [120]. This report provides six focal points on which measures will be taken:

1. Sustainable care through digitalization (more networking, greater transparency, better information).
2. Investment in health professions, including the strengthening of the nursing profession and the academization of the midwifery profession.
3. Sustainable and effective disease control.
4. Health literacy through prevention and health promotion.
5. Strengthening care in the long term, especially in hospitals and care for the elderly.
6. Assuming international responsibility.

In the following, two examples of sustainable change are discussed: (1) the innovative NEUSTART project of the Robert-Bosch Foundation and (2) the Common Good Economy launched by Christian Felber.

NEWSTART: Changes in the Health Care System in Germany

In order to create sustainable change in companies, employees must be involved at an early stage. In order to bring about lasting change in the health care system in Germany, citizens must be involved at an early stage. For this reason, the Robert-Bosch Stiftung invited citizens to participate in its health care reform project "Neustart." In this unprecedented project, citizens and experts were able to provide impetus for an innovative and sustainable healthcare system in Germany, with an eye on the next 20 years. The focus is on a health care system that is patient-oriented, multi-professional, quality-driven, and open to innovation (http://www.bosch-stiftung.de).

This project involves three activities in parallel: Citizens' Dialogues, Expert Discussions, and Health Policy Panels. For example, on May 25, 2019, about 500 randomly selected people representing a cross-section of the population (age, education, gender) debated their ideas for reforming the healthcare system in Cologne, Rostock, Fürth, Kiel, and Freiburg. Out came six main areas of interest: Digitization, Financing, Quality of Care, Common Good, Prevention and Education, and Organization of Healthcare. While a number of the ideas are practicable, a few had more of an idealistic value. The commitment of the participants was greater than expected. Two citizen meetings in forums were followed by discussions with experts. Here, citizens were able to discuss their ideas directly with the experts, which was fruitful for both sides. The aim of the project is to have developed concrete proposals by the time of the 2021 federal elections in order to provide politicians with a working basis for future decisions in the health sector (http://www.bosch-stiftung.de).

Economy of the Common Good

Christian Felber from Vienna thinks about a reorganization of the economy and developed the exciting approach of the Common Good Economy. The focus is not on competition with other companies, but on the greatest possible common good. Companies commit themselves to act in a socially responsible, democratic, ecological, and solidarity-based way [121]. What started like a crazy idea in 2010 has today found great popularity among companies. Worldwide, more than 2000 organizations participate. Felber has received many awards for the development of this alternative economic model, such as the "Courage for Sustainability" award from Zeit-Wissen in 2017, and was named a successful model by Top 100 Changemaker Business in 2019.

Felber presents a Common Good Matrix in which companies assess themselves on human dignity, solidarity, ecological sustainability, social justice, and democratic co-determination as well as transparency. An extensive table on this examines the above-mentioned aspects in relation to suppliers, financial backers, employees, customers, and the social environment. For example, plus points (+70) are awarded if the organization shows solidarity with service providers or fellow companies and minus points for hostile takeovers (−200) or blocking patents (−100). The democratic idea is that companies that are successful in the sense of the common good matrix receive legal advantages [121].

Against the background of the urgently sought-after employees in the health care sector, the common good economy is also a thoroughly attractive model. Because the young employees of Generation Y and Z are enthusiastic about this idea. They specifically look for employers who represent their values. The positive effects of the Common Good Economy on employee retention and recruitment were demonstrated by Mischkowski and his colleagues [122] in their study.

15.7 Crisis Management as a Secret of Success

"Samira Pfefferkorn, Code Red" sounds in the middle of the night in Samira's bedroom. A check of the bracelet on her wrist confirms: this is not a dream! Immediately Samira is wide awake. "I'm ready" Samira announces. The crisis tool of her hospital is activated and provides a short report of the events while Samira gets dressed.

ACTUAL SITUATION: "Programmed bots have gained access to the hospitals software and manipulated data. Information exchanged between external network partners is affected. Currently no interference with patient data registered."

BACKGROUND: "Tino from the research department noticed the exuberantly positive feedbacks of some network partners yesterday, which he found suspicious. Together with Isabelle from data protection, trolls and sock puppets could be spotted. The suspicion that bots were also used has just been confirmed. A first wave of negative criticism on all departments of our clinic was launched around 23:52 from servers worldwide."

TO-DO: "Crisis team has already been informed via crisis tool. First meeting via videocall with extra secure line is scheduled for 00:06. Fresh coffee is ready for you in the kitchen. You have three minutes until the call."

Okay, Samira thinks and goes to the bathroom. Her toilet bowl reports "noticeably high adrenaline levels" and Samira comments "then everything is working properly." Shortly she brushes her hair and then sits with her coffee in the study simulation, which was activated automatically in the living room. As the call begins all the members of the crisis team appear in front of her in a holographic semicircle. Samira looks into worried, sleepy, chipper, and grumpy faces. "Good," begins the Supervisor, Isabelle, "anyone else in their pajamas?" With that, she immediately puts a smile on a few faces. The humorous intro at a tense situation turns out to be a nice wake-up greeting in the middle of the night. Isabelle summarizes the events and initial interventions, then hands off to the head of the crisis team, deputy hospital director Chloé Dubois. Chloé thanks Isabelle and Tino for their nighttime efforts and quick response to this attack and then turns to Isabelle "are patient records or medical technology affected?" "Not so far, the firewall is stable." Glancing at the digital crisis manual, Chloé asks the group "are there any questions at this time, or does everyone know what to do?" When there's no response, Chloé shares responsibilities by name so that the auditory types are also served informatively. "Isabelle works with her team to contain the hacker attack, Roland from Corporate Communications gets the press on board and Sylvia is responsible for internal communications with all employees, I ask Tino and Samira to analyze all company-related events that coincide with the appearance of the trolls' first activities, everyone else works on their tuned-in to-dos and posts an update every 30 minutes. The next call is at 1:20." Chloé takes another look at everyone in the round individually and says goodbye with "together we'll get this done."

No sooner had Samira ended the call than Tino answered her with the words: "I thought I'd come to you, I haven't tidied up," he grinned mischievously at her. "How do we proceed, Tino?" "Well" Tino starts "I suggest I check the data, when exactly in which departments were attacked and you list change processes to these data. That way we can find out which processes we installed ourselves and what we're being led to believe from the outside." Samira nods, "okay, then let's work on the same platform of the crisis tool. I'll access your data immediately then." 1:19 "Secure line for next video call is prepared"

When this message reaches Samira and Tino, they look at each other in amazement from their laptops. Time has flown by.

1:20. Chloé now appears in the virtual round, made up as we know her, and asks everyone for a quick update. Isabelle begins. Everyone looks to her remarks at the currently reported information in the crisis tool, which continues to update throughout her report. Her team works diligently. "The troll's activities have been stopped, as well as the sock puppet attacks. We are currently working on tracking down the originator. About 60% of the bots attacks have been stopped, my team is working on the rest. With any luck, we'll have it done by 6:30. The attacks began 11 days ago. However, a first scout was installed earlier." Here Tino interjects "the first scout in our network was located on 12/15/2032." Chloé concludes, "then there are 4 weeks between the first scout and the attacks. Do we know if it's the same handwriting?" Tino feeds in his data. A series of long-chain cryptic characters emerge for all to see. Isabelle lays her ascertained data over it and says "Yes, unique, same sender. The pattern looks more like personal revenge than a digital attack on our hospital's reputation."

Sylvia informs that she has played all internal channels with the information of the hacker attack and will also give each employee the possibility of a personal conversation, if that is necessary. She had developed a short video with the most important data and posted it to each employee. So far, she said, she has had 12 responses to note, but no further queries. "The night shift responded immediately, and in 4 hours the early shift staff will respond. I expect a great response there."

Roland from Corporate Communications played a press release and short video to all national media and the same in English for the international press. "The national news ticker first broke the news 4 minutes ago. A virtual press conference is scheduled for 7:00."

Samira and Tino appear in a joint recording, as if they were sitting together at a desk, with Tino virtually fading in. Samira starts "Okay, so far we have the following information: all departments are affected by the attack, with the exception of the outpatient clinic. At the time of the first scout, we were interviewing 9 people from other hospitals. 14 days before the first attack we have the employment contracts with the surgeon Christopher Weller from New Zealand, Paul Smith from London, head of the outpatient clinic, and Tino Klahan from Thailand, who is sitting here next to me and is in charge of the research center." Tino speaks up, "I assure you I have no old corpse in my cellar. Until we have some concrete leads, we'll keep looking for connections and check in with Christopher and Paul at 7:00 when they start their shift."

Chloé addresses Sylivia, "Why don't you send a message to Christopher and Paul that I expect them in my office at 7:00 on this matter." Sylvia nods. "Merci à tous" slips out Chloé before translating "thank you all very much. Roland, you can go to bed now and continue in the morning. Isabelle, Tino, and Samira, may I ask you to keep the ball rolling?" All three nod. "Merci,"

Chloé thanks them again. Then the next call at 6:00 will do, unless there is news."

At 7:33, Sylvia reports to all employees that the cause has been determined and the danger has passed and no sensitive data has been compromised at any time.

At 7:45 Roland informs the press that the spook is over, the perpetrator has been arrested and reported. Since a victim-offender settlement was being sought, no names were mentioned.

What happened?

The quiet and polite Paul Smith had a love affair with a woman at his last workplace in London, who did not want to accept the separation. For Paul also a reason to move to Berlin. This woman had clearly overestimated her PC hacking skills. It almost felt like she wanted to be found. She wanted to harm the hospital that had "taken Paul away from her." That's why she had left out attacking the outpatient clinic where Paul works during the attacks.

Currently, Paul and his ex-girlfriend are having a discussion with the help of leadership trainer Tabea Groß. She will have to pay for the damage caused and psychological support to regulate her emotions is a must. Paul will continue to work with Tabea Groß in order to learn to distance himself more clearly so he has not to flee after every unhappy love affair. The judiciary has been informed and will work with all parties involved on a meaningful perpetrator-victim reconciliation.

Crises Are Getting Bigger

▶ At the crossroads of life there are no signposts
Charlie Chaplin

Progress through technology and globalization also brings new vulnerabilities. Previously, natural disasters or industrial accidents could trigger a crisis. Globalization allows epidemics to spread more quickly, as the COVID-19 virus taught us in 2020. The advantages of technical networking bring with them the disadvantage that security gaps can be used for attacks, for example, to paralyze entire hospitals. For example, the hospitals Fürstenfeldbruck and Fürth [123, 124] had to bitterly experience how a hacker attack affected the entire clinic process. Terrorist attacks also pose a threat.

A troll is a person who deliberately uses provocations in the network to thwart the network partner in question and undermine his or her trust. Sock puppets, however, are invented, copied, or stolen identities that are used to influence opinion formation on the net. Sock puppets often act friendly at first until they have hacked into the other person's network and spread out. They only start hostilities when they are sure of their success and have caused a lot of damage in the other person's network. Bots are machines that work according to an algorithm and act independently without being controlled by humans. We know them, for example, as automatic vacuum cleaners that conquer households [125].

For Germany, there are crisis teams organized by the Federal Ministry of the Interior. "Staff work means a coordinated and rehearsed procedure of a fixed number of participants. This includes, for example, certain reporting and communication channels or chains of command. Staff work is practised regularly" (http://www.bmi.bund.de).

In the case of companies, we speak of organizational resilience to describe the ability to deal with risks, resistance, crises, and the unknown. Organizational resilience can be divided into five levels of maturity. While level O denotes an organization with neither a risk management nor a crisis management organization in place, level 5 has fully explored risk scenarios that have also been trained. Depending on the initial situation, companies need a different approach in the crisis [126]. For example, it is necessary to clarify how quickly critical processes must be functional again so that minimum operations can be achieved. The maximum tolerated downtime is described as *recovery time objective (RTO)*.

What Is a Crisis?

Crises come unexpectedly and are usually experienced as unpleasant or even forced. They lead to process interruptions and thus mark a turning point in development that produces new decision-making situations. While for Merten [127] crisis is a disruption of habit, Sandhu [128] describes it as a social constant that every company experiences at some point. Crises are characterized by time pressure, existential threat, ambiguity (i.e. initially no clear cause–effect mechanism visible), and the fact that they come unexpectedly [129].

In a study, Hansen et al. [131] show that successful companies no longer just do well financially, but also have the well-being of their employees in mind, as well as the community in which the company is located ([131]: 89). In this volume, Mary Jo Kreitzer describes how to develop a healthy organization in her chapter "Well-being at work produces important measurement results."

This broader perspective replaces the idea that an organization is only beholden to its shareholders, i.e. the board of directors. Especially in times of crisis, it pays off if all stakeholders have already been considered as equal stakeholders. When a company is in crisis, not only shareholders and board members have the right to be informed, but also employees, customers, suppliers, the community, and so on.

What Does Successful Crisis Management Need?

Instead of wasting energy worrying about the future, it is important to plan ahead as much as possible. Active crisis management includes four basic criteria [132]:

1. Managing Issues

    Managing issues refers to questions and problems of social interest that harbor conflict potential. In the best case, an organization addresses this proactively and thus preventively. For example, if universities conduct animal experiments, it is important not to deny them, but to regularly highlight their social benefits.

2. The crisis manual

    When nerves are on edge in a crisis, people often act in a fear-driven and thus irrational manner. In order to be able to ensure a regulated process in an emergency, companies fall back on the crisis manual, which they have already developed and also train regularly. The crisis manual lists responsibilities, processes, and communication chains, as well as contact details and guidelines.

3. The crisis unit

    The crisis team, which is convened immediately, is now faced with many tasks, some of which are already regulated in the manual. The composition of the crisis unit is based on the organization chart of the company and always works interprofessionally. The management of the crisis unit is supported by all its members. It brings together the organization's key decision-makers, such as the organization's management and board of directors. In addition, depending on the focus of the crisis, other people may also be involved, such as quality managers, IT officers, heads of the departments concerned, press officers, caretakers, gatekeepers, research managers, etc. It is important that a personnel separation is made between those who are responsible for solving the crisis and those who communicate internally and externally.

4. Crisis communication

    Crisis communication, especially with authorities and journalists, is of particular importance. It must be clear to all members of the crisis team that only one person (the face of the crisis) shares information with the media. It can be dangerous if all members of the crisis team pass on different information about the causes and the processing status to the press. In this case, the communication monopoly applies to the person in charge, in order to signal continuity and reliability.

    Crisis communication is not a skill that can be learned overnight. Practice and preparation for possible crisis situations pay off here. When dealing with the media, it is important to be brief, crisp, and precise and to adhere to the following three-step process ([132]: 29):

    (a) Emotional entry
    (b) Maximum three arguments
    (c) Target set

The company appoints one or two people to maintain communication with the media during the crisis, the so-called face of the crisis. The time pressure and open outcome of the situation demand a high level of communicative competence. Silence has a negative effect on public confidence and salami tactics in offering information have had their day. It is now necessary to proactively seek dialogue instead of seeing journalists as enemies. Therefore, information must be truthfull and free of contradictions [127]. While in traditional crisis management the communication focus was on the sender with the motto "tell and preach," in the postmodern crisis communication focuses on the public with the task of "understanding, connecting, and integrating" [133].

A basic understanding of media logic pays off [134]. The formation of society's opinion is a great good and is significantly influenced by the preparation of information by journalists. Journalists thus construct realities, the effects of which can in turn influence the crisis [127].

Decisive factors for the choice of the "face of the crisis" are the disposal of authority (i.e. an important person of the company), the ability to communicate empathically, authentically, and congruently, showing reliability [135]. Especially important is the ability to apologize. The correct process for doing this is in six steps: (1) apologize, (2) explain what went wrong, (3) take responsibility for it, (4) express remorse, (5) formulate a sincere offer on how to repair the damage, and (6) ask for forgiveness [136].

Releasing false information in a crisis is a mistake. Thus, there are a number of disinformation strategies, such as manipulation or setting a false context, that should be avoided [137].

The ongoing maintenance and updating of the website and social media platforms must be managed as well as the agreement on communicative responsibilities (who is allowed to create editorial texts and who releases them?). In case of emergency, a so-called dark site must be set up. Here, the crisis is reported on the first homepage page. For internationally operating companies, reliable contacts to political stakeholders, associations, authorities, and influencers are necessary [138].

Even with professional preparation and implementation of crisis communication, it can happen that communication takes on a momentum of its own. A misunderstood sentence can lead to a media mudslinging that is difficult to recover from. If sentences are taken out of context or heavily abbreviated (motto: we only have 1 minute of airtime), then they can take on a different meaning. The clothing of the crisis speaker or the location of a recording can also create incongruities that send double messages. All of this cannot always be controlled, but it can always be put into the right picture. Such dynamics must be analyzed at the end of the crisis in order to learn from them. Unfortunately, they are not completely avoidable.

Media Training

The importance of professional communication takes on additional weight in a crisis. It is therefore recommended that all potential members of a crisis team train in dealing with the media. It is important to put yourself in the journalists' shoes and ask yourself what the public wants to know. And not all journalists are the same, as Julia Drews [134] was able to work out in her study on journalists' expectations of communication with authorities in times of crisis. Thus, journalists with economic interests in times of crisis are significantly more interested in getting advice from authorities on how to cope (88%) than journalists without economic interests (65.7%). As daily newspapers have a much higher interest in retaining their readership (80%) than online media (47%), they also have to orient their information much more towards their customers. This supposed freedom of the online media can lead to sharper formulations or provocations in crises.

CAVE: Experienced journalists can get anyone to talk! They have developed a variety of techniques to do this, such as the ambush interview, the undercover investigation, the particularly empathetic interview, provocation or fictional description [139]. Therefore, the crisis team must have internalized the three C's of crisis [138]:
Concern: Expressing sympathy for those affected.
Commitment: The company takes responsibility for the crisis.
Control: The company repairs the damage and keeps you informed about the status.

The power of language must be used effectively, especially in times of crisis. Formulations, metaphors, and selected frames have a high potential impact [140]. A negative example is the word "asylum tourism," which CSU politician Markus Söder used in 2018 to "protect" Bavaria from further asylum seekers. A positive example was provided by Ursula von der Leyen in her speech to the European Commission on 26.03.2020. She swore Europe to joint action against the coronavirus. After von der Leyen had criticized the isolation of individual states, she called for Europe to oppose the coronavirus together, "with one big heart and not 27 small ones" [141].

Internal and external communication is the be-all and end-all in times of crisis. This is where it pays off if companies have continuously invested in leadership skills and successful communication. Unprofessional communication and the inability of an emergency task forced to work respectfully as a team can easily turn a crisis into a disaster. Language is a sharp instrument. Underestimating its power would be a leadership mistake.

Crisis Management

Making actionable and sensible decisions is central to crisis management. The Management Rhythm Method has been developed for structured decision-making, which usually takes place in several cycles. It takes place in six steps: Facts, Options, Risks, Decisions, Execution, and Check (success control), in short FORDEC [142].

The larger the company, the more difficult it is to get all the relevant people together in a short time. Especially if there are several external locations, as is the case with hospital chains or larger care services. Here, a digital toolbox can be used as a precaution. Instead of losing valuable time at the beginning of a crisis, all those involved can access the toolbox, in which the most important processes for possible crises are already pre-installed. The chemical company Currenta, with sites in Leverkusen, Krefeld and Dormagen, has developed such a technology for itself. With the digital toolbox, all those involved can be coordinated without losing time, and all tasks can be presented transparently and their completion can be tracked and viewed by everyone. In its close communication with journalists, Currenta provides its own visual material and receives journalists with selected friendliness as crisis partners who are to be taken seriously. For example, a rain-protected meeting point is offered at the factory gate, with electricity, coffee, water and, if necessary, an umbrella: "not a superfluous service, but an expression of good preparation and sovereinty" ([143]: 72).

Currenta's self-developed crisis tool is a mobile app that is designed for speed and clearly captures all the essentials. Everyone involved has 20 minutes to respond. It contains clear checklists with clear instructions for the parties involved, which can be immediately accepted and executed as an order. Also integrated is an "Easy Publish" system, which clearly presents the entire situation in a few simple steps and prepares it in simple text modules for the media. The crisis tool contains checklists of all kinds, such as what may and may not be done or which words may not be used. This mobile clarity can help in crises to focus on the essentials and avoid mistakes [143].

Perception in the Crisis

When people are under pressure, distortions of perception regularly occur. Here, a distinction can be made between individual and organizational distortions of perception. Individual means the leadership personality, who, for example, hides the approach of the crisis through wishful thinking or a strong striving for harmony [129].

Enzler Denzler and Schuler [130] identify three crisis types here: the cognition type, the social type, and the order type. In a crisis, the cognition type is able to separate factual and personal interests well and appears rational and action-oriented. He does not like it when his train of thought is interrupted and can react aggressively.

For the social type, a breach of trust is a serious violation of his values and is particularly hard for him in a crisis. Always striving to please everyone, he focuses above all on the people and their suffering in the crisis, which may go beyond the limits of what he can cope with himself.

Order structure types suffer more than the other two types from the loss of control that a crisis brings with it. Here, the fear of losing one's own position is in the foreground. In a crisis, he does without advisors and tries in particular to regain control through structures and likes to resort to checklists and the crisis manual.

In organizational perception bias, the people of the company follow their typical corporate culture and thus their collective pattern [129]. Each organization has its own taboo topics and correspondingly developed avoidance behavior. The phenomenon of groupthink can also distort perception; for example, if members experience themselves as invulnerable with their organization, the threat of crisis may be blanked out for a long time.

When organizational perceptual biases are added to individual ones, it can create institutionalized blindness [144].

Structural circumstances and political corporate processes can also lead to perception distortion. If, for example, the structure stipulates that certain departments work separately and do not relate to each other. Then the first signs of crisis experienced by all departments cannot be seen as a common phenomenon at an early stage and thus identified as a crisis. Political processes mean corporate policy and thus, for example, the question of what may be called a crisis in an organization at all and can be passed on to the public [129].

Technical Assistance in the Event of Disasters

If it's not just a crisis, but disasters that befall the population, there are several warning apps that can be easily installed on your mobile phone, such as PEMAEA, EU-Amber, Hurricane Hound, or FEMA. PEMAEA stands for the Pan-European Emergency App and interconnect the different 112 Apps in Europe. EU-Amber is an App for missing people report in Europe. In the USA the App Hurricane Hound warns for hurricanes and FEMA informs about all kinds of weather events possible and stands for Federal Emergency Management Agency. FEMA provides also storm preparedness tips and resources.

All of these alert apps provide people and professionals like health care rescuers, firefighters, or police the ability to get real-time information from the surrounding area to provide immediate first aid.

Taking Responsibility

Mastering crises means taking responsibility. It is a matter of stepping out of the pool of whining (I can't do anything) and bathing in the pool of influence (I do what I can). This turns influencing into an attitude that needs to be learned and practiced. Instead of putting energy into defensive processes (I'm not responsible for that), it's about focusing on what's possible (what do I need to be responsible for?). The ability to take responsibility is expressed especially in times of crisis. In order to act responsibly, four prerequisites are necessary: (1) autonomy (self-determination), (2) authority (legitimate power to exert influence), (3) professional knowledge, and (4) interpersonal competence. Then the sense of control (self-efficacy conviction) can develop, which makes it easier to take action [145].

In crises, organizations tend to look for a "savior." This can be dangerous. For example, when a company is on the verge of bankruptcy, a charismatic leader is often sought to "fix it." Here we must warn against narcissists who like to offer themselves in such situations. The lack of humility of narcissistic personalities can be the company's undoing, since only one's own success is celebrated, not cooperation with others. Especially in times of crisis, a crisis team is needed that is capable of working as a team and where everyone can rely on each other. Of course, someone needs to take the lead, but this person must not feel the need to bask in success alone [74].

Responsibility also always means looking beyond one's own nose and not only at one's own advantage. The Federal Ministry of Health, Germany also emphasizes the importance of international responsibility for the health of all [120]. From the unculture of looking away ("environmental sinners are the others") to a culture of looking (actively keeping one's own ecological footprint small).

Responsibility in healthcare also means leaving professional group egos behind in order to enable genuine teamwork. Let us recall the communication studies from the operating theatres, which prove that hierarchy-dominated behavior promotes errors and teamwork reduces them. Instead of seeking power over someone (*power over* corresponds to the old leadership model), sharing power with each other (*power to* corresponds to a modern understanding of leadership in the sense of empowerment). The young generations Y and Z seem to be ready to take on this responsibility, because they demand team play. For them, "leading for a period of time" is an appealing concept, which always puts them in new roles and promotes working at eye level. In addition, they reject dominant leadership, which is based solely on positional power. A study in which over 18,000 people from 19 countries took part was able to prove this (http://www.insead.edu).

Responsible action also means political commitment. The smallest contribution here would be membership in a professional association. It can also be more and actively influence corporate policy or show civic commitment to health policy. Political commitment helps to get out of the "them on top" mindset and strengthens one's own potential for influence. Especially in times of crisis, knowledge of corporate and health policy is very helpful.

15.8 The Future of Human Resources Development: Bold And Innovative

> ▶ If we take the future seriously, then we have to stop leaving it to others, but become active ourselves.
> *Jane Goodall*

Globalization and digitization are driving complexity. While medical knowledge was still doubling every 50 years in 1950, it was only doubling every 7 years in 1980 and every 3.5 years in 2010. By 2020, it is estimated that all medical knowledge worldwide will double every 73 days. Knowledge expansion is happening faster than we humans are able to adapt effectively [146]. Thus, it makes little sense to pack healthcare training more fully in terms of content or to construct extensive continuing education for every new innovation. Rather, it is necessary to learn to acquire the new knowledge oneself, to reflect on it and to integrate it into everyday professional life. This requires permanent adaptation and the ability to adjust to changes in permanent mode.

Communication as a Revenue-Relevant Factor

While professional competences have been propagated as the most important basis of knowledge in health care for many years, the so-called soft skills have rather been devalued as nice-to-have but not life-saving. However, the fact that precisely these skills of communication, reflection, emotion control, network competence, or collaboration form the central means of transport for any professional intervention has been criminally neglected. Today we know that the main cause of treatment failures can be traced back to poor communication [43, 44].

Technical Competence and Emotional Intelligence as Future Winners

The red educational thread of the future for successful personnel development in the healthcare sector relies not only on technical competence, but above all on emotional intelligence. Whether it is a question of introducing changes or managing crises, emotional competence plays a decisive role. Emotional intelligence plays an important role in team success [147]. For example, Oldhafer and her colleagues declare the typical phase models for change management processes in healthcare companies to be outdated. They uncover the secret power of emotions in change processes and developed the 6C theory. This theory is based on six key capabilities that organizational leaders and employees need if they are to successfully implement change: curiosity, compassion, courage, creation, calmness, and cooperation. Above all, as an imagined seventh C, is communication, which connects all aspects [148].

The explosion of digitalization with the emergence of vast amounts of data, networks, and robots will turn the entire healthcare system upside down. In the future, a large part of the population will work in technical professions that do not even exist today. This will create a high demand for qualifications, which must always be accompanied by the teaching of ethical knowledge (see below).

For all employees in the health care sector, training in communication, reflection, ethics, and responsibility is recommended. This forms a good basis for the next trainings in interprofessional cooperation, networking, and generational knowledge. With this knowledge, the basis is finally created for learning transition and crisis management.

Leadership Competence as a Sustainable Success Factor

Positional power and dominance-oriented leadership was yesterday. This outdated understanding of leadership required employees to adapt and sometimes even submit. However, employees experience the greatest satisfaction when they have room for maneuver and can participate in decision-making.

Innovative leadership concepts include emotionally intelligent (and thus relationship-based) leadership, coaching and culturally sensitive leadership, self-directed teams, temporary leadership, and interprofessional collaboration in which robots are also valued as colleagues.

The internationally successful LEO leadership training therefore focuses on decentralized decision-making and empowerment. Here, managers learn how to develop the competencies of their employees responsibly and how to manage change processes in an emotionally intelligent way. In addition, they reflect on their own unhealthy leadership behavior and say goodbye to it in peer coaching.

Personnel Development as Shaping the Future

Human resources development in the healthcare sector can therefore prepare itself for new challenges. The future is already here, but the necessary qualification of the personnel is still missing.

The development of leadership skills is no longer directed at specific individuals, but must include all employees who want to take on leadership and management tasks on a temporary basis. Blended learning formats that can be selected on a modular basis are suitable for this purpose.

The increase in digitalization must be combined with ethical competences in order to always consider crucial questions of user autonomy. Therefore, each technology module needs an integrated part for the reflection of social, personal, and organizational questions.

The lucky circumstance that communicative competence and interpersonal cooperation not only reduce treatment errors, but also reduce staff turnover and promote the health of employees is reason enough to place more emphasis on these competencies in the future. The mistake of degrading communication as a soft skill *to a nice to have and* overvaluing professional competence as the most important *must-have* must not be repeated. In order to prevent this, appropriate training in personal and interprofessional communication is needed, which is integrated into the initial training of the various health care professions and is an obligatory part of the interprofessional modules. Interprofessional case studies are recommended here, in which students learn with, from, and about each other. In this way, a common understanding can be developed at an early stage, in which the perspectives of other professions can either be considered or consulted when decisions are made. In order to promote genuine togetherness in everyday professional life, bonuses should only be awarded to exemplary teams, because ultimately every special achievement by an individual person is due to the support of colleagues. This is because a bonus to individual leaders for a specific annual performance devalues teamwork and thwarts interprofessional collaboration.

Due to globalization, the mixing of people from different cultures will continue to increase. This makes the integration of foreign employees necessary and requires cultural competence [149, 150].

Physiological Knowledge as a Basic Competence

The physiology of thought and judgment processes must become the foundation of all health professions. Understanding about the effect of positive and negative thoughts for our body is an important basis for healthy working and healthy leading. This is because it explains why whining and complaining are harmful, why uncollegial collaboration ompacts error rates, and why relationship-based working makes you satisfied. Controlling these thoughts can be positively influenced by certain forms of stress management, such as HeartMath® training [149–151].

Academization of the Nursing Profession as a Basis for Fair Interprofessional Cooperation

For fair interprofessional cooperation, some health care professions, such as nursing, need an academic degree as an initial qualification in order to be able to bring the necessary competences of scientific thinking and research into the professional discussion of interprofessional teamwork. With the communication at eye level that this makes possible, treatment errors in the interprofessional team can be reduced at the same time.

The many years of experience with nurses studied at University must suffice as proof that a course of study does not get lost in theories, but qualifies for practice. The political concern in Germany that academically qualified nursing staff prefer activities that are far removed from patients has proved to be unfounded. The research results of international hospitals, most of which work with graduated nurses, impressively demonstrate that the costs of care errors, patient falls, and injuries with cannulas have been reduced, while job satisfaction has increased and a committed working climate in nursing increases the appreciation of one's own professionalism [152].

Meaningful Activities as Motivation Drivers

The younger generations' increasing need for meaningful work, varied tasks, and sustainable processes requires new methods and focuses of personnel development. The primary incentive will no longer be driven by money, but by meaning and satisfying teamwork. Thus, all procedures and customary structures in health care facilities must be reconsidered and, if necessary, questioned if they turn out to be meaningless rituals. Work with patients must no longer be devalued by leaving patient-related tasks to beginners and non-patient-related tasks to the more advanced. Satisfaction through relationship-based work with patients and colleagues is a great good and must not be objectified in functional actions. The success of the concept of Relationship-Based Care speaks for itself (Wessels et al. in this volume). Here, all processes are oriented first to a good relationship with oneself, then to a good relationship with colleagues, and only then to a good relationship with patients and residents. With Relationship-Based Care, all care processes are systematically reviewed for relational competence and revised if necessary. The result is an increase in satisfaction among all professional groups, as processes run more smoothly and costs can be saved through lower illness rates and fluctuation (www.chcm.com). The meaningful element of satisfying interprofessional cooperation and relationship-based patient care can no longer be underestimated, as it will become one of the greatest attractors for work in the healthcare sector in the future.

Individualized Career Development as a Motivation Driver

The desire of younger generations to fulfill themselves in different areas is increasing. Personnel developers therefore need a broad view when providing career advice. In the future, it will be more common for a medical professional to want to qualify in IT, for example, after a few years in the operating room, in order to live out her tech-savvy side, or for a psychiatric nurse to begin studying sports in order to express her joy in physical performance. Of course, it is quite conceivable that these multi-skilled individuals will one day return to their original profession. For this to happen, there need to be continuous incentives of innovative processes and research findings that want to be implemented. Connections between the different qualifications are also possible. For example, the technology-qualified medical professional can set up new computers in the operating room that can be used to improve procedures. And the sports-qualified nurse can use her knowledge of movement patterns in psychiatry with the staff and patients, both preventively and curatively. This also meets the need for people to put their knowledge to use rather than remain in professionally limited activities. Supporting individualized career paths and using them in a meaningful way will be another task of personnel development. At the Institute for Personalized Medicine (MOLIT), the individualized career development of employees is linked with agile methods and relies on self-managing teams (see Bochum et al., in this book).

Emotional and Crisis Competence for Change Success

In the future, change processes will shape our everyday lives even more than before. Change management and transition competencies are needed for this. Managers must learn to maneuver organizations and teams through the neutral zone so that the obsolete can be left behind and the new can be developed. In order to deal with fears and resistance, superiors need to be well qualified to face these feelings in an emotionally competent manner.

Globalization and networking mean that crises are also becoming bigger. Responsible crisis management can be learned. To this end, a crisis manual must be developed for the entire organization that covers all scenarios and rehearses how to deal with potential crisis events. The potential "faces of the crisis" need intensive media training with sophisticated communication training.

In the future, personnel development will therefore deal much more intensively with individual career paths and identify attractive job offers for those with multiple qualifications. Teaching modules will become more compact and more blended learning. For this, a lot of short videos have to be made, which prepare the knowledge transfer in a practical and appropriate way. Book knowledge will be reduced in favor of instructional films. Thus, personnel development will become more colorful, lively, interactive, and person-centered. Many good reasons to look forward to it.

References

1. Förster A. Mut ist störend. In: Harvard business manager Spezial. 2020;(3):34–5.
2. Tilk S. Mut ist nicht nur was für Junge. In: Harvard business manager Spezial, 2020;2020(3):13.
3. Herrmann P. Mut wurde verlernt. In: Harvard Business manager Spezial. 2020;(3):18–9.
4. Panse W, Stegmann W. Kostenfaktor Angst. 3. Auflage. MI Verlag; 2001.
5. Cumming S, Harris L. The impact of anxiety on the accuracy of diagnostic decision-making. Stress Health. 2001;17:281–6. https://doi.org/10.1002/smi.909.
6. Tewes R. Da hin gehen, wo die Angst ist. Personalentwicklung in der Pflege. Pflegezeitschrift. 2015;68(5):308–11.
7. Handelsblatt. 2014. https://www.handelsblatt.com/finanzen/vorsorge/versicherung/europaweiter-vergleich-jeder-deutsche-zahlt-2219-euro-im-jahr-fuer-versicherungen/9506130.html?ticket=ST-4852887-GayTKtsz5tva6bATcccb-ap6.
8. Abramovic M. Vergeben verlangt Mut. In: Harvard business manager Spezial; 2020;(3):12.
9. Endres H. Nur Mut! In: Harvard business manager Spezial; 2020(3):40–7.
10. Kets de Vries M. Zwischen Mut und Dummheit verläuft ein sehr schmaler Grat. In: Harvard business manager Spezial. 2020;3:48–51.
11. Federal Ministry of Health-Germany. 2019. https://www.bundesgesundheitsministerium.de/themen/gesundheitswesen/gesundheitswirtschaft/gesundheitswirtschaftals-jobmotor.html.
12. Bundesministerium für Inneres: BMWI Gesundheitswirtschaft Fakten & Zahlen. 2018. https://www.bmi.bund.de/DE/themen/bevoelkerungsschutz/krisenmanagement/organisation/krisenmanagement-organisation-node.html;jsessionid=B336D8353657DB3180A385AF655AD52D.1_cid287.
13. Specht F. Studie: Renteneintritt der Babyboomer könnte weniger dramatisch sein als befürchtet. Handelsblatt; 2019. https://www.handelsblatt.com/politik/deutschland/studie-renteneintritt-der-babyboomer-koennte-weniger-dramatisch-sein-als-befuerchtet/25058786.html?ticket=ST-37671932-7azaXKd4TObTbVO0RlRz-ap6.
14. Bernd F. "In jeder Hinsicht betriebssicher." In der Science Fiction stand der Umstieg auf den Elektromotor bereits vor 100 Jahren fest. In: Horstmann T, Döring P, editors. Zeiten der Elektromobilität. Beiträge zur Geschichte des elektrischen Automobils. Berlin: VDE Verlag; 2018. p. 181–8. (Geschichte der Elektrotechnik, Bd.27).
15. Jánszky SG, Abicht L. 2025: So arbeiten wir in der Zukunft. Leipzig: AHEAD Publishing; 2013.

16. Gergs H-J. Die Kunst der kontinuierlichen Selbststeuerung. Acht Prinzipien für ein neues Change Management. Weinheim: Beltz; 2016.
17. Brosinski C, Riddel AJ, Valdez S. Improving triage accuracy: a staff development approach. Clin Nurse Specialist. 2017;31(3):4.
18. https://www.bildung-forschung.digital/de/digitalisierungsstrategie-der-bundesregierung-2529.html.
19. Czeschik C. Blockchain im Gesundheitswesen. 2018. https://e-health-com.de/thema-der-woche/blockchain-im-gesundheitswesen/551b1e7047172eaf7fc5889ffbabadf7/.
20. Schiller K. SimplyVital Health setzt auf Blockchain. 2017. https://blockchainwelt.de/simplyvital-health blockchain-connectingcare-health-nexus/.
21. Ruß A, Schumacher K, Reithinger N. MoreCare: Gemeinsam Pflegen in der Mobilen Rehabilitation : das Pflegeassistenzsystem MoreCare, Abschlussbericht : Laufzeit des Vorhabens: 01.01.2016–31.12.2018. Berlin: Deutsches Forschungszentrum für Künstliche Intelligenz; 2019. https://doi.org/10.2314/GBV:1067512195.
22. Bundesministerium für Gesundheit. 2017. ePflege. Kommunikations- und Informationstechnologie für die Pflege. 2017_BMG_ePflege_Abschlussbericht_final.pdf.
23. Pfannstiel M, Krammer S, Swoboda W, editors. Digitale Transformation von Dienstleistungen im Gesundheitswesen IV. Impulse für die Pflegeorganisation. Springer/Gabler: Berlin; 2019.
24. Rosengreen D. 2017 Building Motivational Interviewing Skills: A practitioner Workbook. New York: The Guilford Press.
25. Jánszky SG, Abicht L. 2030: Wieviel Mensch verträgt die Zukunft? Leipzig: AHEAD Publishing; 2018.
26. Bendel O. Pflegeroboter. Berlin: Springer/Gabler; 2018.
27. Lill F. "Hallo, wie geht es Ihnen?" Die Zeit online 1/29. 2017. https://www.zeit.de/2017/01/pflegeroboter-japan-krankenpflege-terapio.
28. Pu L, Moyle W, Jones C. How people with dementia perceive a therapeutic robot called PARO in relation to their pain and mood: a qualitative study. J Clin Nurs. 2020;29(3–4):437–46.
29. Forsa. Politik- und Sozialforschung GmbH. Service-Robotik: Mensch-Technik-Interaktion im Alltag: Ergebnisse einer repräsentativen Befragung. Berlin: Deutschland; 2016. https://www.bmbf.de/files/BMBF_forsa_Robotik_FINAL2016.pdf.
30. Monti A, Coleman C. Future health: seven visions of the future of healthcare. 2016. http://tgr.ph/futureofhealth oder https://www.telegraph.co.uk/wellbeing/future-health/healthcare-predictions/?WT.mc_id=tmgspk_shto_1511_AnLNWSGYPbN4&utm_source=tmgspk&utm_medium=shto&utm_content=1511&utm_campaign=tmgspk_shto_1511_AnLNWSGYPbN4.
31. Telgheder M. KI im Krankenhaus. Wie der Essener Radiologe Felix Nensa mit KI die Diagnostik verändert. 2019. Handelsblatt 22.03.2019. https://www.handelsblatt.com/unternehmen/it-medien/ki-im krankenhaus-wie-der-essener-radiologe-felix-nensa-mit-ki-die-diagnostik veraendert/24092852.html?ticket=ST-1372760-RLVVcRA4VKgASM eZAGne-ap2.
32. Aruba Networks. Internet of things—IoT heading for mass adoption by 2019 driven by better-than expected business results. 2017. https://news.arubanetworks.com/press-release/arubanetworks/iot-heading-mass adoption-2019-driven-better-expected-business-results.
33. Schnall S, Harber K, Stefanucci J, Proffitt D. Social support and the perception of geographical slant. J Soc Psychol. 2008;44(5):1246–55.
34. McCraty R. New frontiers in heart rate variability and social coherence research: techniques, technologies, and implications for improving group dynamics and outcomes. Front Public Health. 2017;5:267. https://doi.org/10.3389/fpubh.2017.00267.
35. Plass D, Vos T, Hornberg C, et al. Entwicklung der Krankheitslast in Deutschland: Ergebnisse, Potenziale und Grenzen der Global Burden of Disease-Studie. Deutsches Ärzteblatt 2014;111(38): 629–38.
36. Insead. n.d. https://www.insead.edu/sites/default/files/assets/dept/centres/emi/docs/generations-series-brave-newworkplace.pdf.
37. Koloroutis M. Beziehungsbasierte Pflege. Ein Modell zur Veränderung der Pflegepaxis. Bern: Huber; 2011.

38. Koloroutis M, Abelson D, editors. Advancing relationship-based cultures. Minneapolis: Creative Health Care Management; 2017.
39. McCormack B, McCance T. Person-centred practice in nursing and health care. Theory and practice. West Sussex: Wiley Blackwell; 2017.
40. McCormack B, van Dulmen S, Eide H. Person-centred healthcare research. West Sussex UK: Wiley Blackwell; 2017.
41. Eide T, Cardiff S. Leadership research: a person-centred agenda. In: McCormack B, van Dulmen S, Eide H, editors. Person-centred healthcare research. West Sussex: Wiley Blackwell; 2017. p. 95–115.
42. Steck M, Simshäuser U, Niederberger M. Arbeitgeberattraktivität aus Sicht der Generation Z: Eine quantitative Befragung zur Bedeutung gesundheitsrelevanter Dimensionen im Betrieb. Prävention und Gesundheitsförderung. 2019;14(3):212–7. https://doi.org/10.1007/s11553-019-00703-w.
43. Hannawa Annegret (2018) SACCIA- Sichere Kommunikation. Berlin: De Gruyter Kluge, 2012, Korrekt ist de Heer & Kluge
44. Nagpal K, Arora S, Vats A, Wong HW, Sevdalis N, Vincent C, Moorthy K. Failures in communication and information transfer across the surgical care pathway: interview study. BMJ Qual Saf. 2012;21(10):843–9.
45. WHO. https://www.who.int/news-room/detail/13-09-2019-who-calls-for-urgent-action-to-reduce-patient-harm-in healthcare.
46. Thistlethwaite J. Interprofessional education: a review of context, learning and the research agenda. Med Educ. 2012;2012(46):58–70. https://doi.org/10.1111/j.1365-2923.2011.04143.x.
47. Ronner M. Treffende Pointen zu Geld und Geist. Thun: Ott Verlag; 2000.
48. Fassier T, Azoulay E. Conflicts and communication gaps in the intensive care unit. Curr Opin Crit Care. 2010;16(6):654–65. https://doi.org/10.1097/MCC.0b013e32834044f0.
49. Azoulay E, Timist J-F, Sprung CL, et al. Prevalence and factors of intensive care unit conflicts: the conflicus study. Am J Respir Crit Care Med. 2009;180:853–60.
50. Lingard L, Espin S, Whyte S, Regehr G, Baker GR, Reznick R, et al. Communication failures in the operating room: an observational classification of recurrent types and effects. Qual Saf Health Care. 2004;13:330–4.
51. Chowdhury SA, Habib L. Improved documentation and record management: a necessity to prevent medical errors in health care system. Int J Med Sci. 2015;2(11):1–3.
52. De Heer G, Kluge S. Kommunikation in der Intensivmedizin. Medizinische Klinik-Intensivmedizin und Notfallmedizin. Berlin: Springer; 2012. p. 1–6. https://doi.org/10.1007/s00063-011-0060-3.
53. Gurvits TV, Shenton Martha E, Hokama H, Ohta H, Lasko N, Gilbertson M, Orr S, Kikinis R, Jolesz FA, McCarley R, Pitman RK. Magnetic resonance imaging study of hippocampal volume in chronic, combat-related posttraumatic stress disorder. Biol Psychiatry. 1996;40(11):1091–9. https://doi.org/10.1016/S0006-3223(96)00229-6.
54. Bremner DJ, Randall P, Vermetten E, Staib L, Bronen RA, Mazure C, Capelli S, McCarthy G, Innis R, Charney D. Magnetic resonance imaging-based measurement of hippocampal volume in posttraumatic stress disorder related to childhood physical and sexual abuse—a preliminary report. Biol Psychiatry. 1997;41(1):23–32.
55. Winch G. The squeaky wheel. New York: Walker; 2011.
56. Marchant N, Lovland LR, Jones R, Piche Binette A, Gonnevaud J, Arenaza-Uriquijo EM, Chètelat G, Villeneuve S. Repetitive negative thinking is associated with amyloid, tau, and cognitive decline. Alzheimers Dement. 2020;16:1054–64.
57. Alon C, editor. Stress resilience. Cambridge: Elsevier; 2020.
58. Bauer J. Das Gedächtnis des Körpers. Wie Beziehungen und Lebensstile unsere Gene steuern. München: Piper Verlag 2018.
59. Engert V, Smallwood J, Singer T. Mind your thoughts: associations between self generated thoughts and stress-induced and baseline levels of cortisol and alpha-amylase. Biol Psychol. 2014;103:283–91.

60. Linz R, Singer T, Engert V. Interactions of monetary thought content and subjective stress predict cortisol fluctuations in a daily life experience sampling study. Sci Rep. 2018;8(1): 15462.
61. Pössel P, Mitchell AM, Harbison B, Fernandez-Botran GR. Repetitive negative thinking, depressive symptoms, and cortisol in cancer caregivers and noncaregivers. Oncol Nurs Forum. 2019;46(6):E202–10.
62. Weintraub K. Stress hormone cortisol linked to early toll on thinking ability. Periodical. Sci Am Mind. 2019;30(1):4–6.
63. Aloe L, Rocco ML, Bianchi P, Manni L. Nerve growth factor: from the early discoveries to the potential clinical use. J Transl Med. 2012;10:239.
64. Balasubramanian S, Jacobo M, Wahlquist Amy E. Induction of salivary nerve growth factor by yogic breathing: a randomized controlled trial. Int Psychogeriatr. 2015;27(1):168–70.
65. Obholzer A, Roberts VZ. The troublesome individual and the troubled institution. In: Obholzer A, Roberts VZ, editors. The unconscious at work: individual and organisational stress in human services. London: Routledge; 2019. p. 129–38.
66. Obholzer A, Roberts VZ. The unconscious at work: individual and organisational stress in human services. London: Routledge; 2019.
67. Kanning UP. Selbstwertdienliches Verhalten und soziale Konflikte im Krankenhaus. Gruppendynamik. 1999;30(2):207–29.
68. Halton W. Some unconscious aspects of organizational life. In: Obholzer A, Roberts V, editors. The unconscious at work: individual and organisational stress in human services. London: Routledge; 2019. p. 11–8.
69. Hamel G, Michelle Z. Build a change platform, not a change program. McKinsey Journal. 2014. https://www.mckinsey.com/business-functions/organization/our-insights/build-a-change-platform-not-a change-program.
70. Tewes R. Verhandlungssache. Verhandlungsführung im Gesundheitswesen. Berlin: Springer; 2011.
71. Jullien F. Die stillen Wandlungen. Berlin: Merve Verlag; 2010.
72. Waleczek H, Hofinger G. Kommunikation über kritische Situationen im OP- Schwierigkeiten, Besonderheiten, Anforderdungen. In: Hofinger G, editor. Kommunikation in kritischen Situationen. Frankfurt/Main: Verlag für Polizeiwissenschaft; 2012. p. 151–68.
73. Pattni N, Arzola C, Malavade A, Varmani S, Krimus L, Friedman Z. Challenging authority and speaking up in the operating room environment: a narrative synthesis. Br J Anaesth. 2019;122(2):233–44.
74. Hinterhuber H. Die 5 Gebote für exzellente Führung. Frankfurt: Frankfurter Allgemeine Buch; 2010.
75. Petri L. Concept analysis of interdisciplinary collaboration. Nurs Forum. 2010;45(2):73–82.
76. Reeves S, Lewin S, Espin S, Zwarenstein M. Interprofessional teamwork for health and social care. Oxford: Wiley-Blackwell; 2010.
77. Cough J. Collaboration between physicians and nurses: essential to patient safety. Nursing Forum. 2008;26(2):1–2.
78. Kim M, Barnato AE, Angus DC, Fleisher LF, Kahn JM. The effect of multidisciplinary care teams on intensive care unit mortality. Arch Intern Med. 2010;170(4):369–77.
79. Jacobson P. Evidence synthesis for the effectiveness of interprofessional teams in primary care. Ottawa: Canadian Health Services Research Foundation; 2012.
80. Virani T. Interprofessional collaborative teams. Ottawa: Canadian Health Services Research Foundation; 2012. https://doi.org/10.1136/bmjqs-2012-000886.
81. Meuerling L, Hedman L, Sandahl C, Felländer-Tsai F, Wallin CW. Systematic simulation–based team training in a Swedish intensive care unit: a diverse response among critical care professions. Br Med J Qual Saf. 2013;22:485–94.
82. Rosa H. Resonanz. Eine Soziologie der Weltbeziehung. Suhrkamp: Berlin; 2018.
83. Hibbeler B. Ärzte und Pflegekräfte: Ein chronischer Konflikt. Deutsches Ärzteblatt. 2011;108/41:B-1814/C 1794.

84. Chioccio F, Paule L, Due J-N. Informational role self-efficacy: a validation in interprofessional collaboration contexts involving healthcare service and project teams. BMC Health Serv Res. 2016;16:153.
85. Josi R, Bianchi M, Brand S. Advanced practice nurses in primary care in Switzerland: an analysis of interprofessional collaboration. BMC Nurs. 2020;19:1.
86. Mafuba K, Kupara D, Cozens M, Kudita C. Importance of role-clarity: a critique of literature. Learn Disabil Pract. 2015;18(8):28–31.
87. Furseth PA, Taylor B, Kim SC. Impact of interprofessional education among nursing and paramedic students. Nurse Educ. 2016;41(2):75–9. https://doi.org/10.1097/NNE.0000000000000219.
88. McGettigan P, McKendree J. Interprofessional training for final year healthcare students: a mixed methods evaluation of the impact on ward staff and students of a two-week placement and of factors affecting sustainability. BMC Med Educ. 2015;15:185. https://doi.org/10.1186/s12909-015-0436-9.
89. Seitz T, et al. Rückgang von Empathie der Medizinstudierenden im Laufe des Studiums – was ist die Ursache? Z Psychosom Med Psychother. 2017;63:20–39.
90. Joas H, editor. George H. Mead: Gesammelte Aufsätze. Berlin: Suhrkamp TB Wissenschaft; 1987.
91. Igde F, Sahin M. Changes in empathy during medical education: an example from Turkey. Pak J Med Sci. 2017;33(5):1177–81. https://doi.org/10.12669/pjms.335.13074.
92. Mandel ED, Schweinle WE. A study of empathy decline in physician assistant students at completion of first didactic year. J Phys Assist Educ. 2012;23(4):16–24. 9p. 4 Charts.
93. Wimmers P, Stuber M. Assessing medical students' empathy and attitudes towards patient centered care with an existing clinical performance exam (OSCE). Procedica Soc Behav Sci. 2010;2:1911–3. https://doi.org/10.1016/j.sbspro.2010.03.1008.
94. Batt-Rawden SA, Chisolm MS, Anton B, Flickinger TE. Teaching empathy to medical students: an updated, systematic review. Acad Med. 2013;88(8):1171–7. https://doi.org/10.1097/ACM.0b013e318299f3e3.
95. Kebe NNM, Chioccio F, Jean-Marie B, Fleury M-J. Variables associated with interprofessional collaboration: a comparison between primary healthcare and specialized mental health teams. BMC Fam Pract. 2020;21:4.
96. Wei H, Corbett RW, Ray J, Wei TL. A culture of caring: the essence of healthcare interprofessional collaboration. J Interprof Care. 2019;8:1–8.
97. Fox S, Gaboury I, Chiocchio F, Vachon B. Communication and interprofessional collaboration in primary care: from ideal to reality in praxis. Health Commun. 2019;3:1–11.
98. Tewes R. Interprofessionelle Kommunikation will gelernt sein. Heilberufe. 2015;67(1):20–2.
99. Gilles I, Filliettaz SS, Berchtold P, Peytremann-Brideyaux I. Financial barriers decrease the benefits of interprofessional collaboration within integrated care programs: results of a nationwide survey. Int J Integr Care. 2019;19(S1):1–2.
100. Mertens F, Gendt D, Anneleen, Deveugele M, Hecke V, Ann, Pype P. Interprofessional collaboration within fluid teams: community nurses' experiences with palliative home care. J Clin Nurs. 2019;28(19–20):2680–3690.
101. Miller KL, Kontos P. The intraprofessional and interprofessional relations of neurorehabilitation nurses: a negotiated order perspective. J Adv Nurs. 2012;68(11):1016–102.
102. Clausen C, Cummins K, Dionne K. Educational interventions to enhance competencies for interprofessional collaboration among nurse and physician managers: an integrative review. J Interprof Care. 2017;31(6):685–95.
103. Vittadello F, Mischo-Kelling M, Wieser H, Cavada L, Lochner L, Naletto, Carla F, Verena, Reeves S. A multiple-group measurement scale for interprofessional collaboration: adaptation and validation into Italian and German languages. J Interprofess Care. 2018;32(3):266–73.
104. Bookey-Basset S, Markle-Reid M, McKey C, Akhtar-Danesh N. A review of instruments to measure interprofessional collaboration for chronic disease management for community-living older adults. J Interprofess Care. 2016;30(2):201–10.

105. Samuelson M, Tedeschi P, Aarendonk D, Gronewegen P. Improving Interprofessional Collaboration In Primary Care: Position Paper Of The European Forum For Primary Care. Quality of Primary Care. 2012;20: 303–12.
106. Laschinter H; Smith LM. The influence of authentic leadership and empowerment on new-graduate nurses' perception of interprofessional collaboration. Journal of Nursing Administration. 2013;43(1):24–9.
107. Jung K. Krankenhäuser brauchen eine integrierte Personalentwicklung. Stand und Perspektiven einer integrativen Personalentwicklung an den Universitätsklinika Deutschland, Österreichs und der Schweiz. 2010. https://docplayer.org/6381118-Krankenhaeuser-brauchen-eine-integrierte-personalentwicklung.html.
108. Zurmehly J. The relationship of educational preparation, autonomy, and critical thinking to nursing job satisfaction. Journal of Continuing Education in Nursing. 2008.
109. Swanson J, Tidwell C. Improving the culture of patient safety through the magnet journey. OJIN Online Journal Issues in Nursing 2011;16(3):1. Manuscript 1. http://nursingwolrd.org.
110. Gokenbach V, Drenkard K. The outcomes of magnet environments and nursing staff engagement: a case study. Nursing Clinics of North America. 2011;46(1):89–105.
111. Kelly Lesly A, McHugh Mathew D, Aiken Linda H. Nursing outcomes in Magnet and Non-Magnet hospitals. Journal of Nursing Administration. 2011;41(10):428–33.
112. Jayawardhana J, Welton JM, Lindrooth R. Adoption of national quality froum safe practices by Magnet hospitals. Journal of Nursing Administration. 2011;41(9):350–6.
113. Lake ET, Shang J, Klaus S, Dunton NE. Patient falls: Association with hospitals Magnet status and nursing unit staffing. Research in Nursing & Health 2010;33(5):413–25.
114. Mark BA, Huges LC, Belyea M, et al. Changes in transformation leadership and empirical quality outcomes in a finnish hospital over a two-year period: a longitudinal study. Journal of Nursing Management. 2007;15(3):256–63.
115. Tewes R. Zukunft der Personalentwicklung in der Pflege. In: Tewes/Stockinger: Personalentwicklung in Pflege- und Gesundheitseinrichtungen. Berlin: Springer; 2014. p. 215–40.
116. Schuss U, Blank R. Qualitätsorientierte interprofessionelle Kooperation (QuiK) Pflegefachkräfte und Mediziner im Fokus. Bern: Hogrefe; 2018.
117. Hargie O. Skilled interpersonal communication. 6th ed. London: Routledge; 2017.
118. Mink J, Mitzkat A, Milhaljevic A, Trierweilter-Hauke B, Götsch B, Schmidt J, Krug K, Mahlter C. The impact of an interprofessional training ward on the development of interprofessional competencies: study protocol of a longitudinal mixed-methods study. BMC Med Educ. 2019;19:48. https://doi.org/10.1186/s12909-019-1478-1.
119. Bridges W, Bridges S. Managing transitions. Erfolgreich durch Übergänge und Veränderunsprozesse führen. 4. Auflage ed. München: Vahlen; 2018.
120. Bundesministerium für Gesundheit. Agenda für mehr Nachhaltigkeit in Gesundheit und Pflege. Ressortbericht des Bundesministeriums für Gesundheit zur Umsetzung der Deutschen Nachhaltigkeitsstrategie vom. 2019;27(5):2019. https://www.bundesgesundheitsministerium.de/fileadmin/Dateien/5_Publikationen/Ministerium/Berichte/Ressortbericht-gesundheit-und-pflege-data.pdf.
121. Felber C. Gemeinwohl-Ökonomie. Wien: Deuticke; 2014.
122. Mischkowski NS, Funcke S, Kress-Ludwig M, et al. Die Gemeinwohl-Bilanz – Ein Instrument zur Bindung und Gewinnung von Mitarbeitenden und Kund*innen in kleinen und mittleren Unternehmen? NachhaltigkeitsManagementForum. 2018;26:123–31. https://doi.org/10.1007/s00550-018-0472-0.
123. Reich S. Computervirus legt Klinik lahm. Rettungswagen können Krankenhaus wieder anfahren. 2019.
124. FAZ. Hacker-Angriff schränkt Betrieb im Klinikum Fürth ein. 2019. https://www.faz.net/aktuell/wirtschaft/hacker-angriff-schraenkt-betrieb-imklinikum-fuerth-ein-16534082.html.
125. Bruno G. Digitaler Angriff auf die Reputation. In: Meißner J, Schach A, editors. Professionelle Krisenkommunikation. Basiswissen, Impulse und Handlungsempfehlungen für die Praxis. Wiesbaden: Springer Gabler; 2019. p. 105–17.

126. Washausen J, Meißner J. Reifegrade organisationaler Reslienz. In: Meißner J, Schach A, editors. Professionelle Krisenkommunikation. Basiswissen, Impulse und Handlungsempfehlungen für die Praxis. Wiesbaden: Springer Gabler; 2019. p. 3–16.
127. Merten K. Krise, Krisenmanagement und Krisenkommunikation. In: Thießen, editor. Ansgar: Handbuch Krisenkommunikation. Wiesbaden: Springer; 2014. p. 155–76.
128. Sandhu S. Krisen als soziale Konstruktion: zur institutionellen Logik des Krisenmanagements und der Krisenkommunikation. In: Thießen, Ansgar: Handbuch Krisenkommunikation. Wiesbaden: Springer; 2014. p. 95–118.
129. Schreyögg G, Ostermann S. Krisenwahrnehmung und Krisenbewältigung. In: Thießen A, editor. Handbuch Krisenmanagement. Wiesbaden: Springer; 2014. p. 119–39.
130. Enzler Denzler R, Schuler E. Krisen erfolgreich bewältigen. Wie Führungskräfte in Wirtschaft und Politik Schicksalsschläge überwinden. Berlin: Springer. 2018.
131. Hansen M, Ibarra H, Peyer U. 100 best-performing CEOs in the world. A scorecard of leaders who deliver long-term success. In: Harvard business review; 2013. https://hbr.org/2013/01/the-best-performing-ceos-in-the-world.
132. Immerschitt W. Aktive Krisenkommunikation. Erste Hilfe für Management und Krisenstab. Wiesbaden: Springer Gabler; 2015.
133. Falkmeier J, Heide M. On dropping the crisis communication tools. From plans to improvisations. In: Rogonijaru A, Wolstonhome S, editors. Current trends in international public relations. Bucharest: Tritonic; 2009. p. 403–18.
134. Drews J. Risikokommunikation und Krisenkommunikation. Kommunikation von Behörden und die Erwartungen von Journalisten. Wiesbaden: Springer; 2018.
135. Kappe B. Das Gesicht der Krise. In: Meißner J, Schach A, editors. Professionelle Krisenkommunikation. Basiswissen, Impulse und Handlungsempfehlungen für die Praxis. Wiesbaden: Springer Gabler; 2019. p. 985–94.
136. Jiménez F. So entschuldigen Sie sich richtig. Psychologie. Hg. v. Die Welt Online. 2016. https://www.welt.de/gesundheit/psychologie/article154375065/So-entschuldigen-Sie-sich-richtig.html. Zugegriffen 26 Mar 2020.
137. Schulz C, Neelson M. Das Risiko der Desinformation. In: Meißner J, Schach A, editors. Professionelle Krisenkommunikation. Basiswissen, Impulse und Handlungsempfehlungen für die Praxis. Wiesbaden: Springer Gabler; 2019. p. 95–104.
138. Fink A. Krisenkommunikation im internationalen Kontext. In: Meißner J, Schach A, editors. Professionelle Krisenkommunikation. Basiswissen, Impulse und Handlungsempfehlungen für die Praxis. Wiesbaden: Springer Gabler; 2019. p. 171–87.
139. Messer B. Der Nutzen von Medientrainings für Krisenmanagement und Kommunikation. In: Meißner J, Schach A, editors. Professionelle Krisenkommunikation. Basiswissen, Impulse und Handlungsempfehlungen für die Praxis. Wiesbaden: Springer Gabler; 2019. p. 201–13.
140. Schach A. Die Macht der Sprache. In: Meißner J, Schach A, editors. Professionelle Krisenkommunikation. Basiswissen, Impulse und Handlungsempfehlungen für die Praxis. Wiesbaden: Springer Gabler; 2019. p. 235–47.
141. Von der Leyen U. Rede vor der Europäischen Kommission anlässlich der Coronakrise am. 2020. https://ec.europa.eu/germany/news/20200326-von-der-leyen-coronavirus_de. Accessed 26 Mar 2020.
142. Koulalis J, Schäfer C. Der Werkzeugkasten des Krisenmanagements. In: Meißner J, Schach A, editors. Professionelle Krisenkommunikation. Basiswissen, Impulse und Handlungsempfehlungen für die Praxis. Wiesbaden: Springer Gabler; 2019. p. 55–62.
143. Brückner J. Einbindung der Krisenkommunikation ins Krisenmanagement. In: Meißner J, Schach A, editors. Professionelle Krisenkommunikation. Basiswissen, Impulse und Handlungsempfehlungen für die Praxis. Wiesbaden: Springer Gabler; 2019. p. 63–74.
144. Smith D. Crisis management—practice in search of a paradigm. In: Smith D, Elliot D, editors. Key readings in crisis management. Systems and structures for prevention and recovery. London: Routledge; 2006. p. 1–12.
145. Tewes R. Pflegerische Verantwortung. Bern: Huber; 2002.

146. Densen P. Challenges and opportunities facing medical education. Trans Am Clin Climatol Assoc. 2011;122:48–58.
147. Luca J, Tarricone P. Does emotional intelligence affect successful teamwork? Meeting at the crossroads; 2001. p. 367–76.
148. Oldhafer M, Schneider S, Beil E, Schmidt C, Nolte F. Change Management in Gesundheitsunternehmen. Die geheime Macht der Emotionen in Veränderungsprozessen. Wiesbaden: Springer/Gabler; 2019.
149. Tewes R. Das Stress-war-gestern Programm. Pflegezeitschrift. 2018;71(9):29–31.
150. Tewes R. Teamtraining zur Integration ausländischer Mitarbeiter. Pflegezeitschrift. 2018;71(10):38–41.
151. Tewes R. Biofeedback und HeartMath-Training. Pflegezeitschrift. 2015;68(8):500–4.
152. Tewes R, Ulrich L. Nursing Leadership: Führungspraxis. Studienbrief der Fern-Hochschule Hamburg; 2020.

GPSR Compliance

The European Union's (EU) General Product Safety Regulation (GPSR) is a set of rules that requires consumer products to be safe and our obligations to ensure this.

If you have any concerns about our products, you can contact us on ProductSafety@springernature.com

In case Publisher is established outside the EU, the EU authorized representative is:

Springer Nature Customer Service Center GmbH
Europaplatz 3
69115 Heidelberg, Germany

Batch number: 08823208

Printed by Printforce, the Netherlands